A Companion to Specialist Surgical Practice

Series Editors

O. James Garden
Simon Paterson-Brown

ENDOCRINE SURGERY

FOURTH EDITION

Edited by

Tom W.J. Lennard

MD LRCP MRCS FRCS(Ed) FRCS

Professor of Breast and Endocrine Surgery and
Head of School of Surgical and Reproductive Sciences
University of Newcastle upon Tyne
Newcastle upon Tyne, UK

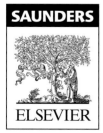

Edinburgh   London   New York   Oxford   Philadelphia   St Louis   Sydney   Toronto   2009

SAUNDERS
ELSEVIER

First edition 1997
Second edition 2001
Third edition 2005
Fourth edition 2009
Reprinted 2009

ISBN 9780702030161

British Library Cataloguing in Publication Data
A catalogue record for this book is available from the British Library

Library of Congress Cataloging in Publication Data
A catalog record for this book is available from the Library of Congress

Notice

Knowledge and best practice in this field are constantly changing. As new research and experience broaden our knowledge, changes in practice, treatment and drug therapy may become necessary or appropriate. Readers are advised to check the most current information provided (i) on procedures featured or (ii) by the manufacturer of each product to be administered, to verify the recommended dose or formula, the method and duration of administration, and contraindications. It is the responsibility of the practitioner, relying on their own experience and knowledge of the patient, to make diagnoses, to determine dosages and the best treatment for each individual patient, and to take all appropriate safety precautions. To the fullest extent of the law, neither the Publisher nor the Editors assumes any liability for any injury and/or damage to persons or property arising out of or related to any use of the material contained in this book.

The Publisher

ELSEVIER your source for books, journals and multimedia in the health sciences

www.elsevierhealth.com

Working together to grow libraries in developing countries

www.elsevier.com | www.bookaid.org | www.sabre.org

ELSEVIER   BOOK AID International   Sabre Foundation

The Publisher's policy is to use paper manufactured from sustainable forests

Printed in China

Commissioning Editor: Laurence Hunter
Development Editor: Elisabeth Lawrence
Project Manager: Andrew Palfreyman
Text Design: Charlotte Murray
Cover Design: Kirsteen Wright
Illustration Manager: Gillian Richards
Illustrators: Martin Woodward and Richard Prime

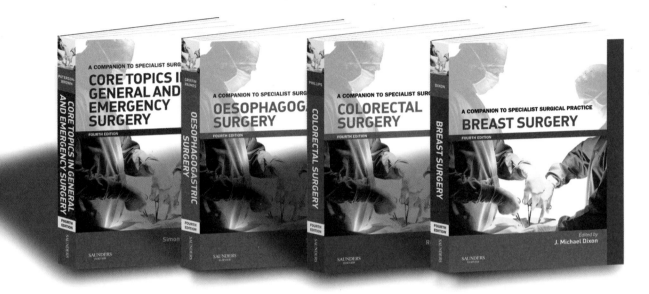

A COMPANION TO SPECIALIST SURGICAL PRACTICE

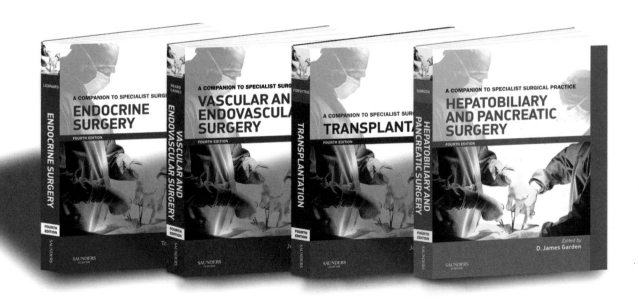

ENDOCRINE SURGERY

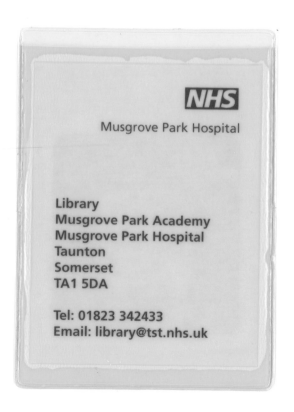

Contents

Contributors   vii

Series preface   ix

Editor's preface   xi

Acknowledgements   xi

Evidence-based practice in surgery   xiii

1   **Parathyroid disease**   1
William B. Inabnet, James A. Lee, Jean-François Henry and Frédéric Sebag

2   **The thyroid gland**   39
Gregory P. Sadler and Radu Mihai

3   **The adrenal glands**   73
Richard D. Bliss and Tom W.J. Lennard

4   **Familial endocrine disease: genetics, clinical presentation and management**   99
Stephen G. Ball, Paul Brennan and Tom W.J. Lennard

5   **Endocrine tumours of the pancreas**   121
Robin M. Cisco and Jeffrey A. Norton

6   **Gastrointestinal carcinoids**   147
Göran Åkerström, Per Hellman and Ola Hessman

7   **Clinical governance, audit and medico-legal aspects of endocrine surgery**   177
Barnard J. Harrison and Anthony E. Young

8   **The salivary glands**   191
Steven J. Thomas and Zenon Rayter

Index   215

Contributors

Göran Åkerström, MD, PhD
Professor and Head of Endocrine Surgery
University Hospital
Uppsala, Sweden

Stephen G. Ball, BSc, MB, BS, PhD, FRCP
Senior Lecturer
University of Newcastle;
Honorary Consultant
Endocrine Unit
Newcastle Hospitals NHS Trust
Newcastle upon Tyne, UK

Richard D. Bliss, MB, FRCS
Consultant Surgeon
Royal Victoria Infirmary
Newcastle upon Tyne, UK

Paul Brennan, MS, PhD
Honorary Clinical Lecturer
Institute of Human Genetics
International Centre for Life
Newcastle upon Tyne, UK

Robin M. Cisco, MD
Postdoctoral Fellow
Stanford University Medical Center
Stanford, CA, USA

Barnard J. Harrison, MB, BS, MS, FRCS, FRCS(Ed)
Consultant Endocrine Surgeon
Royal Hallamshire Hospital
Sheffield, UK

Per Hellman, MD, PhD
Associate Professor and Consultant Surgeon
University Hospital
Uppsala, Sweden

Jean-François Henry, MD
Professor of Surgery and Chairman
Department of Endocrine Surgery
University Hospital La Timone
Marseilles, France

Ola Hessman, MD, PhD
Consultant Surgeon
University Hospital
Uppsala, Sweden

William B. Inabnet, MD, FACS
Chief, Section of Endocrine Surgery
Columbia University

College of Physicians and Surgeons
New York, NY, USA

James A. Lee, MD
Endocrine Surgery Fellow
Columbia University Medical Center
New York, NY, USA

Tom W.J. Lennard, MD, LRCP, MRCS, FRCS(Ed), FRCS
Professor of Breast and Endocrine Surgery
Head of School of Surgical
and Reproductive Sciences
University of Newcastle upon Tyne
Newcastle upon Tyne, UK

Radu Mihai, MD, PhD, FRCS Gen Surg (Eng)
Consultant Endocrine Surgeon
John Radcliffe Hospital
Oxford, UK

Jeffrey A. Norton, MD
Professor of Surgery
Chief of General Surgery and Surgical Oncology
Stanford University Medical Center
Stanford, CA, USA

Zenon Rayter, MS, FRCS
Consultant Surgeon
Bristol Royal Infirmary
Bristol, UK

Gregory P. Sadler, MD, FRCS(Ed), FRCS Gen Surg (Eng)
Consultant Endocrine Surgeon
John Radcliffe Hospital
Oxford, UK

Frédéric Sebag, MD
Assistant Surgeon
Department of Endocrine Surgery
University Hospital La Timone
Marseilles, France

Steven J. Thomas, BDS, FDSRCS, MB, BCh, PhD, FRCS
Consultant Senior Lecturer
Department of Oral and Dental Science
University of Bristol Dental School
Bristol, UK

Anthony E. Young, MA, MChir, FRCS
Consultant Surgeon
St Thomas' Hospital
London, UK

Series preface

Since the publication of the first edition in 1997, the *Companion to Specialist Surgical Practice* series has aspired to meet the needs of surgeons in higher training and practising consultants who wish contemporary, evidence-based information on the subspecialist areas relevant to their general surgical practice. We have accepted that the series will not necessarily be as comprehensive as some of the larger reference surgical textbooks which, by their very size, may not always be completely up to date at the time of publication. This Fourth Edition aims to bring relevant state-of-the-art specialist information that we and the individual volume editors consider important for the practising subspecialist general surgeon. Where possible, all contributors have attempted to identify evidence-based references to support key recommendations within each chapter.

We remain grateful to the volume editors and all the contributors of this Fourth Edition. Their enthusiasm, commitment and hard work has ensured that a short turnover has been maintained between each of the editions, thereby ensuring as accurate and up-to-date content as possible. We remain grateful for the support and encouragement of Laurence Hunter and Elisabeth Lawrence at Elsevier Ltd. We trust that our aim of providing up-to-date and affordable surgical texts has been met and that all readers, whether in training or in consultant practice, will find this fourth edition an invaluable resource.

O. James Garden MB, ChB, MD, FRCS(Glas), FRCS(Ed), FRCP(Ed), FRACS(Hon), FRCSC(Hon)

Regius Professor of Clinical Surgery, Clinical and Surgical Sciences (Surgery), University of Edinburgh, and Honorary Consultant Surgeon, Royal Infirmary of Edinburgh

Simon Paterson-Brown MB, BS, MPhil, MS, FRCS(Ed), FRCS

Honorary Senior Lecturer, Clinical and Surgical Sciences (Surgery), University of Edinburgh, and Consultant General and Upper Gastrointestinal Surgeon, Royal Infirmary of Edinburgh

Editor's preface

This Fourth Edition brings the subject of endocrine surgery up to date comprehensively. Most, if not all, of the contributors were at the Montreal 2007 International Association of Endocrine Surgeons' Meeting and have been able to incorporate the very latest advances in the relevant chapters. Advances in imaging of endocrine tumours, using positron emission tomography technology, have been significant and no doubt there will be more to come in the years ahead. The ability to find small functioning tumours and interpret their likely pathology and morphology continues to be an aspiration for all of us involved in treating patients with endocrine surgical disease and that dream becomes closer and closer.

Minimally invasive approaches to most endocrine tumours are now in widespread practice and this book details when that is appropriate and outlines the optimal approach.

The science of molecular genetics and diagnostics has also advanced in recent years, enabling us now to get presymptomatic diagnoses in some of the predisposition syndromes that occur in endocrine disease. The endocrine surgeon will need to understand work and collaborate closely with colleagues in planning prophylactic surgery for these patients. Finally, we are now well and truly in the era of multidisciplinary team working and there can be no better example of this than in endocrine surgery.

All of the chapters in this book reflect the multidisciplinary approach to the subject, with up-to-date information on cytopathology, assays of hormones, localisation techniques, anaesthetic requirements, input from genetics and, of course, histopathology and adjuvant treatments. It is hoped that this book will therefore be of value to all of those disciplines, but most particularly to the surgeon who will be charged in managing the final pathway for these fascinating and sometimes challenging patients.

Acknowledgements

I would like to record my thanks to all of the contributors for their updates and their hard work in producing this comprehensive but very readable volume. As before, I would like to dedicate this book to the memory of John Farndon, a close friend to many of us and a mentor for me, and a man who advanced the science and clinical aspects of endocrine surgery enormously.

Tom W.J. Lennard
Newcastle upon Tyne

Evidence-based practice in surgery

Critical appraisal for developing evidence-based practice can be obtained from a number of sources, the most reliable being randomised controlled clinical trials, systematic literature reviews, meta-analyses and observational studies. For practical purposes three grades of evidence can be used, analogous to the levels of 'proof' required in a court of law:

1. **Beyond all reasonable doubt**. Such evidence is likely to have arisen from high-quality randomised controlled trials, systematic reviews or high-quality synthesised evidence such as decision analysis, cost-effectiveness analysis or large observational datasets. The studies need to be directly applicable to the population of concern and have clear results. The grade is analogous to burden of proof within a criminal court and may be thought of as corresponding to the usual standard of 'proof' within the medical literature (i.e. $P < 0.05$).
2. **On the balance of probabilities**. In many cases a high-quality review of literature may fail to reach firm conclusions due to conflicting or inconclusive results, trials of poor methodological quality or the lack of evidence in the population to which the guidelines apply. In such cases it may still be possible to make a statement as to the best treatment on the 'balance of probabilities'. This is analogous to the decision in a civil court where all the available evidence will be weighed up and the verdict will depend upon the balance of probabilities.
3. **Not proven**. Insufficient evidence upon which to base a decision, or contradictory evidence.

Depending on the information available, three grades of recommendation can be used:

a. Strong recommendation, which should be followed unless there are compelling reasons to act otherwise.
b. A recommendation based on evidence of effectiveness, but where there may be other factors to take into account in decision-making, for example the user of the guidelines may be expected to take into account patient preferences, local facilities, local audit results or available resources.
c. A recommendation made where there is no adequate evidence as to the most effective practice, although there may be reasons for making a recommendation in order to minimise cost or reduce the chance of error through a locally agreed protocol.

Strong recommendation

Evidence where a conclusion can be reached 'beyond all reasonable doubt' and therefore where a **strong recommendation** can be given.

This will normally be based on evidence levels:

- Ia. Meta-analysis of randomised controlled trials
- Ib. Evidence from at least one randomised controlled trial
- IIa. Evidence from at least one controlled study without randomisation
- IIb. Evidence from at least one other type of quasi-experimental study.

Expert opinion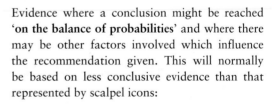

Evidence where a conclusion might be reached 'on the balance of probabilities' and where there may be other factors involved which influence the recommendation given. This will normally be based on less conclusive evidence than that represented by scalpel icons:

- III. Evidence from non-experimental descriptive studies, such as comparative studies and case–control studies
- IV. Evidence from expert committee reports or opinions or clinical experience of respected authorities, or both.

Evidence in each chapter of this volume which is associated with either a strong recommendation or expert opinion is annotated in the text by either a **scalpel** or **pen-nib** icon as shown above. References associated with **scalpel** evidence will be highlighted in the reference lists, along with a short summary of the paper's conclusions where applicable.

1

Parathyroid disease

William B. Inabnet, James A. Lee,
Jean-François Henry,
Frédéric Sebag

Part 1
Parathyroid disease, syndromes and pathophysiology

William B. Inabnet
James A. Lee

Introduction

Hyperparathyroidism is a disease characterised by elevated serum calcium and inappropriately elevated parathyroid hormone (PTH) levels, that occurs with a prevalence of 3/1000 in the general population.[1] The modern era of treating parathyroid disease began in 1925, when Mandl performed the first parathyroidectomy in a patient with severe bone disease. Early in the history of hyperparathyroidism, patients presented with advanced clinical disease, including fractures, skeletal deformities, kidney stones and kidney failure. The discovery of the peptide PTH in the early 1970s coupled with the development of a chemical analyser to measure calcium permitted the biochemical diagnosis of hyperparathyroidism much earlier in the disease course.[2]

 During this era, bilateral neck exploration was the standard approach, resulting in a cure rate ranging from 92 to 96% when performed by a skilled surgical team.[3,4]

Over the last 20 years, the treatment of hyperparathyroidism has experienced a dramatic change with the development of new technology to permit accurate preoperative localisation of abnormal glands, and intraoperative confirmation of the completeness of parathyroid resection.

Embryology and anatomy

In order to successfully diagnose and treat disorders of the parathyroid glands, a keen understanding of parathyroid embryology and anatomy is essential. The parathyroid glands are small, brownish-tan glands located in the space around the thyroid gland. During the fifth week of fetal development, the inferior parathyroid glands arise from the dorsal aspect of the third pharyngeal pouch.[5] Following development of the thymus from the ventral aspect of the third pharyngeal pouch, the inferior parathyroid glands and thymus descend in a caudal and medial direction to rest in the inferior neck and thorax respectively. The superior parathyroid glands arise from the dorsal wing of the fourth pharyngeal pouch and descend in a caudal direction with the thyroid gland.[5]

Because of the longer pathway of descent, the inferior parathyroid glands have a higher variability of location compared with the superior parathyroid glands, an observation that is important during parathyroid surgery.

In an autopsy series of 503 human subjects, Akerstrom et al showed that four parathyroid glands were present in 84% of cases, whereas 3% of patients had only three glands and 13% had supernumerary glands.[6] The presence of missed hyperfunctioning supernumerary glands is an important but infrequent cause of persistent hyperparathyroidism and should be considered in all cases of persistent disease. In 80% of cases, the location of the inferior and superior glands is symmetrical when compared with the glands on the contralateral side of the neck.[6] The superior parathyroid glands are most commonly found immediately superior to the junction of the recurrent laryngeal nerve and the inferior thyroid artery and can be located inside the thyroid gland in 0.2% of cases.[6]

 Approximately 50% of inferior parathyroid glands are located in the vicinity of the inferior pole of the thyroid gland and about 30% are found in the thyrothymic ligament.

Calcium and parathyroid hormone (PTH) regulation

The parathyroid glands play a central role in regulating serum levels of calcium through a complex feedback loop involving PTH, serum ionised calcium levels and vitamin D. The key organ systems involved in this process include the parathyroid glands, gastrointestinal tract, kidneys and skin. Although multiple factors influence parathyroid function, it is now clear that calcium is the single most potent stimulator of PTH release. Calcium-sensing receptors (CSRs), which are located on the surface of the parathyroid chief cells and are coupled with a G-protein receptor, are able to detect minuscule changes in serum levels of extracellular ionised calcium.[7,8] When serum levels of calcium decrease the CSRs are activated, thereby stimulating the synthesis and release of PTH.[9] In primary hyperparathyroidism (PHP), the set point of the CSRs is adjusted upwards, probably through a mutation of unknown aetiology, causing the parathyroid chief cell to 'believe' that serum calcium levels are low when in fact they are not. As a result of this alteration in the CSR set point, the parathyroid chief cell increases production of PTH, ultimately leading to

hypercalcaemia. Calcium-sensing receptors are also present on other tissues such as the kidneys and gastrointestinal tract, where calcium homeostasis is influenced.[8,10,11] In the kidney, the CSRs regulate renal calcium excretion and influence the transepithelial movement of water and other electrolytes.[8] In the gastrointestinal tract, CSRs are present in the gastrin-secreting G cells and acid-secreting parietal cells, thereby providing a molecular link between hypercalcaemia and acid hypersecretion.[10] These facts also underscore the complexity of calcium homeostasis in influencing cellular function throughout the body.

PTH is an intact 84-amino-acid peptide with amino and carboxy terminals.[12] Production of PTH begins in the endoplasmic reticulum of the parathyroid chief cells as a 115-amino-acid molecule, which undergoes a series of cleavages before being released from the cytoplasm as the biologically active (1–84) PTH molecule. The circulating (1–84) PTH molecule, which has a half-life of 3–5 minutes in patients with normal renal function, is initially cleaved in the liver, yielding an inactive C-terminal fragment, which is ultimately cleared by the kidneys.[12,13] The N-terminal fragment is the part of the peptide that is responsible for the biological activity of PTH on peripheral tissues.

PTH acts directly on the kidneys, bone and gastro-intestinal tract to activate several intracellular second messengers, including cyclic AMP and calcium.[14,15] In the kidneys, PTH increases serum calcium levels by acting on the renal tubule to increase resorption of calcium and to increase the hydroxylation of 25-hydroxyvitamin D to the biologically active 1,25-dihydroxyvitamin D.[15] PTH also stimulates the renal tubular secretion of phosphate and bicarbonate. In the bone, PTH acts on osteoblasts and osteoclasts to increase bone turnover, thereby providing a large source of calcium for the extracellular space.[16]

Vitamin D is a fat-soluble vitamin that is prevalent in dairy products. After being absorbed by the gastrointestinal tract, it is hydroxylated in the liver to become 25-hydroxyvitamin D, which in turn is hydroxylated in the kidneys to become 1,25-dihydroxyvitamin D. The latter plays an important role in calcium homeostasis by increasing the resorption of phosphorus in the kidneys and increasing the absorption of calcium from the gastrointestinal tract. Calcitonin, which is synthesised by the parafollicular C cells of the thyroid gland, acts as the physiological antagonist to PTH. Calcitonin decreases serum levels of calcium by decreasing bone turnover and in fact can be used to treat patients in hypercalcaemic crisis.[17]

Primary hyperparathyroidism

Incidence

Early in the history of PHP, patients presented with manifestations of severe hypercalcaemia and advanced disease, but the true incidence of hyperparathyroidism was not known due to the inability to routinely measure serum calcium levels. The development of the automated serum chemical analyser and the practice of widespread biochemical screening permitted the detection of mild increases in serum calcium levels, thereby allowing earlier recognition of abnormalities in calcium homeostasis.

Multiple factors influence the incidence of PHP, including the region of the world under evaluation, the nutritional status of the studied population, iatrogenic factors and the availability of routine biochemical screening.

 In the 1970s, there was a dramatic fivefold increase in the incidence of PHP, largely due to the 'catch-up' effect of identifying patients who had PHP prior to the development of the automated calcium analyser.[1] During the 1980s, the incidence of PHP in North America actually decreased as the impact of the 'catch-up' effect levelled off.[18]

The number of patients with a history of irradiation to the head and neck region for benign disorders decreased in the 1980s, which may also have contributed to the decreased incidence of PHP, as head and neck irradiation is a known risk factor for parathyroid hypersecretion.

PHP occurs more frequently in women than men, but the overall incidence increases with age in both sexes. In North America, the incidence of PHP in the general population is 4.3/1000, whereas in Europe the incidence is 3/1000.[1,18] In women aged between 55 and 75 years, the incidence of PHP is 21/1000.[1] Possible explanations for the increased incidence with age include the lower rate of biochemical screening in patients less than 50 years of age and the increased use of bone density measurements in

postmenopausal women as a routine part of healthcare screening. The detection of osteopenia and/or osteoporosis that is out of proportion to age-matched controls often leads the clinician to measure serum calcium and PTH levels, thereby identifying hyperparathyroidism as the cause of increased bone loss. Vitamin D deficiency also influences the true detected incidence of PHP as this condition may cause serum calcium levels to be normal in patients with hyperparathyroidism. For example, the incidence of vitamin D deficiency in southern Europe is high, leading to an underestimation of the true incidence of hyperparathyroidism in this region of the world.[1]

Clinical manifestations

The clinical presentation of patients with PHP is highly variable, ranging from none to profound symptoms of hypercalcaemia, such as excessive thirst, dehydration, kidney stones, muscle weakness and pathological fracture. Generally, the clinical manifestations of PHP can be broadly classified by organ system (Box 1.1). Since many of these symptoms overlap with other clinical conditions, particularly in the elderly, the diagnosis of hyperparathyroidism is often delayed until hypercalcaemia is recognised on biochemical screening. Often the presence of a classic symptom, such as nephrolithiasis, will lead the astute clinician to assess the patient for PHP. By far, fatigue is one of the most common symptoms of hyperparathyroidism, being present in >80% of patients.[18] Numerous studies have shown that a high percentage of patients that are thought to be asymptomatic actually have occult symptoms attributable to PHP.[18]

There are numerous medical conditions that are associated with and/or exacerbated by PHP, including hypertension, diabetes, pancreatitis, nephrolithiasis, gout and peptic ulcer disease.

Diagnosis

Prior to the 1970s and the advent of routine serum calcium measurements as part of the basic metabolic profile, the diagnosis of PHP was made primarily on clinical findings. Walter St Goar immortalised this constellation of findings in the mnemonic 'bones, stones and groans'. However, with routine serum calcium measurements, an elevated serum calcium level has become the most common presentation.

Box 1.1 • Symptoms of primary hyperparathyroidism classified by organ system

Gastrointestinal
- Nausea/vomiting
- Epigastric pain
- Pancreatitis
- Peptic ulcer disease
- Anorexia
- Weight loss
- Constipation

Cardiovascular
- Hypertension
- Shortened Q–T interval, wide T wave
- Bradycardia
- Heart block
- Lethal arrhythmias

Renal
- Renal colic
- Polyuria/oliguria/anuria
- Thirst/dehydration
- Renal failure

Neuropsychiatric
- Anxiety
- Headaches
- Dementia/paranoia
- Confusion
- Depression
- Muscle weakness
- Hyporeflexia
- Ataxia
- Coma

Miscellaneous
- Visual changes
- Band keratopathy
- Conjunctivitis
- Myalgia
- Pruritus

PHP is confirmed by elevated serum calcium and serum PTH levels and can be suggested by other laboratory values (see below):

- **Elevated serum calcium.** While a useful screening tool, many conditions can lead to inaccuracies in the measured total serum calcium levels. For example, hypoalbuminaemia and acidosis can create 'normal' serum calcium levels. Given these variables, many groups favour measuring the ionised serum calcium level instead. Monchik found in a number of series that an elevated serum ionised calcium correlated better with the presence of PHP as confirmed by surgery.[19]

- **Elevated serum PTH.** Current antibody-driven assays for serum intact parathyroid hormone (iPTH) levels are highly accurate.

- **Chloride:phosphate ratio.** A recent retrospective study suggests that a chloride:phosphate ratio ≥33 is indicative of PHP in both hypercalcaemic as well as normocalcaemic patients.[20]

- **Hypercalciuria.** The presence of hypercalciuria rules out benign familial hypercalcaemic hypocalciuria, which can mimic PHP.

- **Hypophosphataemia.** Due to the decreased resorption of phosphate by the renal tubule, phosphate levels decrease in approximately 50% of patients with PHP.

Normocalcaemic hyperparathyroidism

There is a small subset of patients with PHP who present with normal or only intermittently elevated calcium levels. Mather first described normocalcaemic hyperparathyroidism in 1953 in a woman who presented with osteitis fibrosa cystica. Since that time, this variation of PHP has been an infrequent but recognised entity. While still uncommon when compared with hypercalcaemic PHP, recent population studies have shown that this variant of the disease may be more prevalent than previously believed and that improved screening may help identify mildly symptomatic or asymptomatic patients.[21]

The exact biochemical mechanisms of normocalcaemic PHP remain elusive. Some investigators postulate that the normocalcaemic variant of PHP represents an early or preclinical phase that progresses to typical hypercalcaemic PHP.[22,23] Others have found distinct differences in the biological response to PTH in patients with normocalcaemic vs. hypercalcaemic hyperparathyroidism. For example, Maruani et al found that patients with normocalcaemic hyperparathyroidism displayed a resistance to the renal and bony effects of PTH as measured by a lower fasting urine calcium excretion and renal tubular calcium resorption, as well as lower values of markers of bone turnover.[24]

 While most patients with normocalcaemic PHP present with nephrolithiasis, recent data show that other classic constitutional symptoms are just as prevalent in normocalcaemic patients as in hypercalcaemic PHP patients, suggesting that there is a larger unidentified population with PHP.[25,26]

The majority of patients with normocalcaemic PHP present with renal calculi and hypercalciuria. However, the most common cause of renal calculi and hypercalciuria is idiopathic hypercalciuria (IH). To further confound the matter, some variants of IH have elevated PTH levels. It is vitally important to distinguish between these two entities since surgical parathyroidectomy effectively cures normocalcaemic PHP, whereas postsurgical IH patients continue to form stones.[25]

Many tests are helpful in differentiating between the two diseases, but none has been shown to be conclusive enough to be used in isolation. The best diagnostic yield is to use two or more tests in combination:

- **Thiazide administration.** Administration of thiazide diuretics leads to a decrease in urinary calcium excretion. Patients with normocalcaemic PHP will have persistently elevated PTH levels, whereas those with IH will have a normalisation of PTH.[27]
- **Phosphate deprivation.** After restricting phosphate to 350 mg/day and administering 650 mg of aluminium hydroxide four times a day (while on a normal calorie and normal calcium diet), serum calcium and phosphorus levels are checked every day for 4 days. Patients with subsequent hypercalcaemia or persistent hypercalciuria usually have normocalcaemic PHP. This test is no longer used routinely.
- **Calcium loading test.** After administration of either 350 or 1000 mg of oral calcium, serum calcium and urine calcium are measured. Patients with normocalcaemic PHP have a significant increase in serum calcium (due to increased intestinal absorption) and an increase in urine calcium excretion, whereas intestinal absorption of calcium varies widely in patients with IH.[28] In a recent study, after administration of 1 g of oral calcium, the combined parameters of (i) circulating PTH nadir (pg/mL) × peak calcium concentration (mg/dL) and (ii) relative PTH decline/relative calcium increment diagnosed normocalcaemic PHP with 100% sensitivity and 87% specificity.[29] Furthermore, calcium loading suppressed urinary cAMP[28] but did not suppress PTH levels below 70% of baseline.[19]
- **Serum ionised calcium.** An elevated ionised calcium, in conjunction with an elevated PTH, is increasingly gaining acceptance as an excellent means of distinguishing normocalcaemic PHP from IH.[19]

As mentioned previously, the mainstay of treatment for normocalcaemic PHP is operative parathyroidectomy.

Hypercalcaemic crisis

Hypercalcaemia is seen in approximately 0.5% of the general population and up to 5% of the hospital population.[30,31] The majority of cases of hypercalcaemia are classified as mild to moderate (<12 mg/dL or 12–14 mg/dL respectively), and the patient is asymptomatic. This group responds to dietary measures and treatment of the underlying aetiology. However, a subset of patients will present in hypercalcaemic crisis, with serum calcium >14 mg/dL, and are severely symptomatic. These patients require hospitalisation and aggressive reduction of serum calcium. Fortunately, except in cases of malignancy, treatment for hypercalcaemia is typically successful.

Since the calcium ion plays a crucial role in membrane potentials throughout the body, the symptoms of hypercalcaemia are varied and potentially life-threatening. The classic presentation of severe hypercalcaemia includes acute confusion, abdominal pain, vomiting, dehydration and anuria. In addition, patients may develop lethal arrhythmias due to decreased conduction velocities and shortened refractory periods, which manifest on an electrocardiogram as a prolonged P–R interval, a shortened Q–T interval, and arrhythmia. Hypercalcaemic crisis is the most extreme form of hypercalcaemia and is defined as severe hypercalcaemia in association with profound dehydration and obtundation.[32] At serum calcium levels of 15–18 mg/dL, coma and cardiac arrest may occur.

The most common aetiology of hypercalcaemia in non-hospitalised patients is PHP, while malignancy accounts for almost two-thirds of the hypercalcaemic inpatient population. It is crucial to identify the underlying cause of hypercalcaemia in order to effectively and definitively address the acute event. Box 1.2 lists the differential diagnoses for hypercalcaemia. The treatment of severe hypercalcaemia revolves around aggressive rehydration, increasing renal excretion of calcium, blunting of calcium release from skeletal stores, and treating the underlying cause of the hypercalcaemia.[33]

The primary goal of treatment is to achieve adequate volume resuscitation, which in turn increases calcium excretion in the kidneys.[33,34] Patients are invariably dehydrated due to poor oral intake and

Malignancy
- Solid tumour (parathyroid hormone-related peptide mediated): lung, kidney, squamous cell carcinoma of head/neck/oesophagus/female genital tract
- Metastases (osteoclastic lesions): breast, prostate
- Haematological: multiple myeloma, lymphoma, leukaemia

Hyperparathyroidism
- Primary hyperparathyroidism
- Familial: multiple endocrine neoplasia (MEN) types 1 and 2, benign familial hypocalciuric hypercalcaemia, idiopathic hypercalcaemia of infancy
- Lithium

Increased bone turnover
- Vitamin A intoxication
- Thiazide diuretics
- Hyperthyroidism
- Immobilisation
- Paget's disease

Excess vitamin D
- Vitamin D intoxication
- Increased 1,25-dihydroxylated vitamin D: granulomatous disease

Renal failure
- Milk alkali syndrome
- Secondary hyperparathyroidism
- Aluminium intoxication

Miscellaneous
- Addisonian crisis
- Laboratory error: haemoconcentration, hypoproteinaemia

vomiting. The resultant decrement in glomerular filtration rate leads to a decrease in renal excretion of calcium. Typically, 200–500 mL/h of normal saline is given to maintain urine output above 100 mL/h, with the caveat that comorbidities may limit the rate of resuscitation. Using normal saline lends substrate for the resultant natriuresis. Once the intravascular volume is restored, loop diuretics such as furosemide may be given to enhance calciuresis by inhibiting calcium resorption in the thick ascending limb of the loop of Henle. During the resuscitative phase, the patient must be monitored closely for signs of fluid overload, hypokalaemia and hypomagnesaemia. Serum calcium levels can be reduced by 1.6–2.5 mg/dL within 24 hours by volume repletion and loop diuretic administration alone.[32] However, when serum calcium exceeds 12 mg/dL or hypercalcaemia is caused by malig-nancy, intravenous fluids and diuretics alone are usually insufficient to normalise calcium levels.

Numerous agents are available to blunt the release of calcium from bone resorption and treat the underlying disease.[32–34] Table 1.1 provides an overview of agents available to combat hypercalcaemia and their relative strengths and weaknesses.

- **Bisphosphonates: pamidronate 60–90 mg i.v.** Bisphosphonates are pyrophosphate analogues that are concentrated in areas of high bone turnover and inhibit osteoclast activity. Endogenous phosphatases cannot hydrolyse the central carbon–phosphorus–carbon bond, making this drug stable in vivo. Bisphosphonates should be given intravenously due to their poor absorption by the gastrointestinal tract. In the USA, only etidronate (first generation) and pamidronate (second generation) are approved for use in treating hypercalcaemia. Pamidronate has widely supplanted etidronate as the bisphosphonate of choice due to its faster onset, increased duration of action, increased efficacy and minimal adverse effect on mineralisation. One dose of intravenous pamidronate normalises serum calcium for 10–14 days in 80–100% of patients with hypercalcaemia of malignancy. Newer, more potent generations of bisphosphonates may replace pamidronate as the standard as more clinical data become available.[35]
- **Calcitonin: salmon calcitonin 4–8 U/kg s.c./i.v.** Calcitonin diminishes osteoclast activity and increases calciuresis within minutes of administration. However, the duration of action is limited to only a few days. Calcitonin therapy only rarely results in normocalcaemia. Tachyphylaxis limits the long-term use of calcitonin. Currently, calcitonin is used primarily as an immediate hypocalcaemic agent that temporises until the more sustained effects of other agents begin.
- **Gallium nitrate: 200 mg/m² i.v. q.d. for 5 days.** Gallium nitrate inhibits bone resorption by reducing the solubility of hydroxyapatite crystals. This drug induces a normocalcaemia within 2–3 days that lasts for 5–6 days in approximately 75% of patients. The use of gallium nitrate has been limited by its nephrotoxicity, the need for continuous infusion and lack of clinical data.

Table 1.1 • Treatment of hypercalcaemia

Treatment	Onset	Duration	Effectiveness (% normalised)	Advantages	Disadvantages
First-line therapy					
Normal saline	Hours	During use	0–10	Almost always dehydrated	Congestive heart failure Hypokalaemia/hypomagnesaemia
Loop diuretic	Hours	2–6 hours	0–10	Fast onset	Electrolyte abnormalities Dehydration
Bisphosphonates					
Etidronate (first-generation)	1–2 days	5–7 days	30–80	Intermediate onset	Hyperphosphataemia 3-day infusion
Pamidronate (second-generation)	1–2 days	10–14 days	70–100	High potency Prolonged duration	Fever (20%) Hypophosphataemia/hypocalcaemia Hypomagnesaemia
Calcitonin (salmon)	Hours	2–3 days	10–20	Intermediate onset Fast onset Bridge until intermediate-action drugs take effect	Tachyphylaxis Flushing Nausea/vomiting
Second-line therapy					
Plicamycin	1–2 days	Days	75–85	High potency	Hepatocellular necrosis Bleeding (decreased clotting factors) Thrombocytopenia Renal failure Electrolyte abnormalities Hypocalcaemia
Gallium nitrate	Day 6	7–10 days	75–82	High potency	5-day infusion Contraindicated in renal failure Hypophosphataemia Anaemia Nausea/vomiting Rare hypotension
Glucocorticoids	5–7 days	Days to weeks	Variable	Oral therapy Cidal effect on haematological and breast cancers	Only effective in vitamin D excess or granulomatous disease Immunosuppression Cushing's syndrome
Phosphates					
Oral	24 hours	During use	Variable	Low toxicity High potency Rapid action	Only effective in hyperphosphataemia Severe hypocalcaemia Organ damage Potentially lethal
Intravenous	Hours	1–2 days	Variable		

- **Plicamycin: 25 μg/kg.** Plicamycin is an osteoclast cytotoxin originally used in chemotherapy. Due to its serious side-effects (hepatic, renal and bone marrow toxicity), plicamycin is reserved for patients who fail bisphosphonate therapy. Since toxicities are related to the frequency and total dosage, administration is limited to one dose with additional dosing only if hypercalcaemia recurs.
- **Glucocorticoids: prednisone 40–100 mg p.o. q.d. or hydrocortisone 200–300 mg i.v. for 3–5 days.** Glucocorticoids are used primarily to augment the effect of calcitonin or in diseases associated with vitamin D excess (i.e. granulomatous diseases, vitamin D toxicity and multiple myeloma). Glucocorticoids increase calciuresis, decrease intestinal absorption of calcium and have a direct tumoricidal effect on certain haematological malignancies as well as breast cancer.
- **Oral inorganic phosphate: phosphate 1–1.5 g p.o. q.d.** Oral inorganic phosphate has a limited effect in normalising serum calcium in patients who are hypophosphataemic by increasing calcium uptake by bone and intestinal absorption of calcium. Intravenous phosphate is one of the swiftest means to reduce serum calcium levels. However, it can cause fatal hypocalcaemia and severe organ failure by calcium phosphate precipitation. As such, intravenous phosphate is reserved for life-threatening hypercalcaemia, and even then must be used with extreme caution.
- **Dialysis.** This is the treatment of choice for patients with hypercalcaemia and renal or heart failure. Dialysis may also be considered in hypercalcaemic patients who fail standard therapies. Haemodialysis and peritoneal dialysis can remove up to 250 mg of calcium/hour. Care must be taken to avoid the hypophosphataemia that often accompanies dialysis.

The underlying cause of hypercalcaemic crisis must always be addressed as part of the definitive management.[33] In patients with an elevated PTH level and clinical factors suggestive of PHP, parathyroidectomy is the fastest way to decrease PTH levels and consequently serum calcium levels. Therefore, expedient operative intervention should always be considered in this subgroup of patients.[36]

 In contrast, patients with malignancy-associated hypercalcaemic crisis typically present at advanced or terminal stages of their disease with a mean survival of only months. In this setting, discussion with the patient and family regarding end-of-life decisions will be appropriate.

Imaging and localisation

In the hands of experienced surgeons, bilateral neck exploration for PHP cures 95% of cases.[37,38] Furthermore, prior to recent advances in imaging technology, the sensitivity of localisation studies was approximately 60–70%.

 Given these facts, the National Institutes of Health released guidelines in 1990 for the treatment of PHP that included the recommendation that preoperative localisation was not indicated.[39]

Localisation studies were to be limited to re-operative cases. However, the advent of rapid intra-operative PTH assays and the highly sensitive and specific sestamibi scan (see below) have rekindled interest in preoperative localisation for directed unilateral exploration – the so-called focused approach.

Most patients with PHP have a single adenoma, while entities such as multiple adenoma and four-gland hyperplasia are considerably less frequent.

 In a meta-analysis comprising 6331 patients (excluding familial hyperparathyroid cases) with PHP, Denham and Norman found that 87% had single adenomas, 9% had four-gland hyperplasia, 3% had multiple adenomas and fewer than 1% had cancer.[40]

These statistics are consistent across the literature.[41] The fact that the overwhelming majority of patients have unilateral disease or bilateral disease that can be identified by unilateral exploration raises the issue of whether bilateral exploration is mandated in every case. Is it reasonable to expose the patient to the increased morbidity of bilateral exploration to identify the less than 3% of people who will have a second adenoma on the contralateral side? These issues have led many endocrine surgeons to investigate the feasibility of preoperative localisation and directed unilateral exploration. This trend, along with the need to localise pathology in re-operative situations, has spurred the refinement of imaging techniques for parathyroid disease. Table 1.2 provides a summary of the current imaging modalities.

Table 1.2 • Imaging methods for localisation in primary hyperparathyroidism

Study	Sensitivity (%)	Specificity (%)	Re-operative sensitivity (%)	False positives (%)	Advantages	Disadvantages
Ultrasound guidance	71–80	80	40	15–20	Inexpensive Fast Morphology No radiation/no i.v. contrast Confirms findings Can combine with fine-needle aspiration (FNA)	Difficulty with posterior areas and mediastinum Operator dependent Cannot detect lesions below 5 mm
Endoscopic ultrasound	71	–	–	–	Posterior/perioesophageal areas	Difficulty with anterior/lateral areas
CT scan with i.v. contrast	46–80	80	–	50	Mediastinum align Retro-oesophageal/retrotracheal areas Can combine with FNA	Difficulty with lower neck around shoulders/thyroid area Previous surgery yields artefact Radiation Needs i.v. contrast
Magnetic resonance imaging	64–88	88–95	50–88	18	Localising ectopic glands Used if scintigraphy fails to localise lesion No i.v. contrast	Expensive Cannot be combined with FNA Compliance sometimes limited by claustrophobia Cannot detect lesions below 5 mm
Thallium–technetium scan	75	73–82	50	25	Wide availability Minimal radiation	Poor anatomical detail Average sensitivity
Technetium–sestamibi scan	90.7	98.8	–	Low	Best localisation modality Minimal radiation Widely available SPECT offers excellent anatomical localisation Not operator dependent	May not identify four-gland hyperplasia or multiple adenomas
Angiography	–	–	60	–	Precise anatomical localisation	Neurological complications
Angiography and venous sampling	–	96–98	91–95	Low	Re-operative localisation	Embolisation
Venous sampling	–	–	80	6–18	Identifies multiple adenoma and four-gland hyperplasia	Dye-induced renal failure

Ultrasound (US)

Ultrasound was one of the first localisation techniques to be widely used. Typically this test is performed with the 7.5- or 10-MHz probes to optimise penetration and resolution. It is fast, non-invasive, non-irradiating and inexpensive. Furthermore, it allows visualisation of the thyroid, carotid, jugular and cervical areas. However, ultrasound is dependent on operator experience and size of pathology (limit is approximately 5 mm). This technique also has difficulty locating abnormalities in the retro-oesophageal, retrosternal, retrotracheal and deep cervical areas. False-positive results (15–20%) are due to muscles, vessels, thyroid nodules, lymphadenopathy and oesophageal pathology.[42,43] Image quality may be limited by patient motion or metallic clips from previous operations. The reported sensitivity of ultrasound is between 71% and 80%, but falls to 40% for re-operative localisation.[44]

Endoscopic US has also been used to evaluate posterior, deep cervical and perioesophageal glands. Endoscopic US correctly identified 12 of 23 adenomas (the remaining 11 were in either the anterior or lateral neck) in one series and had a sensitivity of 71% in another.[45,46] Endoscopic US appears to have a role in localising certain parathyroid lesions for recurrent or persistent hyperparathyroidism.

Given these limitations, US is perhaps most useful when used in conjunction with other modalities. US combined with thyroid scintigraphy has the specific benefits of identifying intrathyroidal adenomas and distinguishing adenomas from thyroid nodules.[47–49] Performing US-guided fine-needle aspiration (FNA) increases the sensitivity of US localisation by confirming the presence of PTH in the mass. Cytological studies of the aspirate are not useful and often cannot even distinguish between thyroid and parathyroid tissue. In one small series, PTH analysis of the aspirate made the diagnosis in 100% of cases.[50] Finally, US provides a useful means to define the depth and singularity of adenomas found by scintigraphy.

Computed tomography (CT)

With the new-generation CT scanners and alterations in technique, the accuracy of CT has improved greatly over the last 5 years. In the past, the limitations of CT were based primarily on the size of the adenoma in that smaller parathyroid adenomas were more difficult to visualise. CT scan had difficulty in localising adenomas in the lower neck (at the level of the shoulders) and close to or within the thyroid. Furthermore, CT scan was inaccurate in differentiating between upper and lower pole glands.[51,52] CT scans with intravenous contrast had sensitivities in the 80% range, but prior operations in the neck can produce artefacts, such as the 'sparkler effect' (seen with surgical clips), which reduce this number.[53] The false-positive rate, at 50%, is higher than in other imaging modalities.[54,55]

The accuracy of CT scanning is largely dependent on the technique utilised, as well as the experience and dedication of the radiologist interpreting the study. Whereas in the past most reports of CT scanning utilised 5-mm cross-sectional cuts, accurate parathyroid CT localisation mandates the use of 2.5-mm cuts as well as a dedicated radiologist committed to conducting the time-consuming review of parathyroid CT scans. Comparing pre- and post-intravenous contrast scans permits identification of parathyroid adenomas due to the increased vascularity of hyperfunctioning parathyroid tissue. Thin-cut parathyroid CT scanning provides precise anatamomical information regarding gland location (anterior, posterior, superior, inferior or mediastinum) as well as information regarding parathyroid gland relationship to the thyroid gland. Thyroid nodules can be differentiated from parathyroid adenomas due to the difference in shape and vascularity. Moreover, parathyroid gland weight can be estimated by determining the volume of the visualised parathyroid gland. Four-dimensional reconstruction is feasible and permits a remarkable appreciation of parathyroid gland location and relationship to surrounding structures. As with US, CT may be used in conjunction with FNA to increase diagnostic yield.[56] In a retrospective review from Columbia and Cornell Universities, we demonstrated that in patients with negative sestamibi localisation, thin-cut CT scanning permitted a focused parathyroidectomy in 66% of patients (in press).

Magnetic resonance imaging (MRI)

MRI is superior to CT scanning in that it does not require intravenous contrast nor is it subject to the 'sparkler effect' or shoulder artefact. On T2-weighted imaging, enlarged parathyroid glands have significantly increased intensity. T2-weighted MRI is an excellent means of localising ectopic glands in patients undergoing re-operation for PHP, although it was less useful for identifying lesions in normal positions. Aufferman et al found that MRI located

79% of ectopic adenomas while localising only 59% of those in the normal anatomical position.[57] Overall sensitivities are in the 50–88% range for re-operative localisation.[58] Despite better sensitivities (64–88%) than CT scanning, MRI has significant drawbacks.[54,55,59,60] This modality cannot image normal glands or adenomas less than 5 mm in size. Furthermore, it has difficulty localising superior parathyroid glands since they lie posterior to the thyroid. False positives can result from thyroid nodules and lymphadenopathy.[61] Finally, MRI is expensive, cannot be combined with FNA, and patient compliance is sometimes limited by claustrophobia. Given all these factors, MRI is best reserved for localisation in re-operation for PHP or when parathyroid scintigraphy is negative or equivocal.[62,63]

Thallium-201–technetium-99 m pertechnetate scan (Tl–99mTc scan)

Tl–Tc scanning is an image subtraction technique that is rapidly being replaced by sestamibi scanning (see below). Tl–Tc scanning relies on the fact that the thyroid and parathyroid tissues (especially hyperfunctioning glands) take up thallium while the thyroid alone takes up technetium. By subtracting the two images, one can localise the parathyroid tumour. The sensitivity of Tl–Tc scanning is 75% for first-time operations and only 50% for re-operations.[64] The false-positive rate is approximately 25% and occurs with metastatic nodal disease and thyroid pathology.[64] Given the average sensitivity and poor anatomical detail of Tl–Tc scanning, this mode has been relegated to second-line imaging status.

Technetium-99 m sestamibi scan (sestamibi scan)

Ever since Coakley et al fortuitously discovered that technetium-99 m sestamibi concentrated in abnormal parathyroid glands, sestamibi scanning has revolutionised the practice of parathyroid surgery, making directed unilateral exploration a reasonable alternative to routine bilateral exploration.[65] Sestamibi is a derivative of technetium that avidly incorporates itself into mitochondria. The large amount of mitochondria in hyperactive parathyroid glands allows more intense labelling of parathyroid tumours relative to the thyroid and surrounding tissue.[66] The radiotracer also washes out much more slowly from the parathyroid than the thyroid. This differential uptake can be accentuated by pretest medical thyroid suppression. Sestamibi exploits these differences in uptake and retention to localise parathyroid adenomas. This radioisotope has a short half-life and produces high-energy photon emission that allows for low doses of radiation and high-definition imaging. Also, sestamibi scanning images both in the anteroposterior and lateral views, which allows for more precise localisation of the pathology.

There are three basic protocols for sestamibi scanning in current use:

- **Single-isotope dual-phase scan.** After intravenous administration of 15–25 mCi of sestamibi, images are taken at 10, 15, 120 and 180 minutes post-injection. A positive scan demonstrates increased uptake of tracer in the thyroid gland and parathyroid adenoma in early phases with washout of tracer from the thyroid gland but not the parathyroid adenoma in the late-phase images. This is the simplest and most widely used protocol. However, two potential pitfalls of this technique are: (i) sestamibi can accumulate and remain in thyroid nodules; and (ii) rapid washout of sestamibi can lead to false-negative results. To counter the first problem, many investigators are experimenting with dual-isotope subtraction scanning. **Figure 1.1** illustrates a typical parathyroid adenoma in the early-phase scan.

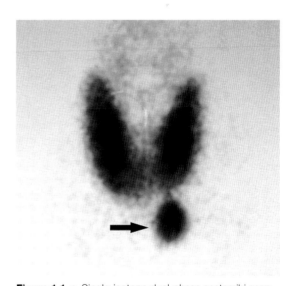

Figure 1.1 • Single-isotope dual-phase sestamibi scan. Sestamibi tracer can be seen concentrating in both the thyroid gland and a left lower pole parathyroid adenoma (arrow) in this early-phase image. Delayed-phase images would demonstrate washout of tracer from the thyroid gland but not the parathyroid adenoma.

- **Dual-isotope subtraction scanning.** Sestamibi and another radioisotope that amasses in the thyroid (such as ^{123}I or thallium chloride) are administered and the two views are subtracted to reveal the parathyroid pathology. Images are taken in both early and late phases. Late-phase imaging helps to exclude false-positive results by allowing more time for thyroid nodules to wash out. Numerous protocols and isotopes are currently being investigated but none has yet proven superior to the rest. **Figure 1.2** demonstrates a dual-isotope subtraction scan. Panel (a) demonstrates ^{123}I tracer uptake in only the thyroid gland. Panel (b) demonstrates an early-phase image with uptake of sestamibi tracer in the right lower parathyroid adenoma (arrow) and parts of the thyroid gland. Panel (c) demonstrates persistent tracer in the parathyroid adenoma (arrow) and washout of tracer from the thyroid gland.

- **SPECT (single-photon emission computed tomography) analysis.** This protocol allows for three-dimensional images to be created, which allows for better anatomical localisation, especially within the mediastinum, without any significant increase in sensitivity.[67,68] While this enhanced anatomical delineation may be useful in re-operative PHP, the significantly increased cost of this modality does not justify its routine use in preoperative localisation. **Figure 1.3** demonstrates a CT-enhanced SPECT scan (CT-SPECT). The top two rows of images mark the parathyroid adenoma on a CT scan (see Figure 1.3). The bottom row of images marks the parathyroid adenoma on SPECT scan (see Figure 1.3).

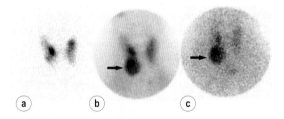

(a)   (b)   (c)

Figure 1.2 • Dual-isotope dual-phase sestamibi scan using both sestamibi and iodine-123. **(a)** The ^{123}I-only scan that delineates the thyroid gland only. **(b)** A right lower lobe parathyroid adenoma (arrow) in the early-phase image with concomitant thyroid uptake of [123]I. **(c)** The same right lower lobe parathyroid adenoma (arrow) with thyroid 'washout' seen in this late-phase image.

Irrespective of the protocol, depending on the series quoted, sestamibi scanning localises parathyroid adenomas in 80–100% of cases and has a specificity of around 90%.[40,69–72]

 The false-positive rate is low and is usually due to thyroid adenomas. The false-negative rate is relatively low, but perhaps the major drawback of sestamibi scanning is that it does not always identify patients with multiple adenomas or four-gland hyperplasia.[68]

The false-negative rate is low and is usually related to small-sized glands or failure to recognise hyperplasia. In a meta-analysis of the English-language literature over the last 10 years, comprising 6331 patients, Denham and Norman found that 87% of patients had a single adenoma that sestamibi scan localised with an average sensitivity and specificity of 90.7% and 98.8% respectively.[40] Sestamibi-guided unilateral exploration led to an average cost saving of US $650 per operation. This study demonstrated that preoperative localisation with sestamibi scan was specific enough to make unilateral exploration both safe and cost-effective. If a single focus of uptake is noted, then unilateral exploration is likely to be successful. If no uptake or multiple areas of uptake are seen then bilateral exploration should be planned. Other radioisotopes, such as [99mTc]-Tetrofosmin and 2[^{18}F]-fluoro-2-deoxyglucose, are currently being evaluated. For the time being, sestamibi scanning remains the standard for non-invasive localisation modalities.

Parathyroid angiography and venous sampling for PTH

Parathyroid angiography involves examination of both thyrocervical trunks, both internal mammary arteries and both carotids with occasional selective superior thyroid artery catheterisation. The highly vascular parathyroid adenomas appear as a persistent oval or round 'stain' on angiography. Glands 4 mm in size or greater may be readily visualised. False positives are typically due to thyroid nodules or inflamed lymph nodes. Due to potentially serious complications like dye-induced renal failure, embolisation and neurological damage, angiography is usually reserved for re-operative localisation. The sensitivity of parathyroid angiography in this situation approaches 60%.[44,73,74]

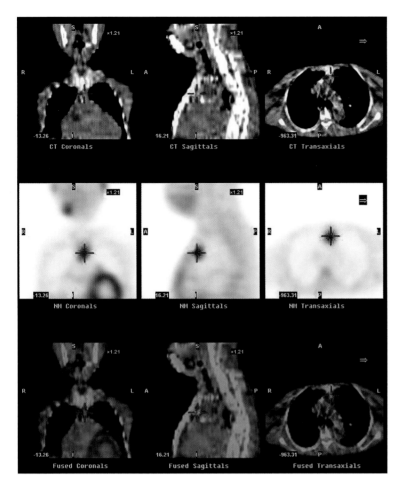

Figure 1.3 • Computed tomography (CT)-enhanced SPECT scan. This image shows a mediastinal parathyroid adenoma identified precisely by SPECT enhancement and CT. The top two rows of images mark the parathyroid adenoma on CT scan (crosshair). The bottom row of images mark the parathyroid adenoma on SPECT scan.

Selective venous sampling for PTH allows for precise localisation of adenomas in the hands of an experienced interventionalist. The venous drainage of the lesion is established when there is a twofold drop in PTH between the sampled blood and the serum PTH. The technique has a sensitivity of 80% and is equally effective in localising mediastinal and cervical adenomas.[43,44,75,76] Venous sampling also allows for the identification of pathology in multiple glands. Venous sampling without concomitant angiography has a false-positive rate of 6–18%.[76]

 When combined, the sensitivity for parathyroid angiography and selective venous sampling for PTH is 91–95%, with a low false-positive rate.[73]

Furthermore, the combination of the two modalities allows for precise localisation of single or multiple adenomas, even in ectopic locations and hyperplasia. However, the significant potential complications limit this study to use in localisation for re-operative PHP.

Pathology

PHP can be caused by single adenomas (87–90%), multiple adenomas (3%), four-gland hyperplasia (9%) or carcinoma (1%). Pathological criteria for differentiation of these entities are not universally accepted. In fact, in a small series of patients with single adenomas reported by Wang et al, none of the patients with histological evidence of hyperplasia in the remaining glands had recurrent or persistent PHP, suggesting that microscopic criteria for identifying pathological lesions are not very accurate. Due to the imprecise nature of histological diagnosis for PHP, frozen section often does not help intraoperative distinction between different lesions.

The best indicators that a gland is abnormal are its size and weight. While normal parathyroid glands weigh 40 mg on average, diseased glands weigh anywhere from 70 mg to 20 g. Indeed, some authors suggest that the only role for frozen section is to determine the weight of the specimen. Numerous markers and special stains have been proposed to aid in differentiation, but none has gained wide acceptance.

Adenoma

The gross appearance of an adenoma is typically large and tan or beefy red. Some authors have described the classic adenoma as a 'little kidney in the neck or mediastinum'.[77] The other glands appear atrophic or normal in size. While normal parathyroids contain predominantly chief cells with scattered oxyphil cells, adenomas contain solid sheets of chief cells, oxyphil cells or a combination of both surrounded by a fibrous capsule. Classically, there is a rim of compressed normal parathyroid surrounding the adenoma, which can be found in 20–30% of patients. **Figure 1.4** demonstrates the characteristic hypercellularity, loss of fat, loss of lobulation and oxyphilic change of adenomatous degeneration. Pleomorphism and multinucleation may be present, but mitotic figures are rare and more strongly associated with carcinoma. There is less stromal fat in adenomas compared with normal parathyroids. Research demonstrates that parathyroid adenomas are typically monoclonal and may have very specific mutations in certain genes, such as the *MEN1* tumour suppressor gene and the *PRAD1* oncogene.[78]

Double adenoma

Although uncommon, this form of PHP may lead to recurrent or persistent PHP if diseased glands are located on the contralateral side of a unilateral exploration. Finding two abnormal glands on one side mandates bilateral exploration.

Hyperplasia

A polyclonal expansion of parathyroid cells is called hyperplasia. This is more typical of familial hyperparathyroidism but may be found in sporadic cases. Grossly, the hyperplasia is typically not uniform. One gland may appear much larger than the rest, giving the false impression of adenomatous disease, but on histological examination each gland is hyperplastic. Microscopically, the chief cells are mainly affected. More so than with adenomas, the absence of parathyroid fat supports the diagnosis of hyperplasia. **Figure 1.5** demonstrates the characteristic hypercellularity, loss of fat, and retained lobulation of parathyroid hyperplasia. Diffuse hyperplasia warrants four-gland exploration with three-and-a-half-gland parathyroidectomy or four-gland excision with autotransplantation.

Carcinoma

A rare finding, parathyroid carcinoma is a difficult diagnosis to make preoperatively and often is a retrospective diagnosis made only after metastatic disease develops. Patients tend to be younger (50s cf. 60s) than in benign disease and there is an equal distribution among men and women. On preoperative evaluation, carcinoma produces a

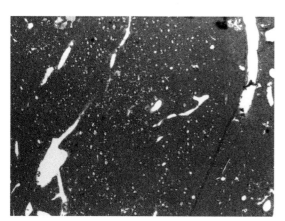

Figure 1.4 • Parathyroid adenoma. This photomicrograph demonstrates the characteristic hypercellularity, loss of fat, loss of lobulation and oxyphilic change of adenomatous degeneration (×40).

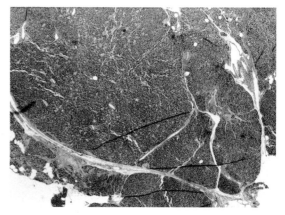

Figure 1.5 • Parathyroid hyperplasia. This photomicrograph demonstrates the characteristic hypercellularity, loss of fat and retained lobulation of parathyroid hyperplasia (×40).

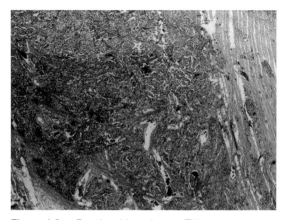

Figure 1.6 • Parathyroid carcinoma. This photomicrograph demonstrates the characteristic thickened fibrous septa, nuclear atypia and capsular invasion of parathyroid carcinoma (×40).

palpable mass in 30–75% of patients (far more frequently than in benign disease) and serum calcium tends to be higher than for adenomatous disease. Furthermore, recurrent laryngeal nerve involvement is suggestive of malignancy. Classic operative findings for parathyroid carcinoma include adherence or invasion into surrounding structures and dense scarring. Typical histological findings include bizarre nuclear atypia, mitotic figures, and capsular or vascular invasion. **Figure 1.6** demonstrates the characteristic thickened fibrous septa, nuclear atypia and capsular invasion. The only definitive criteria for malignancy are metastatic disease (lung, lymph node, liver) and local invasion. There is a recurrence rate of 66%. The 5-year survival is approximately 69%, with death caused by metabolic sequelae of hypercalcaemia.

Secondary hyperparathyroidism (SHP)

Secondary hyperparathyroidism arises when factors other than primary parathyroid disease cause overproduction of PTH. For example, hypermagnesaemia, osteoporosis, rickets and osteomalacia can all cause SHP. By far the most common cause of SHP is chronic renal failure. Indeed, there is such a strong correlation between the two conditions that some call SHP 'renal hyperparathyroidism'. In fact, almost every renal failure patient will develop some form of SHP.

Pathogenesis

Every aspect of renal failure from the decreased renal synthetic function to the metabolic abnormalities to even the treatment contributes to the pathogenesis of SHP. These factors lead to hypertrophy and hyperplastic transformation of the parathyroid gland with subsequent elevation of PTH levels in a futile attempt to normalise serum calcium levels.

Hypocalcaemia and hyperphosphataemia
As outlined previously, hypocalcaemia stimulates PTH secretion in an attempt to normalise levels. Furthermore, phosphate and calcium concentrations are inversely related. As the kidney's ability to excrete phosphates declines and hyperphosphataemia develops, serum calcium levels fall. Further exacerbation of hypocalcaemia comes from the use of calcium-poor dialysates. The consequent decline in calcium levels stimulates PTH overproduction and inhibits the negative-feedback loop.

Decreased synthesis of calcitriol
Calcitriol increases serum calcium by enhancing osteoclast activity and increasing the intestinal absorption of calcium. Calcitriol also acts as part of the negative-feedback loop on the parathyroids to decrease PTH secretion. Decreased renal synthetic function and chronic hyperphosphataemia lead to a reduction in renal 1α-hydroxylase, which in turn leads to a decrement in the conversion of 25-hydroxylated vitamin D_3 (calcidiol) to calcitriol. This dearth of calcitriol not only lowers serum calcium levels leading to increased PTH production, but also dampens an important means of inhibiting the stimulus to secrete PTH.

Bony resistance to PTH
Typically, PTH induces bone resorption with a subsequent rise in serum calcium levels by activating osteoclasts. However, experiments have shown that excessive PTH blunts the mobilisation of calcium from osseous stores.[79]

Changes in PTH set point
The PTH set point is defined as the serum calcium level that decreases PTH levels by 50%.[80] As the set point rises, inhibition of PTH secretion is lost and SHP results. Research suggests that changes in set point may be due to alterations in the expression or sensitivity of the calcium-sensing receptor, but no genetic links have yet been found.[78]

Aluminium intoxication

High aluminium concentrations in renal dialysate and phosphate binders can lead to accumulation in bone. This build-up can lead to osteomalacia, which in turn exacerbates PTH overproduction.

Presentation

As with PHP, many patients are asymptomatic and only come to attention due to serological tests. Symptomatic patients classically present with osseous lesions, pruritus and metastatic calcifications.

Osseous lesions

Bone pain is a common complaint in patients with SHP and is due to increased bone remodelling. Adults tend to develop compression fractures of the axial skeleton, but fractures do occur elsewhere. Children can be afflicted by growth retardation. The classic lesion of hyperparathyroidism is osteitis fibrosa cystica, and this can be seen in up to 30% of patients on dialysis. Caused by increased bone resorption and formation, this lesion leads to a chaotic matrix deposition giving the typical 'woven bone' appearance. This compromised bone is inherently weaker than normal bone and may lead to fractures. Other osseous lesions that may develop include pepperpot skull, osteomalacia and long bone fractures.

Pruritus

Pruritus is found in 85% of patients on haemodialysis and may become so severe as to be disabling. Significant symptomatic relief is achieved after parathyroidectomy.[81]

Metastatic calcification

Metastatic calcification can affect almost any organ system in the body and may be a significant cause of morbidity in patients with SHP. Perhaps the most common site for calcification is in the vasculature. Other typical areas of calcification include the heart, mitral valve, kidneys, gastrointestinal tract and penis. Parathyroidectomy may decrease the severity of metastatic calcification in all organ systems except the vasculature.

Calciphylaxis

This is a rare but severe complication, consisting of soft tissue and vascular calcification that may lead to tissue necrosis. The mottled violaceous lesions can progress to ulcers and gangrene. Calciphylaxis may be present anywhere in the body, but is most common in the extremities. The mortality rate of calciphylaxis is approximately 50%. Patients with a high calcium × phosphorus product are at risk for developing calciphylaxis. The mainstays of therapy include phosphate binders and parathyroidectomy.

Treatment

The initial therapy of SHP is primarily medical and revolves around bringing the serum calcium and phosphate to physiological levels. Normalising these removes the major impetus for PTH overproduction. Non-operative therapy includes calcium supplementation (1500 mg/day), phosphate-poor diets, phosphate binders (<1000 mg/day) and vitamin D supplementation. Other therapies include aluminium-binding agents (desferrioxamine) and haemodialysis with calcium-enriched dialysates. However, hypercalcaemia often complicates these treatment regimens. Newly developed calcimimetics bind to the calcium-sensing receptor and lower parathyroid hormone levels without increasing calcium and phosphate levels. Agents like cinacalcet have been shown to effectively reduce PTH levels in contrast to placebo in randomised double-blind studies.[82] The definitive therapy for SHP is renal transplant, although some patients will develop tertiary hyperparathyroidism postoperatively. Operative parathyroidectomy (four-gland with autotransplantation or three-and-a-half-gland) is indicated in the 5–10% of patients who fail medical management. Other indications include: (1) intractable bone pain; (2) intractable pruritus; (3) fractures; and (4) symptomatic ectopic calcifications.

Tertiary hyperparathyroidism

Tertiary hyperparathyroidism is a rare condition seen in certain patients with chronic renal failure who have resolution of their renal disease, usually due to a kidney transplant. Prior to transplant, a portion of these patients have parathyroid glands that autonomously produce PTH due to the constant hypocalcaemia caused by the hyperphosphataemia of renal failure. Once freed from the metabolic disarray of their renal disease by transplant, a subset will have parathyroids that continue to produce PTH without the normal feedback inhibition, thus producing hypercalcaemia. Approximately 60% of cases of tertiary hyperparathyroidism resolve spontaneously. Therefore, surgical parathyroidectomy is only indicated if there is persistent hypercalcaemia after 12 months or more of observation.

Key points

- PHP occurs more frequently in women than men.
- PHP is confirmed by elevated serum calcium and serum PTH levels.
- The majority of cases of hypercalcaemia are classified as mild to moderate (<12 mg/dL or 12–14 mg/dL serum calcium respectively), and the patient is asymptomatic.
- Hypercalcaemic crisis consists of serum calcium >14 mg/dL and severe symptoms.
- Treatment of severe hypercalcaemia involves aggressive rehydration, increasing renal excretion of calcium, blunting of calcium release from skeletal stores, and treating the underlying cause of the hypercalcaemia.
- Bilateral neck exploration for PHP cures 95% of cases.
- Of patients with PHP, 87% have single adenomas, 9% have four-gland hyperplasia, 3% have multiple adenomas and fewer than 1% have cancer.
- Sestamibi scanning localises parathyroid adenomas in up to 80–100% of cases and has a specificity of around 90%, but results in different series vary considerably.
- The most common cause of SHP is chronic renal failure.

References

1. Adami S, Marcocci C, Gatti D. Epidemiology of primary hyperparathyroidism in Europe. J Bone Miner Res 2002; 17(Suppl 2):N18–23.

2. Heath H 3rd, Hodgson SF, Kennedy MA. Primary hyperparathyroidism. Incidence, morbidity, and potential economic impact in a community. N Engl J Med 1980; 302(4):189–93.

3. Russell CF, Edis AJ. Surgery for primary hyperparathyroidism: experience with 500 consecutive cases and evaluation of the role of surgery in the asymptomatic patient. Br J Surg 1982; 69(5):244–7.

4. Thompson NW, Eckhauser FE, Harness JK. The anatomy of primary hyperparathyroidism. Surgery 1982; 92(5):814–21.

   An excellent overall review.

5. Moore MA, Owen JJ. Experimental studies on the development of the thymus. J Exp Med 1967; 126(4):715–26.

6. Akerstrom G, Malmaeus J, Bergstrom R. Surgical anatomy of human parathyroid glands. Surgery 1984; 95(1):14–21.

7. Brown EM. The pathophysiology of primary hyperparathyroidism. J Bone Miner Res 2002; 17(Suppl 2):N24–9.

8. Goodman WG. Calcium-sensing receptors. Semin Nephrol 2004; 24(1):17–24.

9. Tfelt-Hansen J, Schwarz P, Brown EM et al. The calcium-sensing receptor in human disease. Front Biosci 2003; 8:s377–90.

10. Conigrave AD, Franks AH, Brown EM et al. l-Amino acid sensing by the calcium-sensing receptor: a general mechanism for coupling protein and calcium metabolism? Eur J Clin Nutr 2002; 56(11):1072–80.

11. Hofer AM, Brown EM. Extracellular calcium sensing and signalling. Nat Rev Molec Cell Biol 2003; 4(7):530–8.

12. Hoare SR, Usdin TB. Molecular mechanisms of ligand recognition by parathyroid hormone 1 (PTH1) and PTH2 receptors. Curr Pharm Des 2001; 7(8):689–713.

13. Libutti SK, Alexander HR, Bartlett DL et al. Kinetic analysis of the rapid intraoperative parathyroid hormone assay in patients during operation for hyperparathyroidism. Surgery 1999; 126(6):1145–50; discussion 1150–1.

14. Fujita T, Meguro T, Fukuyama R et al. New signaling pathway for parathyroid hormone and cyclic AMP action on extracellular-regulated kinase and cell proliferation in bone cells. Checkpoint of modulation by cyclic AMP. J Biol Chem 2002; 277(25):22191–200.

15. Brown EM. Extracellular Ca2+ sensing, regulation of parathyroid cell function, and role of Ca2+ and other ions as extracellular (first) messengers. Physiol Rev 1991; 71(2):371–411.

16. Carmeliet G, Van Cromphaut S, Daci E et al. Disorders of calcium homeostasis. Best Pract Res Clin Endocrinol Metab 2003; 17(4):529–46.

17. Austin LA, Heath H 3rd. Calcitonin: physiology and pathophysiology. N Engl J Med 1981; 304(5):269–78.

18. Melton JL. The epidemiology of primary hyperparathyroidism in North America. J Bone Miner Res 2002; 17(Suppl 2):N12–17.

19. Monchik JM. Normocalcemic hyperparathyroidism. Surgery 1995; 118(6):917–23.

20. Boughey JC, Ewart CJ, Yost MJ et al. Chloride/phosphate ratio in primary hyperparathyroidism. Am Surg 2004; 70(1):25–8.

21. Lundgren E, Rastad J, Thrufjell E et al. Population-based screening for primary hyperparathyroidism with serum calcium and parathyroid hormone values in menopausal women. Surgery 1997; 121(3):287–94.

22. Silverberg SJ, Bilezikian JP. "Incipient" primary hyperparathyroidism: a "forme fruste" of an old disease. J Clin Endocrinol Metab 2003; 88(11): 5348–52.

23. Carnaille BM, Pattou FN, Oudar C et al. Parathyroid incidentalomas in normocalcemic patients during thyroid surgery. World J Surg 1996; 20(7):830–4; discussion 834.

Overview of normocalcaemic hyperparathyroidism.

24. Maruani G, Hertig A, Paillard M et al. Normocalcemic primary hyperparathyroidism: evidence for a generalized target-tissue resistance to parathyroid hormone. J Clin Endocrinol Metab 2003; 88(10):4641–8.

25. Siperstein AE, Shen W, Chan AK et al. Normocalcemic hyperparathyroidism. Biochemical and symptom profiles before and after surgery. Arch Surg 1992; 127(10):1157–1160; discussion 1161–3.

26. Wu PH, Wang CJ. Normocalcemic primary hyperparathyroidism with fractures. J Arthroplasty 2002; 17(6):805–9.

27. Parks J, Coe F, Favus M. Hyperparathyroidism in nephrolithiasis. Arch Intern Med 1980; 140: 1479–81.

28. Broadus AE, Dominguez M, Bartter FC. Pathophysiological studies in idiopathic hypercalciuria: use of an oral calcium tolerance test to characterize distinctive hypercalciuric subgroups. J Clin Endocrinol Metab 1978; 47(4):751–60.

29. Hagag P, Revet-Zak I, Hod N et al. Diagnosis of normocalcemic hyperparathyroidism by oral calcium loading test. J Endocrinol Invest 2003; 26(4): 327–32.

30. Greenfield MW. Parathyroid glands. In: Lazar J et al (eds) Surgery: scientific principles and practice, 3rd edn. Philadelphia: Lippincott Williams & Wilkins, 2001; p. 1290.

31. Carroll MF, Schade DS. A practical approach to hypercalcemia. Am Fam Physician 2003; 67(9): 1959–66.

32. Jan de Beur SM LM. Hypercalcemia. In: CW B (ed.) Current therapy in endocrinology and metabolism, 6th edn. New York: Mosby, 1997; p. 552.

33. Bilezikian, JP. Management of acute hypercalcemia. N Engl J Med 1992; 326:1196–203.

34. Edelson GW, Kleerekoper M. Hypercalcemic crisis. Med Clin North Am 1995; 79:79–92.

35. Oura S. Malignancy-associated hypercalcemia [in Japanese]. Nippon Rinsho – Jpn J Clin Med 2003; 61(6):1006–9.

36. Ziegler R. Hypercalcemic crisis. J Am Soc Nephrol 2001; 12(Suppl 17):S3–9.

37. Van Heerden J. Lessons learned. Surgery 1997; 122(6):978–88.

Overview of surgical approach to primary hyperparathyroidism.

38. Weber C, Burke GJ, McGarity WC. Persistent and recurrent sporadic primary hyperparathyroidism: Histopathology, complications, and results of reoperation. Surgery 1994; 116:991.

39. Consensus Development Conference Panel. Diagnosis and management of asymptomatic primary hyperparathyroidism: Consensus Development Conference statement. Ann Intern Med 1991; 114: 593–7.

40. Denham DW, Norman J. Cost-effectiveness of preoperative sestamibi scan for primary hyperparathyroidism is dependent solely upon the surgeon's choice of operative procedure. J Am Coll Surg 1998; 186(3):293–305.

This study is a large meta-analysis that details the pathology of primary hyperparathyroidism in patients undergoing parathyroidectomy.

41. Attie JN, Bock G, August LJ. Multiple parathyroid adenomas: report of thirty three cases. Surgery 1990; 108:1014.

42. Grant C, Van Heerden JA, Charboneau EM. Clinical management of persistent and/or recurrent primary hyperparathyroidism. World J Surg 1986; 10:555.

43. Rodriquez JM, Tezelman S, Siperstein AE et al. Localization procedures in patients with persistent or recurrent hyperparathyroidism. Arch Surg 1994; 129(8):870–5.

44. Miller D, Doppman MD, Shawker MD et al. Localization of parathyroid adenomas who have undergone surgery. Radiology 1987; 162:133–7.

45. Henry JF, Audiffret J, Denizot A et al. Endosonography in the localization of parathyroid tumors: a preliminary study. Surgery 1990; 108(6): 1021–5.

46. Catargi B, Raymond JM, Lafarge-Gense V et al. Localization of parathyroid tumors using endoscopic ultrasonography in primary hyperparathyroidism. J Endocrinol Invest 1999; 22(9):688–92.

47. Casara D, Rubello D, Pelizzo MR et al. Clinical role of 99 mTcO4/MIBI scan, ultrasound, and intra-operative gamma probe in the performance of unilateral and minimally invasive surgery in hyperparathyroidism. Eur J Nucl Med 2001; 28:1351–9.

48. Uden P, Aspelin P, Berglund J et al. Preoperative localization in unilateral parathyroid surgery. A cost-benefit study on ultrasound, computed

tomography and scintigraphy. Acta Chir Scand 1990; 156(1):29–35.

49. De Feo ML, Colagrande S, Biagini C et al. Parathyroid glands: combination of (99m)Tc MIBI scintigraphy and US for demonstration of parathyroid glands and nodules [see comment]. Radiology 2000; 214(2):393–402.

50. Tikkakoski T, Stenfors LE, Typpo T et al. Parathyroid adenomas: pre-operative localization with ultrasound combined with fine-needle biopsy. J Laryngol Otol 1993; 107(6):543–5.

51. Dijkstra B, Healy C, Kelly LM et al. Parathyroid localisation – current practice. J R Coll Surg Edinb 2002; 47(4):599–607.

52. Giuliano M, Gulec SA, Rubello D et al. Preoperative localization and radioguided parathyroid surgery. J Nucl Med 2003; 44:1443–58.

53. Weber AL, Randolph G, Aksoy F. The thyroid and parathyroid glands: CT and MR imaging and correlation with pathological and clinical findings. Radiol Clin North Am 2000; 38:1105–28.

54. Erdman WA, Breslau NA, Weinreb JC et al. Noninvasive localization of parathyroid adenomas: a comparison of X-ray computerized tomography, ultrasound, scintigraphy and MRI. Magn Reson Imaging 1989; 7(2):187–94.

55. Levin KE, Gooding GA, Okerlund M et al. Localizing studies in patients with persistent or recurrent hyperparathyroidism. Surgery 1987; 102(6):917–25.

56. Doppman J, Krudy AG, Marx SJ. Aspiration of enlarged parathyroid glands for parathyroid hormone assay. Radiology 1983; 148:31–5.

57. Aufferman W, Gooding G, Okerlund M. Diagnosis of recurrent hyperparathyroidism: comparison of MR imaging and the other techniques. Am J Roentgenol 1988; 150:1027.

58. Stark D, Clark OH, Moss A. Magnetic resonance imaging of the thyroid, thymus, and parathyroid glands. Surgery 1984; 96(6):1083–90.

59. Kang Y, Rosen K, Clark OH et al. Localization of abnormal parathyroid glands of the mediastinum with MR imaging. Radiology 1993; 189:137–41.

60. Kurbskack A, Wilson SD, Lawson T. Prospective comparison of radionuclide, computed tomography, sonographic, and magnetic resonance localization of parathyroid tumors. Surgery 1989; 106:639.

61. Higgins CB. Role of magnetic resonance imaging in hyperparathyroidism. Radiol Clin North Am 1993; 31(5):1017–28.

62. Fayet P, Hoeffel C, Fulla Y. Technetium-99m-sestamibi, magnetic resonance imaging, and venous blood sampling in persistent and recurrent hyperparathyroidism. Br J Radiol 1997; 70:459–64.

Overview of current state of localisation studies for primary hyperparathyroidism.

63. Gotway M, Reddy G, Webb W et al. Comparison between MR imaging and 99mTc-MIBI scintigraphy in the evaluation of recurrent or persistent hyperparathyroidism: results and factors affecting parathyroid detection. Am J Roentgenol 2001; 166: 705–10.

64. Hewin DF, Brammar TJ, Kabala J et al. Role of preoperative localization in the management of primary hyperparathyroidism. Br J Surg 1997; 84(10):1377–80.

65. Coakley AJ, Kettle AG, Wells CP et al. 99Tcm sestamibi – a new agent for parathyroid imaging. Nucl Med Commun 1989; 10(11):791–4.

66. Sandrock D, Merino MJ, Norton JA. Light and electronmicroscopic analyses of parathyroid tumors explain results of Tl201Tc99m parathyroid scintigraphy. Eur J Med 1989; 15:410.

67. Pattou F, Huglo D, Proye C. Radionuclide scanning in parathyroid diseases. Br J Surg 1998; 85(12):1605–16.

68. McHenry C, Lee K, Saddey J et al. Parathyroid localisation with technetium-99m-MIBI scintigraphy to identify anatomy in secondary hyperparathyroidism. J Nucl Med 1996; 37: 565–9.

69. O'Doherty MJ, Kettle AG. Parathyroid imaging: preoperative localization. Nucl Med Commun 2003; 24(2):125–31.

70. Thule P, Thakore K, Vansant J et al. Preoperative localization of parathyroid tissue with technetium-99m sestamibi 123I subtraction scanning. J Clin Endocrinol Metab 1994; 78(1):77–82.

71. Casas AT, Burke GJ, Mansberger AR Jr et al. Impact of technetium-99m-sestamibi localization on operative time and success of operations for primary hyperparathyroidism. Am Surg 1994; 60(1):12–16; discussion 16–17.

72. Caixas A, Berna L, Hernandez A et al. Efficacy of preoperative diagnostic imaging localization of technetium 99m-sestamibi scintigraphy in hyperparathyroidism. Surgery 1997; 121(5):535–41.

73. Miller DL. Preoperative localization and interventional treatment of parathyroid tumors: when and how? World J Surg 1991; 15:706.

74. Miller DL, Chang R, Doppman J et al. Superselective DSA versus superselective conventional angiography. Radiology 1989; 170:1003.

75. Sugg SL, Fraker DL, Alexander R et al. Prospective evaluation of selective venous sampling for parathyroid hormone concentration in patients undergoing reoperations for primary hyperparathyroidism. Surgery 1993; 114(6):1004–9; discussion 1009–10.

76. Granberg PO, Hamberger B, Johansson G et al. Selective venous sampling for localization of hyperfunctioning parathyroid glands. Br J Surg 1986; 73(2):118–20.

77. Van Heerden J, Farley D. Parathyroid. In: Schwartz S (ed.) Principles of surgery, 7th edn. New York: McGraw-Hill, 1999.

78. Miedlich S, Krohn K, Paschke R. Update on genetic and clinical aspects of primary hyperparathyroidism. Clin Endocrinol 2003; 59:539–54.

79. Rodriguez M, Martin-Malo A, Martinez M. Calcemic response to parathyroid hormone in renal failure: role of phosphorus and its effect on calcitriol. Kidney Int 1991; 40:1055.

80. Felsenfeld A, Rodriguez M, Dunlay R et al. A comparison of parathyroid gland function in haemodialysis patients with different forms of renal osteodystrophy. Nephrol Dial Transpl 1991; 6:244.

81. Demeure M, McGee D, Wilkes W et al. Results of surgical treatment for primary hyperparathyroidism associated with renal disease. Am J Surg 1990; 160:337.

An overview of the treatment of secondary hyperparathyroidism.

82. Block G, Martin K, de Francisco A et al. Cinacalcet for secondary hyperparathyroidism in patients receiving hemodialysis. N Engl J Med 2004; 350(15):1516–25.

Part 2
Operative strategy for the management of parathyroid disease

Jean-François Henry
Frédéric Sebag

Primary hyperparathyroidism

For many years bilateral cervical exploration has been the preferred surgical approach for primary hyperparathyroidism (PHP). When performed by an experienced endocrine surgeon, this procedure is certainly one of the most gratifying of all operations. The success rate is reported to be 95–98%, the morbidity is minimal, the mortality is close to zero and cosmetic results are excellent.[1]

The standard bilateral neck exploration is today challenged by several new minimally invasive techniques. Three main factors have stimulated and allowed these new surgical approaches:

1. The improvement of imaging techniques such as high-resolution ultrasonography and sestamibi scan.
2. The introduction of the quick parathyroid hormone assay (QPTH).
3. The refinement of instrumentation (gamma probe, endoscopic instruments, miniaturised cameras).

Nevertheless, it is imperative to keep in mind the excellent results of conventional parathyroid surgery, which remains the 'gold standard'.

Conventional open parathyroidectomy

Basic principles of parathyroid surgery

Localisation studies may help the surgeon to discover the pathological gland(s) but the success of a standard bilateral exploration is above all based on a thorough knowledge of the anatomy and an understanding of the embryological evolution of the glands. As Cope wrote in 1960, the initial operation is the 'golden opportunity' to cure the patient.

Ideally, the exploration should allow exposure of all parathyroid tissue, i.e. at least four glands, whatever the lesion responsible for the PHP syndrome and the results of preoperative imaging studies. The contribution of frozen section is limited. It has been shown that foci of microscopic hyperplasia observed in biopsy fragments are without functional significance, and such hyperplasia may even lead to the performance of unnecessary excisions causing permanent hypoparathyroidism. Frozen section may help the surgeon to confirm or exclude the presence of parathyroid tissue but it should not be used as grounds for excision of other parathyroid glands.

The pathological nature of the glands is essentially determined from their gross appearance. If the average weight is taken as 40 mg, a gland can only be considered abnormal if above 75 mg. Surgical excision is therefore based on this macrosopic evaluation, which is the more valuable if all the glands have been identified and exposed. However, one must be aware of the risks of devascularisation incurred by too eager a desire to expose a gland.

The excision must be selective. The enlarged gland(s) should be removed in toto and the normal glands preserved. Biopsy of suspected or known carcinomas is strictly contraindicated, and may be responsible for local spread (parathormatosis).

Management of surgical procedure

The operation is usually performed under general anaesthesia but regional anaesthesia[2] and hypno-sedation[3] can also be used.

The patient is positioned on their back with the arms beside the body, the neck in hyperextension. The skin incision is a low transverse cervical incision, one or two fingerbreadths above the heads of the clavicles. The cervical approach is made by separation of the strap muscles in the midline.

The search for superior parathyroid (P IV)

Exposure of the posterior aspect of the thyroid lobe is made by displacing the gland inwards and forwards and retracting the jugulocarotid bundle outwards. The inferior thyroid artery should be preserved. The recurrent laryngeal nerve should be identified.

In 85% of cases this simple exposure allows identification of the normal P IV in its orthotopic site. It 'floats' in a loose fatty setting immediately adjacent to the inferior cornu of the thyroid cartilage, very close to the recurrent nerve and the most cranial branch of the inferior thyroid artery. These structures constitute three basic landmarks in the search for P IV (**Fig. 1.7**).

When a P IV is abnormal, it tends to migrate posteriorly and downwards (**Fig. 1.8**). Therefore, if it is not found in immediate contact with the thyroid capsule, it should be sought beside or behind the oesophagus. Its migration may drag it down very low, well below the inferior thyroid artery, behind whose trunk it crosses during its descent. The lower a P IV, the more posterior it becomes. These adenomas are revealed by their vascular pedicles, whose origin is found at the middle or upper third of the thyroid lobe. They emerge with simple traction on their pedicle. They are closely related to the recurrent nerve, which may be adherent to their capsule, so that their mobilisation calls for prior identification of the nerve and possibly its dissection. If no gland, normal or abnormal,

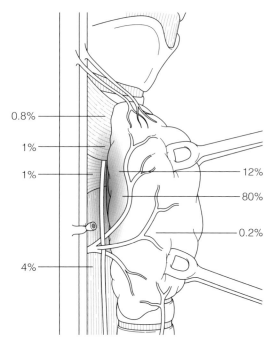

Figure 1.7 • Location of superior parathyroid glands (P IV). The numbers represent the percentages of glands found at different locations in an autopsy study of 503 cases. Adapted from Akerstrom G, Malmaeus J, Bergstrom R. Surgical anatomy of human parathyroid glands. Surgery 1984; 95:14–21. With permission from Elsevier.

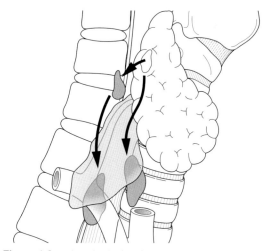

Figure 1.8 • Acquired migration paths of enlarged superior parathyroids (P IV). The enlarged glands tend to migrate posteriorly and downwards. Adapted from Randolph GW, Urken ML. Surgical management of primary hyperparathyroidism. In: Randolph GW (ed.) Surgery of the thyroid and parathyroid glands. Philadelphia: WB Saunders, 2003; pp. 507–28. With permission from Elsevier.

is discovered, the search should be transferred to the perithyroid visceral sheath, carefully exploring the posterior aspect of the lobe from the trunk of the inferior thyroid artery to the superior thyroid pedicle. Particular attention must be devoted to the posterior aspect of the upper pole of the thyroid lobe, where some very flattened adenomas, closely adherent to the surface of the thyroid capsule, may easily pass unnoticed.

If the P IV has not been discovered, the search should be temporarily suspended and transferred to the homolateral parathyroid gland.

The search for inferior parathyroid (P III)

The usual range of position of P III is more extensive than that of P IV (**Fig. 1.9**). The search must be made from the inferior thyroid artery to the inferior thyroid pole, and along the thyrothymic ligament. The P IIIs are rarely posterior and become more anterior the lower they are.

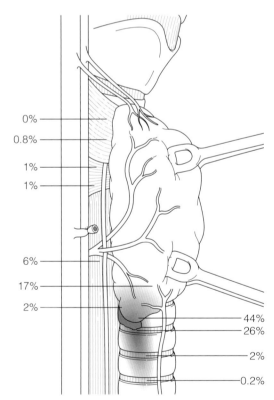

Figure 1.9 • Location of inferior parathyroid glands (P III). The numbers represent the percentages of glands found at different locations in an autopsy study of 503 cases. Adapted from Akerstrom G, Malmaeus J, Bergstrom R. Surgical anatomy of human parathyroid glands. Surgery 1984; 95:14–21. With permission from Elsevier.

The search should first be made at the posterior aspect of the thyroid lobe from the inferior thyroid artery to the lower pole of the lobe. At this site, a normal P III is always situated in front of the recurrent nerve. When it is adenomatous its posterior surface may adhere to the nerve. The exploration must be carried all around the inferior pole of the thyroid lobe, checking its lateral, anterior and inferior aspects in turn. During this dissection one must safeguard the thyroid attachments, i.e. the thyrothymic ligament and the inferior thyroid veins. Then the dissection must be carried as low as possible along the thyrothymic ligaments and the thymus. Nearly 25% of P IIIs are situated along the thyrothymic ligaments or at the upper poles of the thymus.[4,5] Very often they are discovered only after incision of the thymic sheath.

At this stage of the operation, if P III has not been identified, the search should be abandoned and transferred to exploration of the other side. This approach is advised because of the risks of a continued, more aggressive dissection, which may cause devascularisation of a hitherto unperceived normal P III.

Exploration of the second side is made in the same order as the first. The surgeon is fortunate because of the natural symmetry of the glands, though this occurs in only 60% of cases.

Evaluation of the initial bilateral exploration

At the end of this bilateral exploration, the surgeon must decide whether to continue the procedure or not in the light of the number of glands discovered and their pathological or normal appearance.

The exploration can be **abandoned** in two circumstances:

1. **The four glands have been discovered and one or more are abnormal.** A continued search for a supernumerary gland is justified only in cases of familial hyperparathyroidism.
2. **One gland is pathological, the other gland(s) identified are normal, but fewer than four glands have been discovered.** Except in cases of familial hyperparathyroidism the low risk of multiglandular disease that might pass unnoticed does not justify obstinate pursuit of an exploration that risks proving more dangerous than beneficial for the patient. The diagnosis of a solitary adenoma becomes more likely as the number of normal glands found approaches three.

The exploration should be **pursued** in three circumstances:

1. **No gland or fewer than four glands have been discovered and none is pathological.** A probable adenoma remains to be discovered.
2. **Fewer than four glands have been discovered and at least two of these are enlarged.** The surgeon is dealing with a multiglandular disease (MGD). The missing gland(s) must be identified.
3. **All four glands have been discovered but all are normal.** The surgeon must remain convinced of his or her diagnosis and consider the possibility of a probable ectopic supernumerary adenoma.

Continuation of the exploration

The surgeon must keep in mind that: (i) congenital ectopias, in the neck or in the anterior mediastinum, respectively caused by defective or excessive embryological migration, are related to P III (**Fig. 1.10**); and (ii) acquired ectopias in the posterior mediastinum caused by migration affected by gravity, secondary to adenomatous pathology, are essentially related to P IV (Fig. 1.8, Table 1.3).[6] Therefore, it is essential to know whether the missing gland is a P IV or a P III.

If a P IV is absent:

1. Re-explore the juxta-oesophageal regions, as far down as possible in the posterior mediastinum.
2. Remember the defective migration of P IV and explore the superior thyroid pedicle region.

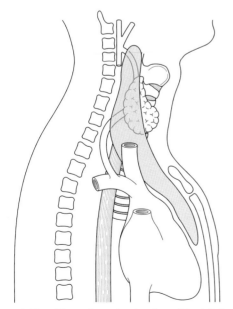

Figure 1.10 • The embryonic migration of the inferior parathyroid gland (P III)–thymus complex results in an extensive area of dispersal of the normal P III from the angle of the mandible to the pericardium.

3. Ligate the superior thyroid pedicle and mobilise the upper pole of the lobe for scrupulous dissection of its posteromedial aspect.
4. Carefully palpate the thyroid lobe to seek an intraparenchymatous parathyroid adenoma.

If a P III is absent:

1. Remember that migration of P III may have been excessive and extend the dissection downwards by performing a thymectomy by the cervical route. The exploration must be made, not by endeavouring to progress downwards, since the space between the manubrium and the trachea is very narrow, but by bringing the thymic lobe upwards by gentle progressive traction, which requires securing several veins. The thymus may thus be exteriorised over 8–10 cm. The elevated thymic lobe must then be dissected since some adenomas are deeply embedded in its substance.
2. Remember the defective migration of P III (undescended gland) and explore the carotid sheath up to the angle of the mandible.
3. Digitally explore the thyroid lobe.

Truly intrathyroid parathyroid adenomas are rare. Most of these so-called intrathyroid adenomas are more or less deeply embedded in a crevice of the thyroid parenchyma. Some other adenomas are hidden just beneath the thyroid capsule and may be revealed by a localised discoloration of the surface of the thyroid, which darkens progressively. Simple incision of the thyroid capsule then allows their dislodgement from their thyroid resting place. Thyroid excision is the last available procedure, but is only indicated when the preoperative investigations suggest an intrathyroid location. Intraoperative ultrasound may be very helpful here.

At the very end of the exploration, and if the abnormal parathyroid sought is still missing, it is very probable that it is not in the neck but in the mediastinum and forms part of the 1–2% of mediastinal adenomas that are virtually inaccessible from the cervical route. This probability will be the greater if four normal parathyroids have been identified in the neck. Median sternotomy should not be done at the same operation for three reasons:

1. The diagnosis should be confirmed.
2. The adenoma should be precisely localised.
3. Left thoracoscopy[7] or anterior mediastinotomy via an incision over and removal of the second

Table 1.3 • Sites, mechanisms and incidence of major ectopias of parathyroid glands III and IV

Site	Parathyroid concerned	Mechanism of ectopia	Incidence (%)
High ectopia in the neck	P III	Embryological: failure of migration	1–2
Anterosuperior mediastinum	P III	Embryological: excessive migration	3.9–5
Posterosuperior mediastinum	P IV	Acquired migration: gravity	4.8
Middle mediastinum	P V*	Embryological: premature fragmentation(?)	0.19–0.3
Intrathyroid	P III, IV, V	Embryological	0.5–3.5

*PV refers to a supernumerary gland.

costal cartilage[8] can be less invasive alternative approaches.

The operation should be halted following a negative cervical exploration, but one cannot spend too much time dissecting the neck carefully at the first operation.

The parathyroidectomy

According to the number of glands discovered and the number of abnormal or normal glands, several typical scenarios can be envisaged.

Solitary parathyroid adenoma (**Fig. 1.11**)

One gland is enlarged and the other gland(s) discovered are normal. This is the commonest situation. The diagnostic test of a single adenoma being one of exclusion, it is the normal appearance of the other glands that leads to the diagnosis of solitary adenoma. The adenoma must be excised, and normal glands preserved.

Sporadic multiglandular disease

When two glands are enlarged and the two other glands are normal, the distinction between double adenoma and hyperplasia may be impossible during the operation. Excision of both enlarged glands is called for; biopsy of the other two grossly normal glands is questionable considering the major risks of hypoparathyroidism due to traumatic biopsies.

When three glands are enlarged, the diagnosis of hyperplasia must be seriously considered. Cases of triple adenomas coexisting with a fourth normal gland are doubtful but when they do occur the fourth normal gland should be preserved.

When all four glands are enlarged (**Fig. 1.12**), in addition to excision of three glands, the fourth, if possible the smallest, should be reduced so as to

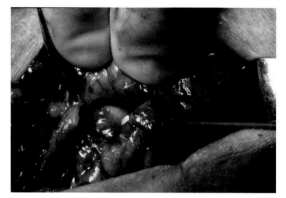

Figure 1.11 • Conventional open parathyroidectomy: left superior parathyroid adenoma and normal inferior parathyroid gland.

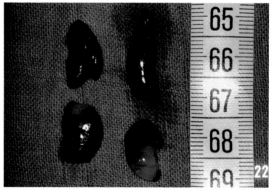

Figure 1.12 • Multiglandular disease: four-gland hyperplasia.

leave in place a fragment of a weight estimated as identical to that of a normal gland, i.e. around 40–60 mg.

In rare cases of water-clear-cell hyperplasia, revealed at operation by the presence of unusually large, chocolate-brown glands, it is advised to save a larger fragment (100–150 mg) because the parathyroid tissue in this entity functions poorly.

The choice of gland to be left in place may, however, be dictated by relations with the recurrent nerve. It is preferable to leave the fragment from the gland farthest from the nerve. The excision should always begin by exposure of the fragment intended to be left in situ. If the fragment appears non-viable, it should be totally resected and the same operation should be done on another gland. Two fragments of smaller size may be left to limit the risks of necrosis and hypoparathyroidism.

Familial hyperparathyroidism

Familial hyperparathyroidism most commonly occurs as a component of multiple endocrine neoplasia type 1 (MEN 1) or type 2A (MEN 2A). It is known to occur also in the absence of other endocrinopathies, when it is apparently unassociated with MEN. The hereditary variants are more difficult to treat than sporadic forms. The glands most often exhibit varying degrees of histopathological disease and the underlying genetic abnormality may be responsible for recurrence in spite of apparently adequate initial surgery.

Primary hyperparathyroidism in MEN 1

The basic principles of parathyroid surgery in patients with MEN 1 include:

1. Obtaining and maintaining normocalcaemia for the longest time possible, avoiding persistent/recurrent hypercalcaemia.
2. Avoiding surgically induced hypocalcaemia.
3. Facilitating future surgery for recurrent disease.

Approaches which have been described as options for patients with hyperparathyroidism in MEN 1 include:

- subtotal parathyroidectomy, leaving a remnant of no more than 60 mg in the neck;
- total parathyroidectomy with immediate autotransplantation of 10–20 1-mm^3 pieces of parathyroid tissue;
- total parathyroidectomy with replacement therapy.

All approaches should be combined with efforts to exclude supernumerary glands and ectopic parathyroid tissue by including resection of fatty tissue from the central neck compartment and thymectomy in all patients.

In a small group of MEN 1 patients with clinically apparent unigland disease, it has been proposed to limit excision of parathyroid tissue to the side of the neck with the enlarged gland.

Selective surgery for hyperparathyroidism in MEN 1 is effectively a palliative procedure for the majority of patients. The underlying disease process predisposes patients to persistent or recurrent disease. Total parathyroidectomy has been reported to have a higher initial 'cure' rate than subtotal resection. Total parathyroidectomy and autotransplantation does carry an increased risk of hypoparathyroidism, of up to 47%.[9,10] Cryopreservation of some resected parathyroid tissue should therefore be considered after total parathyroidectomy. Delayed autotransplantation using cryopreserved parathyroid can be useful in the case of persistent hypoparathyroidism.

A large series of re-operations for persistent and recurrent hyperparathyroidism in MEN 1 patients has been reported.[11] Neck re-exploration resulted in normocalcaemia in 91% of patients, with a rate of 2.1% of permanent injury to the recurrent laryngeal nerve (RLN). Autograft removal was more problematic and resulted in normocalcaemia in 58% of patients. The use of parathyroid autografts does not always simplify subsequent treatment.[12]

Primary hyperparathyroidism in MEN 2A

Before treating hyperparathyroidism in patients with MEN 2A one must rule out a possible coexistent phaeochromocytoma. Hyperparathyroidism in MEN 2A patients is less aggressive than in MEN 1 patients. The main risk of parathyroid surgery in these patients is hypoparathyroidism. Although MEN 2A patients should be considered to have multiglandular disease, most often not all glands are enlarged and aggressive resections are not recommended. Identification of four glands and excision of only macroscopically enlarged glands is associated with a low rate of persistent or recurrent hyperparathyroidism and avoids postoperative hypoparathyroidism. If they look normal, superior glands should be preserved in preference to inferior. Normal inferior glands (which are at higher risk of necrosis during thyroidectomy for medullary carcinoma, lymph node resection and thymectomy) may be preferably autotransplanted. Some authors recommend total parathyroidectomy with autotransplantation in the forearm.[13] The surgeon must bear in mind that permanent hypoparathyroidism can be a worse disease than mild hyperparathyroidism.

Parathyroid carcinoma

Surgery remains the sole therapy for parathyroid carcinoma. The treatment commonly will be determined by two quite different scenarios:

1. **The diagnosis has been established or seriously considered at the first operation.** Severe hypercalcaemia with very high parathyroid hormone (PTH) levels in a patient with a palpable neck tumour are the classic 'at-risk' signs to suggest malignancy. At operation the tumour appears as a grey enlarged parathyroid, often of hard consistency, with a thick capsule with adherence to the surrounding structures. The surgeon must proceed to an en bloc excision of the parathyroid tumour, the thyroid lobe, the other ipsilateral parathyroid, and the recurrent, jugulocarotid and pretracheal lymph nodes. The diagnosis by frozen section is facilitated by this monobloc resection, which will give some idea of the extent of local invasion. Some surgeons remove the lymph nodes only if they are clinically invaded or seen to be so on frozen section. The recurrent nerve should be sacrificed only when it is obviously invaded. The contralateral parathyroids are routinely explored.

2. **The diagnosis is only made postoperatively, from the definitive paraffin section histology.** In equivocal cases, parafibromin immunochemistry may be used to distinguish parathyroid carcinoma from atypical adenoma.[14] The initial operation will usually have been a simple removal of the tumour. It is advisable to re-operate and to resect the structures adjacent to the tumour.[15,16]

Rarely, no obvious evidence of malignancy is found and only the development of recurrences or metastases reveals the true nature of the tumour.

Parathyroid carcinomas are relatively slow growing and should be followed up for life, essentially by clinical evaluation and blood calcium levels. Local recurrences develop in up to 50% of patients. Distant metastases can be expected in 30% of patients.[17] Most authors advocate, wherever possible, an aggressive surgical policy towards recurrences and metastases.[15–17] Residual tumoral tissue in the neck must be removed en bloc, if necessary together with invaded neighbouring organs such as the trachea or muscular wall of the oesophagus. Distant metastases are most often found in the lungs and bones and may or may not be associated with local recurrence. Any subsequent operations are rarely curative. The 1999 National Cancer Data Base Report of 286 patients with parathyroid carcinomas in the USA reported a 5-year survival rate of 86% and a 10-year survival rate of 49% for all patients.[18] The threat to life is related to the degree of hypercalcaemia, so that long-term survival is possible in the presence of metastases if biochemical control is adequate.[15,17]

Parathyroidectomy associated with thyroid excisions

Explorations combining thyroidectomy and parathyroidectomy are frequent. Primary parathyroid exploration is recommended first. Indeed, excision of the thyroid lobe first would lead to section of all the landmarks and moorings used by the surgeon to direct his search for parathyroid tissue. It may also be responsible for an accidental parathyroidectomy, which may pass unnoticed. In cases of a benign thyroid lesion, there should be no hesitation in preserving a layer of thyroid parenchyma so as not to compromise the vascularisation of a normal parathyroid. Excluding MEN 2A patients, definitive hypoparathyroidism is observed in 4.3% of patients who undergo concomitant thyroidectomy and parathyroidectomy.[6]

Overall results of conventional open parathyroidectomy

The immediate operative outcome is usually very straightforward. The plasma calcium returns to normal in 24–48 hours. Nowadays so few patients have bone involvement to a severe degree that significant postoperative hypocalcaemia is relatively uncommon. Preventive treatment for hypocalcaemia is not justified. Apart from hypocalcaemia, the morbidity of parathyroidectomy is mainly represented by laryngeal nerve palsy and haematomas, but this is now reported in only 1% or less of cases.[1] The mortality of parathyroidectomy is very low, close to zero.

PTH levels decrease and are almost undetectable 4 hours after surgery, then begin to return within the normal range on day 1. One month after surgery elevated serum PTH levels are observed in up to 30% of patients despite normalisation of serum calcium levels. In some cases elevated PTH levels are an adaptive reaction to renal dysfunction or vitamin D deficiency.

It has also been recently demonstrated that patients operated on for primary hyperparathyroidism (PHP) show decreased peripheral sensitivity to PTH.[19]

When conventional open parathyroidectomy is done by an expert surgeon, 95–98% of patients become normocalcaemic.[1] With MGD the results are less satisfactory than with solitary adenomas. A multicentre study showed that 20% of MEN 1 patients were still hypercalcaemic immediately after surgery.[20] Therefore, patients with familial PHP must be managed in specialised centres.

Minimally invasive parathyroidectomy (MIP)

In recent years, several new minimally invasive techniques for parathyroidectomy have been developed. These techniques have two common threads:

1. They all have a limited incision when compared with classic open transverse cervical incision.
2. The surgery is targeted on one specific parathyroid gland. In most cases the exploration of other glands is not performed or is limited.

The concept of these limited explorations is based on the fact that 85% of patients will have single-gland disease. Limited parathyroid surgery has been made possible by improvement in preoperative localisation techniques using sestamibi scanning and/or ultrasonography. Nevertheless, whether localisation study results can rule out MGD is questionable, and for most surgeons the risk of missing MGD during a limited parathyroid exploration justifies the systematic use of the quick parathyroid hormone assay (QPTH) assay.

Patients suspected of MGD on imaging studies or patients with familial hyperparathyroidism are not eligible for limited procedures. Therefore, MIP should be proposed only for patients with sporadic hyperparathyroidism in whom a single adenoma has been clearly localised by means of sonography and sestamibi scanning. In addition evidence of associated nodular goitre and history of previous neck operations may contraindicate MIP. Finally suspicion of parathyroid carcinoma is an absolute contraindication for MIP since these tumours require an extensive en bloc excision.

A recent survey from the International Association of Endocrine Surgeons showed that more than half the surgeons responding now performed MIP. Most of these procedures can be performed either under general or regional anaesthesia.

Unilateral neck exploration

Initially the concept of unilateral exploration was based on finding an enlarged gland and an ipsilateral normal gland.[21] Since the introduction of QPTH assay, attempts to identify the ipsilateral gland are no longer made, and in most cases unilateral exploration is focused on one gland alone.

Open minimally invasive parathyroidectomy (OMIP)

This procedure is suitable for day-case surgery.[22] Accurate preoperative localisation is a prerequisite condition for OMIP. The procedure is carried out through a 2- to 4-cm incision. For upper adenomas, the incision is made on the anterior border of the sternocleidomastoid muscle (SCM) and a posterolateral, or 'back-door', approach is used to reach the retrothyroid space. For anterior lower adenomas the incision is made at the suprasternal notch level. This technique when compared with bilateral neck exploration has shown less overall complications (1.2% vs. 3.0%), a 50% reduction in operating time and a substantial reduction in postoperative stay.[22]

Minimally invasive radioguided parathyroidectomy (MIRP)

MIRP is characterised by the use of an intraoperative gamma-probe to direct the dissection according to the level of radioactivity.[23] The operation must be carried out within 3.5 h of the radiopharmaceutical injection. The incision (2–3 cm) is placed according to the expected location of the adenoma as determined by both sestamibi scanning and measurement of gamma emissions on the skin. There is no need to use QPTH measurements. The operation is complete if the excised adenoma has more than 20% of background activity. Gratifying results have been obtained with this technique.[23]

Endoscopic parathyroidectomy

Endoscopic techniques are particularly suitable for parathyroid surgery for several reasons:

1. They are ablative procedures that do not require any elaborate surgical reconstruction.

2. Most parathyroid tumours are small and benign.
3. Reduction in the length of the scar to about 10–15 mm is appealing to many patients.

The first endoscopic removal of enlarged parathyroid glands was from the mediastinum. Thoracoscopy has successfully allowed excision of mediastinal parathyroid adenomas located deep in the anterior mediastinum or in the midde mediastinum.[7]

The three endoscopic neck procedures in most widespread use are:

1. **The pure endoscopic parathyroidectomy.**[24] This technique includes constant gas insufflation and four trocars. A large subplatysmal space is created by blunt dissection. Then the midline is opened and the strap muscles retracted in order to expose the thyroid lobes. A bilateral parathyroid exploration is possible.

2. **Minimally invasive video-assisted parathyroidectomy (MIVAP).**[25] A 15-mm skin incision is made at the suprasternal notch. The cervical midline is opened and complete dissection of the thyroid lobe is obtained by blunt dissection under endoscopic vision. Small conventional retractors maintain the operative space. This gasless procedure is carried out only through the midline incision and also permits a bilateral exploration.

3. **Endoscopic parathyroidectomy by lateral approach.**[26] A 15-mm transverse skin incision is made on the anterior border of the SCM and a back-door approach is used to reach the retrothyroid space. Three trocars (one 10 mm and two 2–3 mm) are inserted on the line of the anterior border of the SCM (**Fig. 1.13**). The working space is maintained with low-pressure CO_2 at 8 mmHg. During this unilateral exploration, one can identify both the adenoma and the ipsilateral parathyroid gland. The lateral approach is applicable in all cases where the parathyroid lesions are located posteriorly.

Other endoscopic techniques, avoiding scars in the neck area, have been proposed but are less commonly used: axillary approach[27] and anterior chest approach.[28]

Depending on the type of access employed, conversion to conventional parathyroidectomy is necessary in 8–15% of cases. The main causes for conversion include difficulties of dissection, capsular ruptures of large adenomas, false-positive results of imaging studies and MGD not detected by preoperative imaging but correctly predicted by QPTH assay results. In experienced hands endoscopic parathyroid techniques are as safe as the standard open procedure. There is virtually no associated mortality. The incidence of recurrent nerve palsy is less than 1%. Insufflation is harmless as long as the procedure is performed under low pressure. Endoscopic operations can be completed in less than 1 hour and the operating time improves dramatically after the first few procedures. Nevertheless, these operations are technically more challenging than standard cervical exploration. Endoscopic techniques have the main advantage of offering a magnified view that permits a precise and careful dissection with minimal risks (**Fig. 1.14**). By direct vision through mini-incisions it is probably more difficult to get an adequate view of structures, and optimal conditions for exploration are not met even if surgeons use frontal lamps and surgical loops.

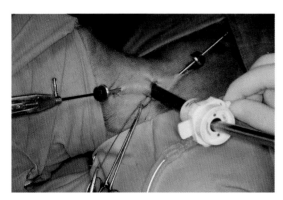

Figure 1.13 • Endoscopic parathyroidectomy by left lateral approach – trocar position.

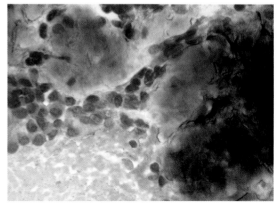

Figure 1.14 • Endoscopic parathyroidectomy by left lateral approach: recurrent laryngeal nerve and superior parathyroid adenoma.

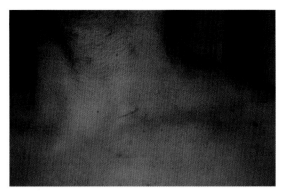

Figure 1.15 • Endoscopic parathyroidectomy by left lateral approach. Cervical scar after 1 week.

 Two studies comparing conventional parathyroid surgery with endoscopic techniques have shown a diminution of postoperative pain and better cosmetic results with endoscopic techniques[29,30] **(Fig. 1.15)**.

MIVAP is also associated with a shorter operative time.[29]

 A prospective randomised trial between MIVAP and OMIP has shown that MIVAP is associated with easier recognition of recurrent laryngeal nerve, lower pain intensity, lower analgesia request rate, lower analgesic consumption, shorter scar length and higher cosmetic satisfaction rate. However, these advantages are achieved at higher costs because of endoscopic tool involvement.[31] Those benefits await confirmation by other randomised studies.

MIP in the broader context

After MIP 95–100% of patients are normocalcaemic.[21–23,32,33]

 Two prospective randomised controlled trials between unilateral and bilateral neck exploration have demonstrated that unilateral exploration provides the same long-term results as bilateral neck exploration.[34,35]

However, it should be kept in mind that these excellent results were obtained in a group of carefully selected patients. In addition the risk of persistent PHP is minimised by the use of intraoperative QPTH assessment.

In contrast to open surgery, the MIP surgeon depends on multiple technologies:

1. The adenoma should be clearly localised before the operation. If the lesion is singular and confirmed by imaging studies, MIP can be advocated. One can choose a lateral or central approach depending on whether the lesion has a posterior or anterior location.
2. The availability of the QPTH assay is of utmost importance. The overall accuracy of intraoperative QPTH monitoring is reported to be 97%.[36] This test may be especially useful when localisation studies are less certain.
3. MIP, and particularly endoscopic techniques, require dedicated instruments.

Demonstrating the advantages of minimally invasive techniques for parathyroid surgery is not easy. Whether MIP is actually less costly than conventional parathyroidectomy is difficult to quantify. Randomised trials have shown that MIP reduces operating time and early symptomatic hypocalcaemia.[34,35] The true advantages of MIP to the patient in terms of comfort and cosmetic results are especially impressive on the first postoperative days.

MIP should not replace conventional parathyroidectomy. Both operations will probably turn out to be complementary to each other in the future. A longer follow-up is needed before one can evaluate the real risk of recurrent PHP following minimally invasive techniques.

Re-operation for persistent or recurrent primary hyperparathyroidism (PHP)

Persistent PHP is defined as the persistence of hypercalcaemia due to hyperparathyroidism in the 6 months following the initial operation. Recurrent PHP refers to the reappearance of hypercalcaemia after 6 months of normocalcaemia.

Analysis of causes of failure

Before undertaking a second exploration of the neck for PHP it is essential to understand the causes of failure of the initial operation. Persistent PHP may be due to a negative exploration or an excision that is inadequate or inappropriate to the lesions discovered. Thus, persistent PHP is nearly always due to technical error during the first operation.

Recurrent PHP constitutes a more complex and controversial problem. The significance of a normocalcaemic interval of at least 6 months between the first operation and the reappearance of hypercalcaemia is debatable. The question is whether this is a true cure of the PHP or a persistent PHP masked by transient return to normal calcaemia. Recurrences may develop after normocalcaemic intervals of several years. In most cases they are seen in patients with familial history of PHP and initially operated on for MGD. The development of a second adenoma in a normal gland, which has been checked at the first operation, is less common and is seen most commonly in patients with history of neck radiation.[37] Persistent PHP is much more commonly observed than recurrent PHP: 80–90% vs. 10–20%.

Carcinoma has a special place among the causes of failed parathyroid surgery. It may be responsible for persistent as well as recurrent PHP. In some cases the recurrence of the carcinoma allows correction of an initial misdiagnosis of an atypical adenoma. Recurrences in situ, probably due to capsular rupture and local spread, are due to carcinomas in most cases but can be seen after removal of a benign lesion (parathormatosis).

Finally, recurrences have been reported in grafts of adenomas or hyperplastic glands implanted in the brachioradialis muscle after total parathyroidectomy. It is not the volume of the implanted tissue that is responsible for the recurrence but its uncontrollable hyperfunctional nature, due either to its autonomy or to the effect of local stimulating factors.

Management

Confirmation of the diagnosis

The diagnosis of PHP can only be raised again after elimination of other causes of hypercalcaemia and fresh confirmation of the biochemical syndrome. Among the many causes of persistent hypercalcaemia after unsuccessful parathyroidectomy, thought should be given to the syndrome of familial hypocalciuric hypercalcaemia (FHH).[38]

Case history

The sporadic or familial nature of the PHP should be determined by searching for a family history or another associated endocrinopathy that may fit into the picture of a MEN 1 or 2A. Study of the operation notes is vital to gain details of the operative

and histology reports from previous operations. This will supply the surgeon with information that is helpful in planning operative tactics (Table 1.4).

Preoperative localisation

While preoperative localisation studies may not seem essential, or even desirable, in the case of a primary bilateral exploration most authors consider that ultrasonography and sestamibi scan should be performed routinely in the work-up for any persistent or recurrent PHP. CT scan and MRI should be reserved for patients in whom the former imaging techniques have failed or when a mediastinal location is strongly suspected. Invasive procedures, including selective venous sampling of PTH or selective angiography, should be performed only if noninvasive procedures are inconclusive. Sometimes, image-guided fine-needle aspiration (FNA) may help distinguish a parathyroid tumour from other structures.

The topographic diagnosis should ideally be established by convergence of the results of at least two different investigations. When used together, imaging techniques correctly identify abnormal glands in nearly 95% of cases.[39–43]

Table 1.4 • Re-operation for persistent-recurrent primary hyperparathyroidism: information supplied from study of case records and surgical implications

Information	Procedure indicated
Familial hyperparathyroidism	Complete exploration of all residual parathyroid tissue
MEN 1 or MEN 2A	Adapt resection to type of familial hyperparathyroidism
Multiglandular lesions	Complete exploration of all residual parathyroid tissue
Three normal glands	Adenoma not found. Re-operation guided by preoperative localisation studies
P III identified (thymus)	Search for homolateral P IV
P IV identified	Search for homolateral P III
Four normal glands in neck; experienced surgeon	Adenoma in major ectopic site: mediastinal site very probable
Cancer suspected or atypical adenoma	Suspect local recurrence and look for visceral or bony metastases
Several normal glands removed	Arrange for cryopreservation

Methods of re-operation

Once the diagnosis has been confirmed, the indications for operation must be discussed. Not every patient needs to be re-operated on. The risks of doing so should be assessed and balanced against those of leaving the patient with PHP. When available, intraoperative ultrasound and gamma-probe may be helpful here. Most surgeons consider that QPTH monitoring is helpful in these patients. The increased rate of recurrent nerve damage in these re-operations calls for precise preoperative assessment of the state of the vocal cords.

According to the case history and the results of localisation studies the surgeon must clearly establish if there is or is not a suspicion of MGD (**Fig. 1.16**). If the lesion sought is a solitary adenoma, an open focused approach can be proposed. Conversely, if there is confirmation or strong suspicion of MGD, revision of the transverse cervicotomy is recommended.

The posterolateral approach ('back-door' approach)

This focused approach should be considered when the adenoma sought has been visualised in a

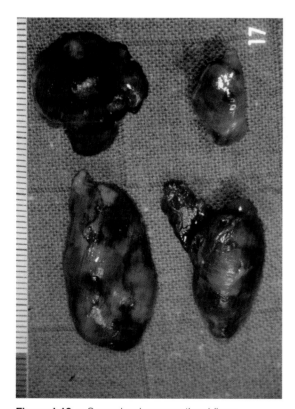

Figure 1.16 • Secondary hyperparathyroidism: four-gland hyperplasia.

posterocervical site: the missing adenoma is probably a P IV. The previous transverse incision is enlarged laterally on the anterior border of the sternocleidomastoid. The approach is behind the muscles and the thyroid, in a zone that is intact or little affected by the previous operation. Search for P IV is made as already described.

The thyrothymic approach ('front-door' approach)

This approach should be considered when the adenoma sought has been visualised anteriorly at the lower pole of the thyroid or along the thyrothymic axis. The missing adenoma is probably a P III. A transverse skin incision is used along the previous cervical incision. The infrahyoid muscles are divided as low as possible allowing direct access to the thyrothymic ligaments. This manoeuvre avoids any dissection between the prethyroid muscles and the thyroid capsule. The search for P III is made as already described.

Revision of the transverse cervicotomy

This long and difficult re-operation is indicated when there is confirmation or strong suspicion of MGD. Search for P IV and P III is made as already described. Ideally all the glands must be identified and assessed. This also involves a search for accessory glands and a bilateral thymectomy. QPTH monitoring and cryopreservation are particularly recommended.

Mediastinal approaches

Most mediastinal adenomas located in the posterior mediastinum or in the anterior mediastinum above the aortic arch can be excised through the neck.[39–43] Only adenomas located deep in the anterior mediastinum or in the middle mediastinum require a thoracic approach. The appropriate approach will be dependent upon careful consideration of localising studies and the depth of the lesion in the mediastinum. Precise localisation can allow a less invasive approach than sternal split: anterior mediastinotomy[8] or left thoracoscopy[7] may be preferable to partial or total sternotomy.

Other focused approaches

These approaches concern glands located in a major ectopic cervical area and not accessible via the previous cervicotomy. The skin incision is placed according to the expected location of the adenoma as determined by imaging studies: undescended glands; or within the carotid sheath in association with the vagus nerve.[44]

Associated procedures

Immediate autotransplantation is debatable, since the hyperfunctional grafts may interfere with assessment of the results of parathyroidectomy. In the presence of persistent PHP it may not be clear whether the source of recurrence is the autograft or residual cervical or mediastinal tissue. Cryopreservation and secondary autotransplantation are essential adjuncts to re-operation for PHP. In cases of postoperative hypocalcaemia, secondary autotransplantation should not be done too soon. Some hypocalcaemic patients regain normocalcaemia after a year. This is the delay, therefore, that seems advisable before considering secondary autotransplantation.

Graft recurrences must be proven before re-operation on the graft site. Hyperfunctioning grafts are sometimes palpable, or may be located by ultrasound or sestamibi scan. In every case, the possibility of recurrence in residual cervical or mediastinal tissue must be eliminated before re-operating on the arm, and Casanova's test may be very helpful.[45]

Results

With experienced parathyroid surgeons, the success rate of re-operations can be as high as 95%.[39–43,46] The overall perioperative morbidity, on average 20%, is much higher than in cases of primary neck exploration. There is a dramatically increased risk of permanent recurrent laryngeal nerve paralysis (up to 10%) compared with initial parathyroid surgery. In up to 20% of cases permanent hypoparathyroidism may result. Transplantation of hyperfunctional tissue can result in recurrent disease in 7–17% of patients. Grafts may fail to function in 6–50% of transplanted tissue, with failure occurring more frequently when using cryopreserved tissue.

Secondary hyperparathyroidism (SHP)

Hyperparathyroidism secondary to uraemia

SHP is present in most, if not all, patients undergoing long-term haemodialysis. Most of them can be managed by prophylaxis and medical therapy. However, between 2.5% and 28% of these patients require surgery because of severe reactive renal hyperparathyroidism, i.e. uncontrolled hypercalcaemia, hyperphosphataemia, high levels of PTH (>500 pg/mL), bone erosions and osteitis fibrosa.

Surgical strategies

The surgical treatment can be considered palliative in nature. Surgery is indicated to treat and prevent the complications of SHP. The underlying disease process, i.e. chronic renal failure, predisposes patients to recurrent disease. Surgery performed in these patients should therefore aim to:

- obtain and maintain correction of hyperparathyroidism for the longest time possible, avoiding persistent disease;
- avoid surgically induced severe hypocalcaemia;
- facilitate future surgery for recurrent disease.

Localisation diagnosis is often considered unnecessary because patients will systematically undergo bilateral neck exploration. However, imaging studies may be performed to reduce the operation time and to detect supernumerary and ectopic glands, of which the incidence (6.5–25%) is increased due to the ongoing stimulation of renal failure.[47,48]

The surgical treatment of SHP is performed by using one of two main techniques:

1. **Subtotal parathyroidectomy (SPTX).**[49] This involves identifying four glands and removing at least three but leaving a parathyroid remnant in the neck (approximately 50 mg). The most diffusely hyperplastic gland should be selected. The main disadvantage of this approach is that a second cervical exploration would be needed if persistent or recurrent SHP occurs.

2. **Total parathyroidectomy + autotransplantation (TPTX + AT).**[50] This involves the resection of at least four glands combined with the transplantation of 10–20 1-mm^3 pieces of parathyroid tissue into individual pockets created in the brachioradialis muscle of the forearm, principally to aid future surgery under local anaesthetic for recurrent disease.

The glands may be markedly enlarged. They are often pale and hard, with fibrosis and calcifications, and may be difficult to distinguish from thyroid tissue or lymph nodes (Fig. 1.16).

To exclude supernumerary glands resection of fatty tissue from the central neck compartment and bilateral thymectomy should also be performed in both techniques.

Theoretically, there should be no difference in outcome in terms of persistent or recurrent hypercalcaemia between these two approaches, as both involve the controlled excision of all parathyroid tissue, but for a remnant in the neck or as grafts in the arm.

The intraoperative selection of the tissue to be left in the neck or the forearm is of particular importance. Neck-remnant or graft-dependent recurrences are observed most often in patients with nodular tissue at initial surgery.[51–53] In practice, this intraoperative tissue selection is easier to perform ex vivo prior to autotransplantation rather than during the parathyroidectomy.

Because parathyroid remnants or grafts can undergo ischaemic necrosis and result in permanent hypoparathyroidism, cryopreservation of 'spare' parathyroid tissue should be performed whenever facilities are available.

Both techniques have advantages and disadvantages (Table 1.5), and no definitive answer can be given to the question of which method is superior.[54–56] Total parathyroidectomy is recommended for patients with four markedly enlarged glands and for patients who are not transplant candidates.[54,55] Subtotal parathyroidectomy is favoured for children, for patients scheduled to receive a renal transplant, and for patients with any normal-sized parathyroid detected at surgery. Total parathyroidectomy alone, without autotransplantation, may also be used in selected patients. These patients will require permanent therapy with oral calcium and vitamin D postoperatively.

Perioperative care

Patients may receive oral calcitriol before operation to decrease the severity and the duration of postop-erative hypocalcaemia. They should undergo dialysis within 1 day of operation and then 48 hours postoperatively or as needed. The risk of bleeding is increased as heparin is used during haemodialysis. Hypocalcaemia is found after subtotal and total parathyroidectomy with autotransplantation in 6.3% and 1.4% respectively.[55] Hypocalcaemia may be severe in patients who have marked bone disease, and this may require intravenous calcium. Prolonged hypocalcaemia should be treated with calcitriol (1–4 µg/day) and oral calcium.

Delayed autotransplantation of cryopreserved tissue may be helpful in correcting hypoparathyroidism but should not be performed within 6 months following surgery. However, the functional results are less good than after immediate autotransplantation of fresh parathyroid tissue.[57,58]

Persistent and recurrent SHP

Persistent or recurrent SHP is encountered in 2–12% of patients. The causes are multiple. First, the initial parathyroidectomy may have been incomplete. It must be expected that an initial resection of no more than three glands will prove to be insufficient. Likewise, the parathyroidectomy may be inadequate if the remnant is too large – more than 60 mg. In both cases, surgical failure accounts for persistent SHP. Recurrent SHP may also be observed after successful subtotal or total parathyroidectomy. Further hyperplasia of parathyroid tissue can occur in the remnant left in the neck or in autografted fragments in the forearm.

It is known that up to 15% of haemodialysis patients have a supernumerary parathyroid gland in the neck or mediastinum.[4,59–61] After removal of four parathyroids, these supernumerary 'missed' glands are capable of causing persistent or recur-

Table 1.5 • Advantages and disadvantages of subtotal parathyroidectomy (SPTX) and total parathyroidectomy + autotransplantation (TPTX + AT) in patients with secondary hyperparathyroidism

Surgical procedure	Advantages	Disadvantages
SPTX	Short or no period of hypocalcaemia postoperatively	Tissue selection not always possible Morbidity of cervical re-operation
TPTX + AT	Tissue selection possible Low morbidity of re-operations on the autografts	Longer period of hypocalcaemia postoperatively Problems in localising the hyperactive tissue: autografts or supernumerary gland? Identification and resection of autografts not always easy (seeding in the muscle)
Both procedures		Do not avoid persistent/recurrent disease due to ectopic supernumerary gland

rent SHP and represent a third cause of surgical failure. During the initial operation, they are usually small and often appear to be embryological rests of parathyroid cells. Most of these glands are associated with the thymus, either in the mediastinum or the neck. Usually without physiological importance, they can develop functional significance because of long-term stimulation over many years in patients with chronic renal failure.

Another cause of recurrent SHP is parathormatosis, in which capsular rupture of the pathological gland causes spillage and inadvertent autotransplantation of cells in the operative site. This tissue will grow and lead to recurrent disease.

In persistent/recurrent SHP, all patients who require re-operation should undergo localisation studies. After TPTX + AT it must be kept in mind that recurrences can occur not only on the grafts but also on supernumerary glands in the neck or the mediastinum. The Casanova test[45] can be used to evaluate whether the origin of recurrence is a residual gland or grafted tissue. The incidence of persistent/recurrent SHP is similar after SPTX and TPTX + AT, namely 5.8% and 6.6% respectively.[55] Cervical re-operations in this setting are more invasive, require greater surgical expertise and are associated with a higher morbidity than the excision of an autograft in the forearm.

Nevertheless, re-operations on autografted parathyroid fragments are not always technically simple. Not all the grafts grow in the same way. Some become hypertrophic whereas others atrophy. Attempts to locate them precisely are difficult because they are embedded in the muscle at varying depths. The volume of the tissue that has to be removed or left is difficult to evaluate. This is particularly true when there is exuberant pseudo-invasive overgrowth that sometimes requires repeated graft resections. In these cases some surgeons prefer to remove all the transplanted tissue as completely as possible. In some cases the problem of persistent or recurrent SHP is no easier to solve after TPTX + AT than after SPTX.[62] Cryopreservation of parathyroid tissue is strongly recommended in re-operations.[58]

Lithium-induced hyperparathyroidism

Approximately 10–15% of lithium-treated patients become hypercalcaemic. This condition is often reversible if lithium is withdrawn. Lithium-induced hyperparathyroidism was first reported in 1973.[63] Hypercalcaemia is generally mild with slight elevation of PTH. It has been suggested that lithium stimulates the entire parathyroid tissue, resulting in hyperplasia,[64,65] but several cases of patients presenting a single adenoma as the cause of hyperparathyroidism have also been reported.[66] Alternatively, it has been suggested that lithium may unmask underlying PHP.[66] For patients who require ongoing treatment with lithium, surgery is indicated.[64–67] The incidence of MGD in this setting contraindicates minimally invasive surgery. Excision should be limited to evidently enlarged glands.

Tertiary hyperparathyroidism

Tertiary hyperparathyroidism is a persistent autonomous hypercalcaemic hyperparathyroidism occurring after kidney transplantation. After renal transplant the hypercalcaemia resolves in 50% of patients in the first month, in 85% in the first 6 months and in 95% after 6 months. However, elevated PTH and abnormal bone biopsy persist in up to 70% of patients with long-term kidney grafts.[68]

Several factors may prevent the involution of the hyperplastic gland after the primary stimulus, i.e. kidney failure, has been removed:

- impaired renal graft function;
- non-suppressible PTH secretion;
- autonomy or slow involution of parathyroid glands;
- insufficient calcitriol conversion by the kidney.[68–72]

Only 0.2–0.3% of all patients with kidney transplants are reported to require parathyroid surgery.[72] Indications for parathyroidectomy are: subacute severe hypercalcaemia (>3 mmol/L) and symptomatic persistent (>2 years) hypercalcaemia. Because transient hypoparathyroidism may provoke reduced graft perfusion which may be a cause of kidney graft deterioration associated with TPTX, one should consider SPTX instead of TPTX + AT.[73] Transplant patients rarely develop recurrent hyperparathyroidism.

Key points

- Bilateral neck exploration is the gold standard in parathyroid surgery.
- In sporadic primary hyperparathyroidism surgical excision is based on macroscopic evaluation: enlarged glands should be removed, normal glands should be preserved.
- In MEN 1 patients subtotal parathyroidectomy or total parathyroidectomy with autotransplantation should be combined with efforts to exclude supernumerary glands.
- In MEN 2A patients the main risk of parathyroid surgery is hypoparathyroidism.
- In patients with parathyroid carcinoma extensive en bloc surgery is recommended at initial operation and in cases of local recurrence or metastasis.
- In primary hyperparathyroidism, 1 month after successful parathyroidectomy, up to 30% of patients have elevated serum PTH levels despite normalisation of serum calcium levels.
- Minimally invasive parathyroidectomy should be proposed only for patients with sporadic primary hyperparathyroidism in whom a single adenoma has been clearly localised by imaging studies.
- The diagnosis of persistent or recurrent primary hyperparathyroidism can only be raised again after elimination of other causes of hypercalcaemia and confirmation of the biochemical syndrome.
- The sporadic or familial nature of primary hyperparathyroidism should be determined for any re-operation for persistent or recurrent hyperparathyroidism.
- In persistent or recurrent primary or secondary hyperparathyroidism all patients who require re-operation should undergo localisation studies.
- In patients with secondary hyperparathyroidism the key to a successful operation is to locate all parathyroid glands (supernumerary glands included) and leave 40–60 mg of viable tissue as a remnant in the neck or as an autotransplant in the forearm.
- After total parathyroidectomy + autotransplantation it must be remembered that recurrences are possible not only in the autografts but also in supernumerary glands in the neck or the mediastinum.

References

1. Van Heerden JA, Grant CS. Surgical treatment of primary hyperparathyroidism: an institutional perspective. World J Surg 1991; 15:688–92.

2. Lo Gerfo P, Kim LJ. Technique for regional anesthesia: thyroidectomy and parathyroidectomy. In: Van Heerden JA, Farley DR (eds) Operative technique in general surgery. Surgical exploration for hyperparathyroidism. Philadelphia: WB Saunders, 1999; pp. 95–102.

3. Meurisse M, Hamoir E, Defechereux T. Bilateral neck exploration under hypnosedation. A new standard of care in primary hyperparathyroidism. Ann Surg 1999; 229:401–8.

4. Akerstrom G, Malmaeus J, Bergstrom R. Surgical anatomy of human parathyroid glands. Surgery 1984; 95:14–21.

5. Thompson NW. The techniques of initial parathyroid exploration and reoperative parathyroidectomy. In: Thompson NW, Vinik AI (eds) Endocrine surgery update. New York: Grune & Stratton, 1983; pp. 365–83.

6. Henry JF, Denizot A. Anatomic and embryologic aspects of primary hyperparathyroidism. In: Barbier J, Henry JF (eds) Primary hyperparathyroidism. Paris: Springer-Verlag, 1992; pp. 5–18.

7. Prinz RA, Lonchina V, Carnaille B et al. Thoracoscopic excision of enlarged mediastinal parathyroid glands. Surgery 1994; 116:999–1005.

8. Schinkert RT, Whitaker MD, Argueta R. Resection of select mediastinal parathyroid adenomas through an anterior mediastinotomy. Mayo Clin Proc 1991; 66:1110–13.

9. O'Riordain DS, O'Brien T, Grant CS et al. Surgical management of primary hyperparathyroidism in multiple endocrine neoplasia type 1 and 2. Surgery 1993; 114:1031–9.

10. Hellman P, Skogseid B, Oberg K et al. Primary and reoperative operations in parathyroid operations in hyperparathyroidism of multiple endocrine neoplasia type 1. Surgery 1998; 124:993–9.

11. Kivlen MH, Bartlett DL, Libutti SK et al. Reoperation for hyperparathyroidism in multiple endocrine neoplasia type 1 (MEN 1). Surgery 2001; 130:991–8.

12. Hubbard JGH, Sebag F, Maweja S et al. Primary hyperparathyroidism in MEN I – how radical

should surgery be? Langenbeck's Arch Surg 2002; 368:553–7.

13. Wells SA, Farndon JR, Dale JK et al. Long term evaluation of patients with primary parathyroid hyperplasia managed by total parathyroidectomy and heterotopic autotransplantation. Ann Surg 1980; 192:451–8.

14. Gill AJ, Clarkson A, Gimm O et al. Loss of nuclear expression of parafibromin distinguishes parathyroid carcinomas and hyperparathyroidism–jaw tumors (HPT-JT) syndrome related adenomas from sporadic parathyroid adenomas and hyperplasias. Am J Surg Pathol 2006; 30:1140–9.

15. Rodgers SE, Perrier ND. Parathyroid carcinoma. Curr Opin Oncol 2006; 18:16–22.

16. Busaidy N, Jimenez C, Habra M et al. Parathyroid carcinoma: a 22-year experience. Head and Neck 2004; 16:716–26.

17. Sandelin K, Tullgren O, Farnebo LO. Clinical course of metastatic parathyroid cancer. World J Surg 1994; 18:594–8.

18. Hundahl SA, Flemming ID, Fremgen AM et al. Two hundred eighty-six cases of parathyroid carcinoma treated in the US between 1985–1995: a national cancer data base report. The American College of Surgeon Commission on Cancer and the American Cancer Society. Cancer 1999; 86:538–44.

19. Nordenstrom E, Westerdahl J, Isaksson A. Patients with elevated serum parathyroid hormone levels after parathyroidectomy showing signs of decreased peripheral parathyroid hormone sensitivity. World J Surg 2003; 27:212–15.

20. Goudet P, Cougard P, Vergès B et al. Hyperparathyroidism in multiple endocrine neoplasia type 1: surgical trends and results of a 256-patient series from Group d'Etude des Néoplasies Endocriniennes Multiples study group. World J Surg 2001; 25:886–90.

21. Tibblin SA, Bondeson AG, Ljunberg O. Unilateral parathyroidectomy in hyperparathyroidism due to single adenoma. Ann Surg 1982; 195:245–52.

22. Udelsman R, Donovan PI, Sokoll LJ. One hundred consecutive minimally invasive parathyroid explorations. Ann Surg 2000; 232:331–9.

23. Norman J, Murphy C. Minimally invasive radioguided parathyroidectomy. In: Van Heerden JA, Farley DR (eds) Operative technique in general surgery. Surgical exploration for hyperparathyroidism. Philadelphia: WB Saunders, 1999; pp. 28–33.

24. Gagner M, Rubino F. Endoscopic parathyroidectomy. In: Schwartz AE, Pertsemlidis D, Gagner M (eds) Endocrine surgery. New York: Marcel Dekker, 2004; pp. 289–96.

25. Miccoli P, Bendinelli C, Conte M. Endoscopic parathyroidectomy by a gasless approach. J Laparoendosc Adv Surg Tech A 1998; 8:189–94.

26. Henry JF. Endoscopic exploration. In: Van Heerden JA, Farley DR (eds) Operative technique in general surgery. Surgical exploration for hyperparathyroidism. Philadelphia: WB Saunders, 1999; pp. 49–61.

27. Ikeda Y, Takami H, Sasaki Y et al. Endoscopic neck surgery by the axillary approach. J Am Coll Surg 2000; 191:336–40.

28. Okido M, Shimizu S, Kuroki S et al. Video-assisted parathyroidectomy for primary hyperparathyroidism: an approach involving a skin-lifting method. Surg Endosc 2001; 15:1120–3.

29. Miccoli P, Bendinelli C, Berti P et al. Video-assisted versus conventional parathyroidectomy in primary hyperparathyroidism: a prospective randomized study. Surgery 1999; 126:1117–22.

30. Henry JF, Raffaelli M, Iacobone M et al. Video-assisted parathyroidectomy via lateral approach versus conventional surgery in the treatment of sporadic primary hyperparathyroidism. Results of a case–control study. Surg Endosc 2001; 15:1116–19.

31. Barczynski M, Cichon S, Konturek A et al. Minimally invasive video-assisted parathyroidectimy versus open minimally invasive parathyroidectomy for solitary parathyroid adenoma: a prospective, randomized, blinded trial. World J Surg 2006; 30:721–31.

32. Miccoli P, Berti P, Materazzi G et al. Results of video-assisted parathyroidectoy: single institution's six years experience. World J Surg 2004; 28:1216–18.

33. Henry JF, Sebag F, Tamagnini P et al. Endoscopic parathyroid surgery: results of 365 consecutive procedures. World J Surg 2004; 28:1219–23.

34. Russell CF, Dolan SJ, Laird JD. Randomized clinical trial comparing scan-directed unilateral versus bilateral cervical exploration for primary hyperparathyroidism due to solitary adenoma. Br J Surg 2006; 93:418–21.

35. Westerdalh J Bergenfelz A. Unilateral versus bilateral neck exploration for primary hyperparathyroidism: five-year follow-up of a randomized controlled trial. Ann Surg 2007; 246:976–80.

36. Irvin GL, Carneiro DM. Rapid parathyroid hormone assay guided exploration. In: Van Heerden JA, Farley DR (eds) Operative technique in general surgery. Surgical exploration for hyperparathyroidism. Philadelphia: WB Saunders, 1999; pp. 18–27.

37. Ippolito G, Palazzo F, Sebag F et al. Long-term follow-up after parathyroidectomy for radiation-induced hyperparathyroidism. Surgery 2007; 142:819–22.

38. Heath H III. Familial benign hypercalcemia – from clinical description to molecular genetics. West J Med 1994; 164:554–62.

39. Shen W, Duren M, Morita E et al. Reoperation for persistent or recurrent hyperparathyroidism. Arch Surg 1996; 131:861–9.

40. Jaskowiak N, Norton JA, Alexander HT et al. A prospective trial evaluating a standard approach to reoperation for missed parathyroid adenoma. Ann Surg 1996; 224:308–22.

41. Thompson GB, Grant CS, Perrier ND et al. Reoperative parathyroid surgery in the era of sestamibi scanning and intraoperative parathyroid hormone monitoring. Arch Surg 1999; 134:699–704.

42. Wadstrom C, Zedenius J, Guinea A et al. Reoperative surgery for recurrent or persistent primary hyperparathyroidism. Aust NZ J Surg 1998; 68:103–7.

43. Mariette C, Pellissier L, Combemale F et al. Reoperation for persistent or recurrent primary hyperparathyroidism. Langenbeck's Arch Surg 1998; 383:174–9.

44. Chan TJ, Libutti SK, McCart JA et al. Persistent primary hyperparathyroidism caused by adenomas identified in pharyngeal or adjacent structures. World J Surg 2003; 27:675–9.

45. Casanova D, Sarfati E, De Francisco A et al. Secondary hyperparathyroidism: diagnosis of site or recurrence. World J Surg 1991; 15:546–54.

46. Lo CY, Van Heerden JA. Parathyroid reoperations. In: Clark OH, Duh QY (eds) Textbook of endocrine surgery. Philadelphia: WB Saunders, 1997; pp. 411–17.

47. Perie S, Fessi H, Tassart M et al. Usefulness of combination of high-resolution ultrasonography and dual-phase dual-isotope iodine 123/technetium Tc 99m sestamibi scintigraphy for the preoperative localization of hyperplastic parathyroid glands in renal hyperparathyroidism. Am J Kidney Dis 2005; 45:344–52.

48. De La Rosa A, Jimeno J, Membrilla E et al. Usefulness of preoperative Tc-mibi parathyroid scintigraphy in secondary hyperparathyroidism. Langenbeck's Arch Surg 2008; 393:21–4.

49. Stanbury SW, Lumb GA, Nicholson WF. Elective subtotal parathyroidectomy for autonomous hyperparathyroidism. Lancet 1960, 1:793–8.

50. Wells SA, Gunnels JC, Shelbourne JD et al. Transplantation of the parathyroid glands in man: clinical indications and results. Surgery 1975; 78:34–44.

51. Tanaka Y, Seo H, Tominaga Y et al. Factors related to the recurrent hyperfunction of autografts after total parathyroidectomy in patients with severe secondary hyperparathyroidism. Jpn J Surg 1993; 23:220–5.

52. Ohta K, Manabe T, Katagiri M et al. Expression of proliferating cell nuclear antigens in parathyroid glands of renal hyperparathyroidism. World J Surg 1994; 18:625–9.

53. Tominaga Y, Tanaka Y, Sato K et al. DNA studies in graft-dependent hyperparathyroidism. Acta Chir Austriaca 1996; 28(Suppl 124):65–8.

54. Takagi H, Tominaga Y, Uchida K et al. Subtotal versus total parathyroidectomy with forearm autograft for secondary hyperparathyroidism in chronic renal failure. Ann Surg 1984; 200:18–23.

55. Rothmund M, Wagner PK, Schark C. Subtotal parathyroidectomy versus total parathyroidectomy and autotransplantation in secondary hyperparathyroidism: a randomized trial. World J Surg 1991; 15:745–50.

56. Gagne ER, Urena P, Leite-Silva S et al. Short- and long-term efficacy of total parathyroidectomy with immediate autografting compared with subtotal parathyroidectomy in hemodialysis patients. J Am Soc Nephrol 1992; 3:1008–17.

57. Tanaka Y, Funahashi H, Imai T et al. Functional and morphometric study of cryopreserved human parathyroid tissue transplanted into nude mice. World J Surg 1996; 20:692–9.

58. Niederle B. The technique of parathyroid cryopreservation and the results of delayed autotransplantation. A review. Acta Chir Austriaca 1996; 28(Suppl 124):68–71.

59. Edis AJ, Levitt MD. Supernumerary parathyroid glands: implications for the surgical treatment of secondary hyperparathyroidism. World J Surg 1987; 11:398–401.

60. Numano M, Tominaga Y, Uchida K et al. Surgical significance of supernumerary parathyroid glands in renal hyperparathyroidism. World J Surg 1998; 22:1098–103.

61. Hibi Y, Tominoga Y, Sato T et al. Reoperation for renal hyperparathyroidism. World J Surg 2002: 26:1301–7.

62. Henry JF, Denizot A, Audiffret J et al. Results of reoperations for persistent or recurrent secondary hyperparathyroidism in hemodialysis patients. World J Surg 1990; 14:303–7.

63. Garfinkel PE, Ezrin C, Stancer HC. Hypothyroidism and hyperparathyroidism associated with lithium. Lancet 1973; 2:331–2.

64. McHenry CR, Racke F, Meister M et al. Lithium effects on dispersed bovine parathyroid cells grown in tissue culture. Surgery 1991; 110:1061–6.

65. Hundley JC, Woodrum DT, Saunders BD et al. Revisiting lithium-associated hyperparathyroidism in the era of intraoperative hormone monitoring. Surgery 2005; 138:1027–32.

66. Awad SS, Miskulin J, Thompson NW. Parathyroid adenomas versus four-gland hyperplasia as the cause of primary hyperparathyroidism in patients with prolonged lithium therapy. World J Surg 2003; 27:486–8.

67. Nordenstrom J, Strigard K, Perkeck L et al. Hyperparathyroidism associated with treatment of manic-depressive disorders by lithium. Eur J Surg 1992; 158:207–11.

68. Sitges-Serra A, Esteller E, Ricart MJ et al. Indications and late results of subtotal parathyroidectomy for hyperparathyroidism after renal transplantation. World J Surg 1984; 8:534–9.

69. Saha HH, Salmela KT, Ahonen PJ et al. Sequential changes in vitamin D and calcium metabolism after successful renal transplantation. Scand J Urol Nephrol 1994; 28:21–5.

70. Straffen AM, Carmichael DJ, Fainety A et al. Calcium metabolism following renal transplantation. Ann Clin Biochem 1994; 31:125–9.

71. Sancho JJ, Stiges-Serra A. Metabolic complications for patients with secondary hyperparathyroidism. In: Clark OH, Duh QY (eds) Textbook of endocrine surgery. Philadelphia: WB Saunders, 1997; pp. 394–401.

72. Fassbinder W, Brunner FP, Brynger H et al. Combined report on regular dialysis and transplantation in Europe. Nephrol Dial Transpl 1991; 6(Suppl):28–32.

73. Schlosser K, Endres N, Celik I et al. Surgical treatment of tertiary hyperparathyroidism: the choice of procedure matters! World J Surg 2007; 31:1947–53.

2

The thyroid gland

Gregory P. Sadler
Radu Mihai

Anatomy and embryology

The thyroid gland is formed by two lobes, one either side of the trachea. A short isthmus connects the lobes across the front of the trachea. Each lobe derives its blood supply from two main arteries. The superior thyroid artery (a branch of the external carotid) enters the superior pole on the anterior surface. The inferior thyroid artery (from the thyrocervical branch of the subclavian artery) enters the lobe midway down the lateral border. Venous drainage is variable but is usually threefold: a middle thyroid vein directly to the internal jugular, superior thyroid veins (running with the superior thyroid artery) and a plexus of veins draining from the inferior aspect of the lower pole. Lymphatic drainage is to local nodes located in the central compartment and thence to the anterior cervical chain.

Embryologically the gland is derived from the median thyroid diverticulum in the floor of the pharynx. It grows downwards between the ventral ends of the first and second pharyngeal arches, the stalk of the diverticulum elongating to become the thyroglossal duct. This duct (later obliterated) extends from the foramen caecum at the base of the tongue to the isthmus, its distal part remaining as the pyramidal lobe of the thyroid. The ultimobranchial bodies, arising from the fourth pharyngeal pouch on each side, become applied to the lateral portion of each thyroid lobe and contribute the parafollicular or C cells. These cells of neural crest origin become secondarily involved with the thyroid, produce calcitonin and may later assume clinical importance as the cells giving rise to medullary thyroid carcinoma.

Investigation of thyroid function

Thyroid hormones and thyroid-stimulating hormone (TSH)

Control of synthesis and release of the thyroid hormones is provided by TSH. This regulatory hormone is released from the anterior pituitary and is the primary growth factor measured when assessing thyroid status. TSH release is regulated via a negative feedback loop provided by the thyroid hormones: thyroxine (T_4) and triiodothyronine (T_3). The higher the levels of T_4 and/or T_3, the lower the levels of TSH. In contrast the lower the levels of T_4 and/or T_3, the higher the level of TSH.

TSH concentration can be measured precisely by a sensitive immunochemiluminometric assay (normal range 0–5 mU/L). Increased TSH concentrations are found in primary hypothyroidism, e.g. autoimmune thyroiditis, and after treatment of thyrotoxicosis by surgery or radioiodine. Suppressed TSH concentrations occur in hyperthyroidism. Thus measurement of TSH is usually all that is needed to establish a biochemically euthyroid state.

The thyroid hormones (T_4 and T_3) are stored in the thyroid gland in colloid. They are bound to thyroglobulin and released in response to TSH. In circulation the hormones are bound to thyroxine-binding globulin (TBG), thyroxine-binding prealbumin (TBPA) and albumin.

The principal metabolic effects of the thyroid hormones are exerted by unbound free T_4 and T_3 (0.03–0.04% and 0.2–0.5% of the total circulating hormones respectively). Because almost all T_4 and T_3 is protein bound, measurement of total hormone concentrations is influenced by conditions that change the serum concentrations of thyroxine-binding proteins. For example, increased concentrations are found in pregnancy and in women taking oral contraceptives, and low concentrations occur in the nephrotic syndrome. Drugs such as salicylates and some antibiotics compete for protein binding.

Radioimmunoassays for free T_4 and T_3 are now readily available and give a precise assessment of thyroid function. T_3 is the more active physiological hormone, with 80% being produced in the periphery by monodeiodination of T_4. Measurement of T_3 is particularly important in T_3 toxicosis when there is a clinical picture of thyrotoxicosis with normal serum T_4 concentrations.

Thyroid antibodies

Thyroglobulin

Antibodies to thyroglobulin, the major constituent of colloid and precursor of thyroid hormones, are found in most people with Graves' disease and virtually 100% of those with Hashimoto's thyroiditis.[1] The presence of such antibodies can interfere with the radioimmunoassay for thyroglobulin leading to falsely elevated results (see below). Measurement of thyroglobulin levels has now become standard in the long-term follow-up and monitoring of patients who have undergone total thyroidectomy and radioiodine ablation therapy for differentiated thyroid cancer.[2]

Thyroid peroxidase

Antibodies to thyroid peroxidase (TPO), previously known as thyroid microsomal antigen, are found in most patients with Graves' disease or Hashimoto's thyroiditis.[3] Raised titres are also detected in patients with postpartum thyroiditis and non-organ-specific autoimmune diseases such as rheumatoid arthritis.

TSH receptor autoantibodies

Most TSH receptor autoantibodies (TRAbs) have a stimulatory action, but in some instances antibodies bind to the receptor and block activity. Measurement of TRAbs is especially valuable in the diagnosis of Graves' disease, being detected in approximately 90% of patients.[4] Neonatal hyperthyroidism may result from transplacental passage of TRAbs.

Calcitonin

Increased serum levels of calcitonin (from the parafollicular or C cells) are found in patients with medullary thyroid carcinoma (MTC).[5]

Measurement of basal or stimulated calcitonin concentrations is employed to assess the completeness of surgical resection of MTC and is valuable in the follow-up and detection of recurrence or metastases after thyroidectomy. Screening for the detection of familial MTC, usually as part of the multiple endocrine neoplasia type 2A (MEN 2A) or 2B (MEN 2B) syndrome, no longer depends on measurement of stimulated calcitonin concentrations.

Identification of germ-line mutations in the RET proto-oncogene on chromosome 10 means that families can be directly tested for the germ-line mutation (replacing biochemical screening; see Chapter 4).[6]

Carcinoembryonic antigen (CEA)

Though CEA is not a direct tumour marker in MTC, when present it is suggestive of a poor prognostic tumour.

Thyroid isotope scanning

Scanning the thyroid gland with either radioactive ^{123}I or technetium pertechnetate (^{99m}Tc) in an attempt to provide a differential diagnosis in euthyroid patients with a solitary nodule should be discouraged. Fine-needle aspiration cytology is the accepted investigation of choice in this group of patients.

When scanning is performed nodules are characterised into those that are non-functioning 'cold' (**Fig. 2.1**), normally functioning 'warm' and hyper-

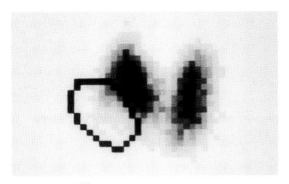

Figure 2.1 • [123]I scan of 'cold' thyroid nodule.

functioning 'hot'. Although the finding of a hot nodule is usually consistent with benign pathology, more than 80% of nodules are cold and only 20% of these will be malignant. Iodine scanning is therefore not helpful in the diagnosis of malignancy and has no significant role in the investigation of euthyroid patients with a solitary nodule. Discrepant imaging is well documented, with hot ^{99m}Tc images being cold on ^{123}I scanning.[7] It has therefore been suggested that all ^{99m}Tc hot scans should be re-evaluated with [123]I.

Isotope scanning is most useful in the investigation of the solitary autonomous toxic nodule (**Fig. 2.2**) or toxic multinodular goitre (**Fig. 2.3**). Iodine scanning is also helpful in the evaluation of patients with metastatic thyroid tumours and in the

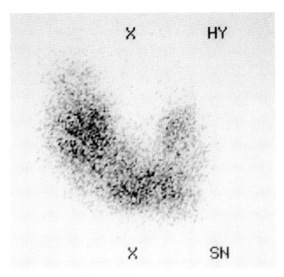

Figure 2.3 • [123]I scan of toxic multinodular goitre.

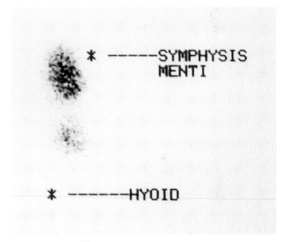

Figure 2.4 • [123]I scan of ectopic submental thyroid.

localisation of ectopic thyroid tissue (**Fig. 2.4**). There is no role for iodine scanning in patients with MTC since C cells do not take up iodine. Alternative isotopes previously employed in the evaluation of patients with MTC – pentavalent dimercaptosuccinic acid (DMSA),[8] thallium[9] and meta-iodobenzyl guanidine (MIBG)[10] – have now been largely superseded by magnetic resonance imaging (MRI) and positron emission tomography (PET) scanning.

Radioiodine uptake

Radioactive ^{123}I is taken into the thyroid gland in an identical manner to inorganic iodine. Measurement of the uptake of an administered dose after 4 and

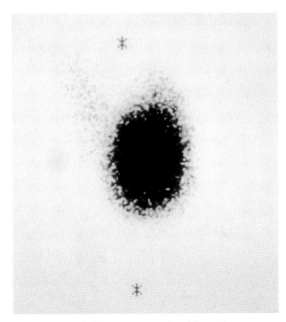

Figure 2.2 • Toxic autonomous thyroid nodule.

48 hours is useful in the assessment of patients with thyrotoxicosis. Increased uptake is seen in most forms of the disorder, with the notable exceptions of thyrotoxicosis due to subacute thyroiditis and after excessive T_4 intake.

Ultrasonography

This technique is operator dependent but capable of identifying impalpable nodules as small as 0.3 mm in diameter. Ultrasonography also discriminates cystic lesions from solid lesions but is not yet reliable in distinguishing benign disease from malignant disease. Cystic nodules constitute 15–25%[11] of all thyroid nodules and when 4 cm or more in diameter may have a malignancy rate of approximately 20% (**Fig. 2.5**).[12]

Computed tomography (CT) and magnetic resonance imaging (MRI)

CT and MRI play an increasingly important part in thyroid disease, particularly in the evaluation of retrosternal goitres and glands producing major pressure effects and distortion of adjacent structures (**Fig. 2.6a,b**).

Fine-needle aspiration cytology (FNAC)

FNAC employs a fine gauge (21 or 23) needle to obtain a thyroid sample suitable for cytological assessment. First used in Scandinavia in the early 1950s,[13] it is now universally accepted as being a

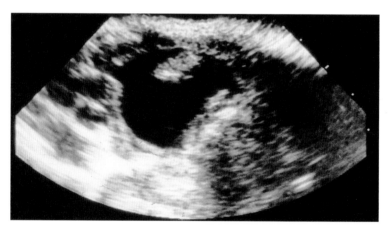

Figure 2.5 • Ultrasound scan of mixed thyroid nodule with cystic and solid component.

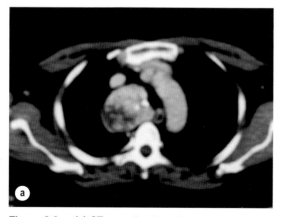
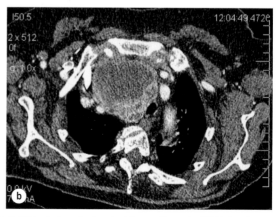

Figure 2.6 • **(a)** CT scan showing a large retrosternal goitre extending below the level of the aortic arch. **(b)** Extensive retrosternal goitre, narrowing the trachea and pushing it well across to the left. The patient presented with significant stridor.

highly accurate, cost-effective method with low morbidity and good patient compliance. In experienced hands the high diagnostic accuracy is such that the method can diagnose colloid nodules, thyroiditis, papillary carcinoma, medullary carcinoma, anaplastic carcinoma and lymphoma.

The major limitation of FNAC is the inability to distinguish benign from malignant follicular neoplasms, this distinction being dependent on the histological criteria of capsular and vascular invasion.[14]

Recently guidelines have been issued such that thyroid cytology should now be reported in a similar fashion to breast cytology. The five cytological categories are summarised in **Table 2.1**.

Lowhagen et al. reported no false-positive results with respect to malignancy and a false-negative rate of 2.2%, which later decreased to zero.[14]

Grant et al. found a false-negative rate of only 0.7% in 439 patients studied and concluded that FNAC was a safe, reliable and accurate means of discriminating between benign and malignant lesions.[15]

Most suspicious lesions on FNAC are follicular tumours, and because of the inability of the technique to provide histological details all such lesions should be resected. An inadequate sample rate of 15% is not uncommon but such a result should not be regarded as being benign but is an indication for repeat aspiration or diagnostic hemithyroidectomy.

Needle core biopsy

Cutting needle biopsy produces a core of tissue suitable for histological examination and has high diagnostic accuracy but has the disadvantages of being a painful procedure with poor compliance. Potential complications include haematoma, tracheal puncture and recurrent laryngeal nerve damage. Lesions less than 3 cm in size may not be amenable to this technique. The technique is most useful in establishing the diagnosis where lymphoma is suspected following FNAC, thus saving the need for an open biopsy. The risk of seeding malignancy along the needle tract has been greatly exaggerated and many if not all of the potential complications can be avoided if ultrasound-guided biopsies are performed rather than freehand.

Developmental abnormalities of the thyroid

Thyroglossal cyst

This condition results from persistence of part of the thyroglossal duct and is usually found as a midline cyst (occasionally more laterally) just below the hyoid bone or above the thyroid cartilage. Less commonly the cyst is found at a higher level above the hyoid bone. The essential diagnostic feature is that of upward movement on swallowing, and because of the attachment of the thyroglossal tract to the foramen caecum, the cyst rises on protrusion of the tongue. These cysts are prone to infection and therefore should be excised. The most appropriate and successful operation is the Sistrunk procedure, with excision of the central portion of the hyoid bone. Malignancy, usually of a papillary type, can occur within the thyroglossal cyst as a primary phenomenon.[16]

Thyroglossal fistula

This results from infection or inadequate removal of a thyroglossal cyst, the opening being found at a lower level in the neck than the original cyst. Careful tracing of the tract to the foramen caecum and excision of the central portion of the hyoid bone achieves complete excision of the fistula.

Lingual thyroid

When the thyroid gland fails to descend it may be found in the back of the tongue close to the foramen

Table 2.1 • Classification of FNA cytology

FNAC category	Cytology
THY 1	Insufficient material
THY 2	Benign (nodular goitre)
THY 3	Suspicious of neoplasm (follicular)
THY 4	Suspicious of malignancy (papillary/medullary/lymphoma)
THY 5	Definite malignancy

caecum. If large it can result in respiratory or swallowing difficulties and haemorrhage. Diagnosis is confirmed by radioactive iodine scanning, and treatment with T_4 can result in shrinkage. Radioactive iodine is an alternative therapeutic measure and excision is rarely necessary.

Ectopic thyroid

Arrested descent of the thyroid results in the gland being found at any point along the line of the thyroglossal tract. In these circumstances this may be the only thyroid tissue present. If this is the case and excision is carried out, then full replacement T_4 dosage is required.

Non-recurrent laryngeal nerve

The embryology of the recurrent laryngeal nerve (RLN) is related to the development of the aortic arches. On the left side the RLN recurs around the sixth aortic arch, which is subsequenly the ligamentum arteriosum. On the right side, the RLN recurs around the fourth aortic arch, which becomes the subclavian artery. The RLN can have a non-recurrent course, a situation nearly always observed on the right side. If the segment of the fourth aortic arch between the origin of the right carotid artery and right subclavian artery disappears, the resulting break in the primitive arterial ring leads to a left-sided aortic arch, with the right subclavian artery being its last branch. In this situation, the right subclavian travels from left to right posterior to the oesophagus or between trachea and oesophagus to reach the right side of the neck (arteria lusoria). The absence of an arterial segment under which the RLN normally forms a loop leads to a non-recurrent laryngeal nerve. In this situation the RLN always passes behind the common carotid artery. This rare anatomical variant should be recognised in order to avoid injury to the NRLN.

Goitre

The term goitre, derived from the Latin *guttur*, meaning throat, is used as a non-specific term to indicate diffuse enlargement of the thyroid gland. A classification of goitre is shown in **Table 2.2**.

Table 2.2 • Classification of goitre

Simple goitre (endemic or sporadic)	Diffuse hyperplastic goitre
	Nodular goitre
Toxic goitre	Diffuse (Graves' disease)
	Toxic multinodular goitre
	Toxic solitary nodule
Neoplastic goitre	Benign
	Malignant
Thyroiditis	Subacute (granulomatous): de Quervain's
	Autoimmune (Hashimoto's)
	Riedel's
	Acute suppurative
Miscellaneous	Chronic bacterial infection (e.g. tuberculosis or syphilis)
	Actinomycosis
	Amyloidosis
	Dyshormonogenesis

Simple goitre

Simple goitre is the result of TSH stimulation, usually secondary to inadequate concentrations of circulating thyroid hormones. In these circumstances, TSH stimulation causes diffuse hyperplasia and an increase in hormone output. Iodine deficiency is a key factor in simple endemic goitre, associated with a low iodine content of water and food.[17] There are 5–10 mg of iodine in the thyroid pool, with a turnover rate of 1% daily. The minimum daily dietary requirements of iodine are therefore small, about 50–100 µg. Endemic goitrous areas are mountainous regions such as the Alps, Andes and Himalayas. In Britain, recognised regions include the Chilterns, Cotswolds, Derbyshire and South Wales.

Iodine deficiency in its most extreme form is associated with congenital hypothyroidism and various degrees of mental impairment. Usually an endemic goitre commences as a soft diffuse enlargement appearing in childhood, which can evolve into a colloid goitre at a later stage when TSH stimulation has diminished. Times of physiological stress, such as puberty and pregnancy, result in increased demands for T_4 and are accompanied by TSH stimulation of the thyroid and diffuse hyperplasia.

The natural history of thyroid stimulation by TSH is such that there are fluctuating levels of stimulation, but eventually active and inactive lobules coexist.

At this stage nodules form, and throughout the thyroid there are changes of hyperplasia, cystic degeneration, haemorrhage, colloid-filled follicles, fibrosis and later calcification. Simple goitre occurring in a non-endemic area is usually described as sporadic, but the nodules of endemic goitre appear earlier. All types of simple goitre occur more often in women.

Environmental factors such as the dietary goitrogen thiocyanate in cassava or vegetables of the brassica family may cause thyroid enlargement.[18] The interaction of environmental goitrogens and iodine deficiency may explain some of the differences in the prevalence of endemic goitre seen with similar degrees of iodine deficiency. Other environmental agents, including calcium and drugs such as the antithyroid agent carbimazole, are capable of acting at various sites within the thyroid gland, and by interfering with the process of hormone synthesis lead to hyperplasia with goitre formation. Paradoxically, excess iodine intake can inhibit proteolysis and release of thyroid hormones, leading to goitre and hypothyroidism.

Deficiency of one or more of the enzymes in the thyroid responsible for T_4 synthesis may be the cause of sporadic goitre. These deficiencies, either complete or partial, are usually genetic and are well illustrated by the dyshormonogenic Pendred's syndrome in which thyroid enlargement progresses to nodular goitre with associated deafness. Severe forms of dyshormonogenesis result in hypothyroidism and cretinism in the infant. Treatment consists of T_4 and thyroidectomy if the goitre produces pressure symptoms or cosmetic concerns.

Prevention and treatment

Prevention of the development of simple endemic goitre can be achieved by the addition of iodine to the diet as, for example, in table salt. Thyroidectomy may be indicated for cosmetic reasons or because of pressure effects if the gland does not regress in the context of satisfactory iodine intake.

Thyroid nodule

Thyroid nodules are common, being a feature of many different thyroid diseases. In a non-goitrous area, the prevalence of palpable thyroid nodules in a population aged 30–59 years can be up to 4.2%.[19]

At adult autopsy the prevalence of thyroid nodules (many less than 1 cm in diameter and impalpable) is much greater, perhaps even as high as 50%.[20] Although the majority of thyroid nodules are benign and include colloid lesions, follicular adenomas, nodular thyroiditis and degenerative cysts, the essential clinical problem, particularly when the lesion is solitary, remains the distinction between benign and malignant diseases.

Clinical assessment

History

Most thyroid nodules are asymptomatic but the acute development of a painful swelling in the thyroid is usually due to haemorrhage into a pre-existing colloid nodule. This is an important condition to recognise as spontaneous resolution, sometimes aided by aspiration, occurs in a few weeks without intervention. Rapid growth of an existing nodule, with discomfort radiating into the face or jaw, may be due to malignancy but this presentation tends to be seen in elderly people with an anaplastic carcinoma. Often malignant nodules may be slow growing and be present for many years before a diagnosis is made.

Thyroid nodules (like most thyroid conditions) occur more often in women, thus a solitary nodule in a man carries a greater risk of malignancy. Young people are particularly at risk for malignancy. A solitary nodule is likely to be malignant in 50% of children under 14 years of age.[21,22] A family history of thyroid or other endocrine disease may be relevant to the diagnosis of MTC in MEN 2A, MEN 2B and non-MEN familial syndromes (see Chapter 4).

Several key environmental and geographic factors require consideration. The incidence of follicular cancer is increased in endemic goitrous areas,[23] for example, whereas iodine-rich regions such as Iceland have an increased incidence of papillary cancer.[24]

Although the association between thyroid carcinoma and a history of head and neck irradiation in children was first recorded in 1950,[25] the true magnitude of the problem was only identified by DeGroot and Paloyan in the Chicago area in 1973.[26] Irradiation also increases the incidence of benign thyroid nodules but the reported risk of malignancy in a palpable nodule found in a previously irradiated thyroid ranges from 20% to 50%. Age at exposure is a significant factor, with the very young (<16 years) being particularly at risk (as demonstrated by the Chernobyl nuclear reactor accident).

High-dose external beam irradiation to the neck for conditions such as Hodgkin's lymphoma may also increase the risk of thyroid malignancy.[27] The latent period for developing post-irradiation tumours ranges from 6 to 35 years. Therapeutic radioiodine used in the treatment of Graves' disease and the administration of diagnostic isotopes are not associated with any increased risk of malignancy.

Examination

A preliminary clinical examination of the patient is directed towards assessment of thyroid status, although most patients with a solitary thyroid nodule will be euthyroid. A nodule in a hyperthyroid patient is highly unlikely to be malignant. Previously much emphasis was placed on the distinction between a clinically solitary nodule and a multinodular gland in the mistaken belief that multinodular goitres were unlikely to contain a malignancy. When a dominant lesion is present within a multinodular gland, the malignancy rate may be virtually identical to that of the true solitary nodule.

A hard fixed nodule is likely to be malignant, but it is not uncommon for papillary lesions to be cystic and follicular lesions to be soft as a result of haemorrhage. A very hard lesion may be an entirely benign calcified colloid nodule. Lymphadenopathy either in the central paratracheal groups or in the lateral deep cervical region is a common finding in papillary and medullary carcinomas and when noted should be treated with a very high index of suspicion clinically.

Although voice change and hoarseness may be non-specific findings, a proven recurrent laryngeal nerve palsy on the side of a palpable thyroid nodule is likely to indicate malignant infiltration. Rarely, direct pressure from a benign lesion can also produce vocal cord paralysis. Although the presence of pressure symptoms and clinical identification of tracheal deviation or retrosternal extension does not aid the distinction of malignant from benign lesion, these features nevertheless will be major considerations in the selection of patients for surgery.

Following this careful clinical assessment, the clinician will have formed an opinion as to the likelihood of malignancy. Further supportive and diagnostic tests are now appropriate. The thyroid status will be confirmed by measurement of T_4 and TSH. Chest X-ray may demonstrate a retrosternal goitre or airway distortion or show evidence of macroscopic metastases. Most calcified thyroid nodules are benign, but some papillary and medullary neoplasms have a characteristic fine stippled or punctate calcification.

Measurement of calcitonin concentration is not currently routinely performed. Hypercalcitonaemia is not absolutely specific for medullary carcinoma but makes that diagnosis highly likely. Occasionally increased concentrations of calcitonin may be seen in patients with carcinoma of the breast, pancreas or lung or in those with carcinoid tumours, phaeochromocytoma and bony metastases. Thyroglobulin measurement, although valuable in the follow-up of patients with malignant tumours, has no value at the time of initial diagnosis of thyroid tumours.

FNAC

FNAC is now considered mandatory is the investigation of the solitary thyroid nodule. This highly accurate and cost-effective technique is the method of choice for achieving a precise diagnosis in most patients with thyroid nodular disease. When a conservative approach to the management of the thyroid nodule is contemplated, a second FNAC some weeks following the initial visit has been shown to increase diagnostic accuracy and reduce the incidence of missed malignancies.[28] Delbridge et al. have shown that proton magnetic resonance spectroscopy (PMRS) analysis of FNAC specimens helps to make the distinction between benign and malignant lesions and thereby reduces unnecessary surgery for patients with benign follicular neoplasms.[29]

Ultrasonography

Ultrasonography has limited diagnostic value in the assessment of thyroid nodules but allows a clear delineation of multinodularity. An apparently solitary nodule may be shown on ultrasonography to be surrounded by small impalpable nodules. Ultrasonography may also be useful in demonstrating the presence of enlarged, non-palpable cervical nodes.

Isotope scanning

Unless the patient has thyrotoxicosis, scintigraphy of the thyroid either with ^{123}I or technetium pertechnetate (^{99m}Tc) has little value in the investigation of the patient with a thyroid nodule.

PET scans

In recent years PET has been increasingly used for the staging of malignant diseases. Such scans can pick up an unexpected thyroid nodule (PET incidentaloma) which can represent a thyroid cancer in up to a quarter of cases. Such nodules therefore warrant further diagnostic work-up along the lines already discussed.

Treatment

Thyroid hormone administration

There is little evidence that the administration of T_4 is capable of reducing the size of benign nodules. The possibility of reducing the size of an incorrectly diagnosed malignant nodule by T_4 is clearly a potential pitfall.

Summary of indications for surgery

Patients in whom there is a suspicion of malignancy (based on clinical features or FNAC) should be considered for surgery. When malignancy is not an issue, surgery should be offered to patients with symptoms of pressure (dyspnoea, choking and dysphagia). Occasionally patients with no pressure symptoms may require surgery on cosmetic grounds. A scheme of management of patients with solitary thyroid nodular disease is shown in **Fig. 2.7**. Clinical features such as characteristics of nodule, lymphadenopathy, recurrent laryngeal nerve palsy, family history and history of irradiation may override cytological findings in the decision for surgery.

Surgery for thyroid nodules

The minimum surgical procedure for adequate treatment of the solitary thyroid nodule is a unilateral *total* lobectomy with removal of the isthmus and pyramidal lobe. In experienced hands this is a relatively safe operation with minimal risk of damaging either the parathyroids or the recurrent laryngeal nerve. A full histological examination of the nodule is permitted with no risk of tumour spillage in the operative field. This surgical procedure completely obviates the need to reoperate and remove a posterior thyroid lobe remnant on the same side if the definitive histology should be returned as malignant or if there should be any benign nodule recurrence at a later date. These are most important benefits compared with the outmoded procedure of unilateral *subtotal* lobectomy.

Frozen section histology can be useful where papillary or medullary thyroid cancer is suspected as confirmation may indicate the need for total thyroidectomy at the initial operation. Frozen section histology is not advocated for follicular lesions (diagnosis of malignancy in this situation is often difficult).[30]

Thyroid cysts

Confirmation of the diagnosis of a thyroid cyst is usually made by fine-needle aspiration and this simple technique can be both diagnostic and therapeutic (**Fig. 2.8**). A full cytological assessment usually requires sampling thyroid tissue adjacent to the cyst to avoid missing a carcinoma in the cyst wall. If a cyst refills it is appropriate to reaspirate but after two or three attempts surgery is likely to be indicated. A large cyst (>4 cm in diameter), a significantly blood-stained aspirate, cytological findings of neoplasia or a history of irradiation are all indications for surgery.

Multinodular goitre

The usual indications for surgery are cosmesis, local pressure symptoms, a dominant nodule increasing in size or showing cytological features that raise the possibility of malignancy, thyrotoxicosis or retrosternal extension (**Fig. 2.9**). The surgical procedure will be tailored to the situation found at operation. Often asymmetrical nodularity is present with one lobe significantly larger than the other; in this situation a unilateral total lobectomy with a subtotal procedure on the opposite side may be indicated.

 More recently, however, there is an increasing trend amongst endocrine surgeons to perform a total thyroidectomy for multinodular goitre, leaving no thyroid tissue in situ.[31]

Retrosternal goitre

Almost all retrosternal goitres arise from growth of the lower half of the thyroid lobes, extending down into a substernal position. The degree of descent of the gland is variable, but when palpable in the neck it is usually classified as substernal, whereas a gland entirely within the chest is intrathoracic.

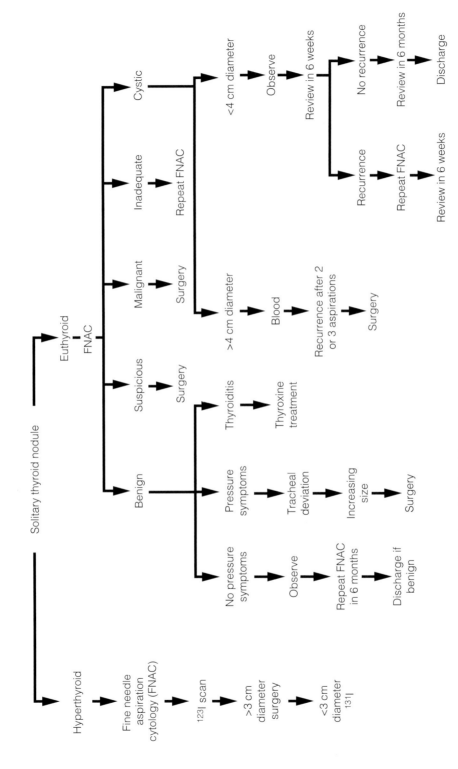

Figure 2.7 • Scheme of management for solitary thyroid nodule.

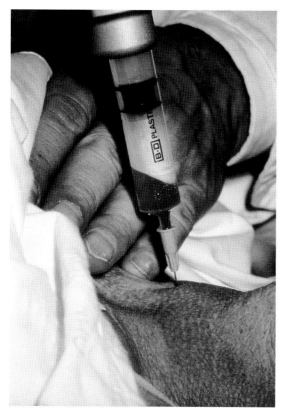

Figure 2.8 • Aspiration of cystic thyroid nodule demonstrating therapeutic as well as diagnostic value of fine-needle aspiration.

Not infrequently a retrosternal goitre may be asymptomatic and found as a coincidental observation on a chest radiograph (**Fig. 2.10**). However, many patients are symptomatic with problems of airway compression, 'asthma', dysphagia and even thyrotoxicosis. Rarely, patients may present with hoarseness of the voice from a vocal cord palsy (a direct effect of pressure from a benign lesion on the recurrent laryngeal nerve). More dramatic pressure effects can lead to superior vena cava compression syndrome (**Fig. 2.11**). The incidence of malignancy in retrosternal glands is probably no different to that of other nodular goitres, but of course a gland behind the sternum is not amenable to palpation or FNAC for diagnosis.

Confirmation of the diagnosis can be made by a combination of plain radiographs and either CT or MRI. The last two investigations will give precise information concerning airway compromise. Respiratory function tests with flow loop studies are also helpful in patient assessment.

The diagnosis of a retrosternal goitre is usually an indication for surgery (**Fig. 2.12**) both to obtain a precise histological diagnosis and to remove the significant risk of progressive airway obstruction resulting from growth of the gland or from haemorrhage into a benign colloid lesion.

Thyroid cancer

Thyroid cancer is rare (3.7–4.7 per 100 000 population), accounting for less than 1% of all malignancies and 0.5% of all cancer deaths.[32–34] Thyroid cancer constitutes an extremely heterogeneous group of tumours, with a wide spectrum of biological behaviour. In most instances if treated appropriately there is a high cure rate with an across-the-board survival rate of >80% at 10 years. Disappointingly, because of the lack of long-term follow-up studies or large randomised trials comparing various procedures, the optimal management for many of these tumours remains controversial.

Molecular biology of thyroid cancer

Thyroid cancer results from complex alterations and disorders of the genetic content of a single cell, which is subsequently inherited by its daughter cells. Several genetic aberrations have been well studied and shown to be implicated in thyroid tumorigenesis.

Oncogenes when activated stimulate tumour growth.[35] Important members of this gene family which play a part in thyroid tumour development include the *Ras* genes,[36] growth factors, such as epidermal growth factor (EGF)[37] (and its receptor EGFr), insulin-like growth factor I (IGF-I), fibroblast growth factor (FGF), TSH, $Gs\alpha$ gene and the *RET* proto-oncogene (see section on familial MTC).

Tumour suppressor genes, especially *p53*,[38] exert an influence on thyroid cell growth by inhibiting tumorigenesis. Mutations in *p53* can lead to its inactivation, which may be important in thyroid tumour initiation and progression, especially leading to anaplastic change. Recently *Ras* mutations have been identified in some aggressive thyroid cancers. This finding raises the possibility that they may be useful as markers of poor prognosis.[39]

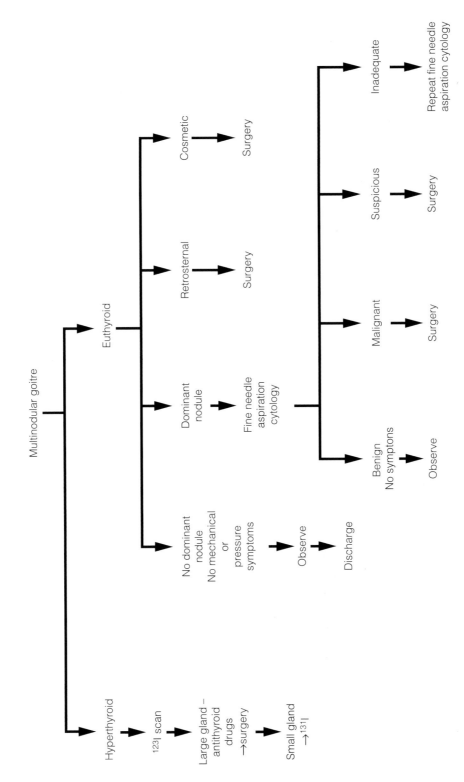

Figure 2.9 • Scheme of management for multinodular goitre.

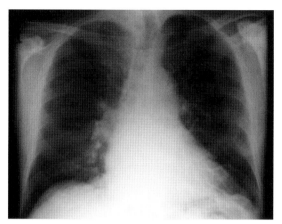

Figure 2.10 • Chest X-ray revealing the incidental finding of a deviated trachea secondary to a previously undiagnosed retrosternal goitre.

Papillary carcinoma

This is the commonest thyroid malignancy, accounting for approximately 70–80% of cancers. It more commonly affects children and young adults and has an increased incidence in iodine-rich areas. Exposure to ionising radiation (as experienced in Chernobyl) or direct irradiation of the neck, particularly in young people, may predispose to thyroid cancer, and approximately 85% of such irradiation-induced tumours are papillary.[26] A rare familial form of the disease has also been described.[40]

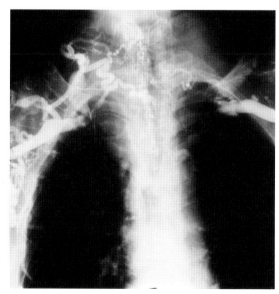

Figure 2.11 • Venogram of a patient with retrosternal goitre producing obstruction of the superior vena cava.

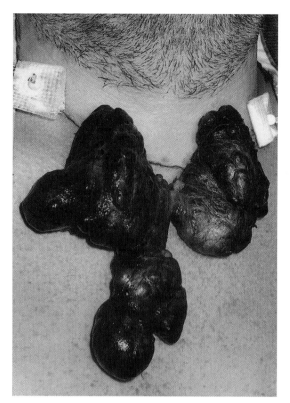

Figure 2.12 • Large retrosternal goitre causing respiratory distress. Specimen resected without the need of a sternotomy.

Pathology

Macroscopically tumours tend to appear as a hard whitish nodule infiltrating the thyroid gland. Papillary cancer is often multifocal (though this is often a microscopic finding and not apparent at surgery). Encapsulation of tumours is unusual (though when this finding is present it is thought to be a good prognostic factor). The tumour has a propensity for early lymphatic spread both within the thyroid and to the paratracheal and cervical lymph nodes. Blood-borne spread to lungs and bones is usually a late feature. Tumours can be divided into three main types based on their size and extent.

Micropapillary cancer

These lesions by definition are less than 1 cm in diameter and usually not clinically obvious. They are most frequently reported as incidental findings following thyroidectomy for other conditions. They readily metastasise to regional lymph nodes and are a common finding at autopsy, being detected in 6–13% of thyroid glands of patients dying from causes other than thyroid disease.

Though the primary tumour is not usually clinically apparent, spread to local cervical nodes may be the presenting feature (the so-called lateral aberrant thyroid). Distant metastatic disease is rare, though deaths have been reported.

 The Mayo Clinic group described four deaths in 396 patients with tumours 1.5 cm or less in diameter,[41] and Noguchi et al. documented two deaths in 867 patients.[42]

Intrathyroidal

These lesions are larger than minimal tumours (i.e. >1 cm) and are situated totally within the thyroid. They have a less favourable prognosis than microcancers.

Extrathyroidal

These tumours are locally advanced, extending through the thyroid capsule, often involving adjacent structures such as the trachea, oesophagus and RLN. The prognosis of this disease type is the least favourable.

Histology

The typical lesion has a mixture of papillary projections and follicular structures. The cuboidal cells with pale abundant cytoplasm have intranuclear cytoplasmic inclusions, nuclear overlapping and grooves (Orphan Annie cells). Psammoma bodies occur and are associated with a high incidence of lymphatic spread. The presence of involved lymph nodes, however, does not seem to adversely affect the prognosis. Follicular, encapsulated, diffuse sclerosing and tall cell varieties of papillary carcinoma have been described and are associated with a poorer long-term prognosis.

Clinical presentation

Clinically, papillary carcinoma usually presents as a hard solitary nodule. Locally enlarged cervical nodes may be present (particularly in children and younger patients). Cystic degeneration of the primary tumour (or metastases) occasionally leads to the mistaken diagnosis of simple thyroid cyst (or branchial cyst in metastases).

Local invasion of the RLN can result in vocal cord palsy, airway symptoms (because of tracheal involvement) and/or dysphagia as a result of oesophageal invasion. Less than 1% of patients at the time of initial presentation will show features of distant metastases. The highest frequency of metastases at initial presentation is seen in children, but ultimately up to 20% of patients develop distant spread.[43]

Follicular carcinoma

This malignancy accounts for 15–20% of thyroid cancers and has a higher incidence in iodine-deficient areas (from chronic TSH stimulation). It can also be caused by previous neck irradiation. The disease has a female to male ratio of 3:1, affecting an older age group than papillary carcinoma (mean age 50 years). A rare familial form also exists (**Fig. 2.13**).[44]

Pathology

Follicular carcinoma is usually encapsulated, solitary and frequently exhibits vascular invasion. Metastatic spread is via the blood stream. In contrast with papillary tumours, lymphatic spread is usually a late phenomenon, seen with advanced tumours. Follicular carcinoma is classified into two types according to histopathological features.

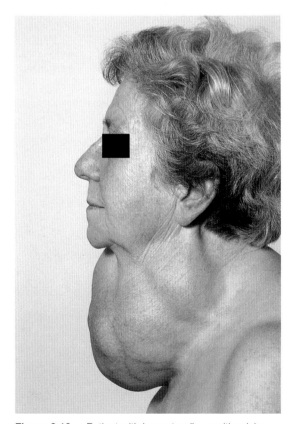

Figure 2.13 • Patient with long-standing multinodular goitre and coexisting follicular thyroid carcinoma.

Minimally invasive cancer

These are the most common follicular malignancy. Tumours exhibit either only slight invasion into the capsule or occasionally just through the capsule, but not widely into the surrounding thyroid. Invasion into capsular blood vessels may also be present.

Widely invasive cancer

This is far less common than minimally invasive cancers. However, it is a more aggressive tumour (diagnosis of which depends on histological confirmation of capsular and angioinvasive features). At surgery, venous extension into the middle thyroid and internal jugular veins may be present. Although most well-differentiated tumours have a well-formed follicular structure, the oxyphilic Hürthle cell lesion is composed mainly of cells with eosinophilic granular cytoplasm, large clear nuclei and trabecular architecture. Some consider this variety to be a particularly aggressive form of follicular carcinoma, with a greater propensity for multifocality and lymph node metastases.[45] Furthermore, therapeutic options in Hürthle cell tumours are limited by the inability of the lesion to concentrate radioactive iodine. They do, however, synthesise thyroglobulin.

Clinical features

Follicular thyroid cancer presents as a discrete solitary thyroid nodule increasing in size. Tumours are usually firm but may be softened by haemorrhage within the lesion. Metastatic disease may already be present at the time of diagnosis, with bone and lung involvement. Cervical lymphadenopathy is not usually present at initial presentation.

In contrast to papillary thyroid carcinoma (where FNAC has a high specificity and sensitivity), follicular carcinoma cannot be diagnosed precisely by FNAC. The cytology report will describe a follicular tumour and only 20% of these will subsequently be identified as follicular carcinoma.

Treatment of differentiated thyroid cancer

There is universal agreement that thyroidectomy is the treatment of choice for patients with differentiated thyroid cancer. The precise extent of the procedure, however, depends upon the type of cancer present and remains controversial.[46] The introduction of guidelines on the management of thyroid cancer in the UK has been demonstrated to increase

Box 2.1 • Treatment goals in thyroid cancer

- Eradicate the primary tumour
- Reduce the incidence of distant or local recurrence
- Facilitate treatment of metastases
- Cure the maximum number of patients
- Achieve all of these objectives with minimal morbidity

the number of patients treated in specialist centres and to decrease the size of the thyroid remnant following thyroid surgery.[47] The treatment goals in the management of thyroid cancer are listed in **Box 2.1**.

Patients with papillary carcinoma can be separated into high- and low-risk groups with regard to risk for recurrence and long-term survival. Several sophisticated prognostic scoring systems have been introduced to identify patients with high-risk tumours and aid comparison between different surgical therapies. The AGES scoring system from the Mayo Clinic considers: Age of patients, histological Grade and Extent and Size of tumour.[48] Most patients being assessed by the scoring system fit into the low-risk group, with an excellent long-term prognosis. Other scoring systems include AMES (Age, Metastasis, Extent and Size) and MACIS (Metastasis, Age, Completeness of resection, Invasion and Size). As a common theme of all these staging/classification systems, the prognosis is influenced by age and sex of the patient and by the size of the primary tumour but not by the lymph node status.

Total thyroidectomy has been advocated for the treatment of differentiated thyroid cancer. This is because of its ability to treat multifocal tumour, decrease local recurrence, decrease distant recurrence, reduce the risk of anaplastic change in remaining remnants, facilitate treatment with ^{131}I and permit postoperative measurements of thyroglobulin concentration for monitoring the patient's subsequent progress.

Papillary carcinoma is usually multifocal, thus unilateral or even near total thyroidectomy may not necessarily remove all disease. It is likely, however, that many small foci of microscopic tumour remaining after less than total thyroidectomy stay dormant and do not necessarily progress and achieve clinical importance. Nevertheless, local tumour recurrence is an extremely serious event, carrying a high risk of death.

Retrospective studies of patients undergoing thyroidectomy have demonstrated a reduced local recurrence rate with total thyroidectomy compared with a subtotal resection.[49]

With respect to mortality risk, it has been shown that high-risk patients have a lower mortality rate at 25 years when treated by bilateral resection than by ipsilateral lobectomy.[45] The rare but life-threatening complication of anaplastic transformation in an inadequately resected papillary carcinoma can be avoided by initial total thyroid clearance.

Most patients with differentiated thyroid cancer present with a unilateral thyroid nodule. In this situation, the minimum primary procedure performed should be total lobectomy on the side of the lesion, isthmusectomy and removal of the pyramidal lobe. If papillary carcinoma is (or has been) confirmed by intraoperative frozen section or preoperative FNAC, a total thyroidectomy is the most appropriate surgical treatment for both intrathyroidal and extrathyroidal tumours.

Thyroidectomy must always include clearance of pretracheal and paratracheal lymph nodes. The thymus should not be disturbed to avoid devascularising the inferior parathyroids often situated within the superior thymic horns. Lymph nodes in the lateral carotid chain group are biopsied and, if they give a positive result on frozen section histology, should be cleared by a modified neck dissection, leaving the internal jugular vein and sternomastoid muscle intact (**Fig. 2.14**). There is no evidence to support the use of the more extensive and mutilating classic block dissection. More extensive extrathyroidal papillary carcinomas, however, may require radical excision of adjacent structures, even including part of the trachea, with construction of a temporary tracheostomy.

Recently the concept of sentinel node assessment has been applied to the operative management of patients with differentiated thyroid cancer, although the precise role of this technique has yet to be defined.

A unilateral total lobectomy and isthmusectomy is adequate for minimal (<1 cm) lesions and the rare encapsulated papillary cancers that generally have an excellent prognosis. The RLN must be identified throughout its course in these procedures so that damage may be avoided. Rarely, is it necessary to sacrifice the nerve to achieve tumour clearance. The incidence of permanent postoperative hypoparathyroidism should be no more than 3%, care being taken to identify the parathyroid glands and leave their blood supply intact.

Currently there is a trend towards recommending routine central compartment lymph node clearance

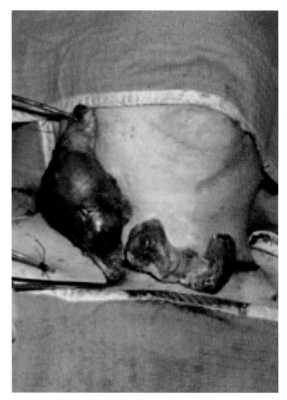

Figure 2.14 • Total thyroidectomy for papillary thyroid cancer with right-sided selective neck dissection to remove involved cervical nodes.

in all patients with preoperative diagnosis of papillary thyroid cancer. This allows better staging of the disease (N0 vs. N1 vs. Nx) and might be more likely to lead to a patient with negative cervical radioactive iodine uptake and undetectable thyroglobulin levels after thyroidectomy and radioactive iodine ablation. Even though the impact on survival has not been demonstrated, these surrogate markers for successful treatment seem appealing to the public and health providers.

Follicular tumours diagnosed on FNAC are treated by total lobectomy, isthmusectomy and removal of the pyramidal lobe. Frozen section is unhelpful, failing to demonstrate capsular or vascular invasion, because of sampling difficulties. If the definitive histology is returned as a minimal lesion, then a unilateral procedure is all that is required. A lesion shown to be frankly invasive requires a total thyroidectomy, either performed within a few days of the initial lobectomy or after a period of 3–4 months. Lymph node dissection is not routinely performed for follicular tumours. A decision to proceed to a total thyroidectomy should not be made at the time of surgery on the basis of the macroscopic appearances of the lesion, in case a patient is subjected to a total thyroidectomy and all its consequences for a benign condition.

Hürthle cell lesions, considered by some to have a bad prognosis, should be treated by total thyroidectomy and central neck node dissection.[43]

Postoperative treatment

Thyroxine (T_4)

Any patient who has undergone total thyroidectomy requires replacement treatment with T_4, and in patients with differentiated thyroid cancer there is compelling evidence for prescribing T_4 to suppress TSH concentrations, which may well influence the biological behaviour of any micrometastases from the tumour.

Thyroglobulin

Measurement of thyroglobulin concentration is a sensitive indicator of residual or recurrent differentiated thyroid cancer after total thyroidectomy and when the patient is on full replacement/suppressive T_4 dosage.[2] This measurement is now performed routinely at each postoperative clinic attendance and has markedly reduced the need for routine serial radioactive iodine scanning.

 Measurement of thyroglobulin concentration may be difficult when there are circulating autoantibodies to thyroglobulin (TgAbs). In these circumstances there is the potential to underestimate the risk or likelihood of metastatic malignancy.[50]

Radioactive iodine

Radioactive iodine is a most useful means of detecting metastatic disease when total thyroidectomy has been performed. However, approximately 20% of patients older than 50 years of age with papillary cancer cannot concentrate ^{131}I.[46] Most follicular carcinomas, with the exception of the Hürthle cell variety, can be imaged by radioiodine. If total thyroidectomy has been performed for differentiated cancer, patients are initially given T_3 20 µg t.d.s. and sent home to await an ^{131}I scan approximately 6 weeks later. T_3 is discontinued 2 weeks before the scan to allow an increase in TSH concentration before administering a therapeutic dose of 150–200 mCi ^{131}I. If there are no metastases or residual remnants of thyroid, the uptake at 24 hours should be less than 1%. It is also useful to obtain a baseline thyroglobulin level when the initial dose of radioiodine is administered.

Patients are then placed back onto T_3 and a second diagnostic radioiodine scan using 1–2 mCi ^{131}I is obtained 3 months later. If this subsequent scan is clear patients can be converted to T_4 150 µg per day (this is then titrated until the TSH level is suppressed below 0.1 iU).

If the second scan is not clear repeated therapeutic doses of ^{131}I are given as necessary until all residual uptake is ablated. The maximum cumulative dose of ^{131}I should be no greater than 800–1000 mCi. Patients whose metastases are visible only on radioiodine scanning despite negative results on chest radiography or tomography have an excellent prognosis.[51] Once the patient is stable and disease free, subsequent follow-up is achieved by a combination of clinical examination and measurement of serum thyroglobulin concentration. Ultrasound examination has also been shown to be a sensitive tool in assessing whether cervical lymphadenopathy is present in the postoperative follow-up of patients.[52] PET scanning may be useful in patients suspected of having recurrent or persistent differentiated thyroid cancer but who fail to demonstrate evidence of disease on radioiodine scanning.[53]

Local radiotherapy and retinoic acid

Radiotherapy may be useful in controlling locally advanced differentiated thyroid cancer, where microscopic or gross disease persists following surgical resection.[54] Similarly radiotherapy has a role in controlling pain from distant bony metastases. Recently attention has been focused on the possibility of redifferentiating tumours that fail to take up radioiodine by administering retinoic acid. Initial studies appear promising but whether this therapy proves to be effective remains to be seen. Haugen et al. have identified retinoic acid receptor isoforms in some thyroid cancers. This offers the possibility of identifying which tumours may respond well to retinoic acid therapy.[55]

Medullary carcinoma

This tumour arises from the thyroid C cells (derived from neural ectoderm). It accounts for approximately 8% of malignant thyroid tumours. In 1959 Hazard et al. described the tumour as a solid, nonfollicular carcinoma with coexisting amyloid.[56] In 1966 Williams, while further defining the histology of the tumour, proposed that the disease arose from the parafollicular or C cells, later shown to secrete calcitonin, a peptide capable of lowering the blood calcium concentration and amenable to measurement by radioimmunoassay.[57,58] MTC is a sporadic tumour in 80% of patients and familial in 20%. The familial syndromes, which are inherited in an autosomal dominant manner with almost complete penetrance but variable expressivity, consist of the MEN 2A and MEN 2B syndromes (**Fig. 2.15**) and the rarer non-MEN familial form.

Pathology

MTC is a solid tumour usually occurring in the upper two-thirds of the thyroid (where the C cells are concentrated). It is often multicentric and bilateral (particularly in the familial form). The typical histological picture is one of infiltrating neoplastic cells invading the thyroid, forming glandular and solid areas with an amyloid stroma. The tumour grows locally but readily spreads by lymphatics to regional nodes (**Fig. 2.16**) and via the bloodstream to distant sites such as liver, lungs and bones. The tumour synthesises and secretes calcitonin, which proves to be a most valuable biochemical and histochemical marker. CEA and calcitonin gene-related peptide (CGRP) are also produced by C cells, but they have little clinical value as tumour markers, though raised CEA levels are thought to be associated with a poorer long-term prognosis.

Clinical features

As with most thyroid tumours, the disease typically presents as a mass in the neck, often with enlarged cervical and mediastinal lymph nodes. Involvement of adjacent organs and the recurrent laryngeal nerve may cause respiratory or swallowing difficulties and

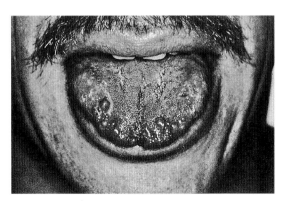

Figure 2.15 • Tongue of patient with multiple endocrine neoplasia type 2B syndrome showing ganglioneuromas.

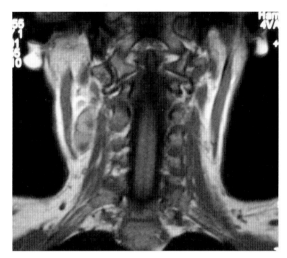

Figure 2.16 • MRI scan demonstrating right-sided cervical lymphadenopathy in a patient with medullary thyroid cancer.

voice changes. Sporadic disease has a peak incidence at 40–50 years of age, whereas inherited familial disease is usually seen at a younger age. Diarrhoea is often a prominent clinical feature, but the ability of this tumour to secrete a range of hormones and peptides, including calcitonin, prostaglandins, 5-hydroxytryptamine and adrenocorticotropic hormone, can give rise to a range of clinical syndromes, which may include Cushing's syndrome.

Although the familial varieties of the disease can present in an identical clinical manner to sporadic disease, genetic screening for *RET* mutations allows detection of the condition at a preclinical stage before there is histological or macroscopic evidence of the disease.

Diagnosis

Clinical assessment and the taking of a careful family history are fundamental to establishing a precise diagnosis. When there is a high index of suspicion, FNAC and measurement of serum calcitonin concentration usually provide confirmation. Even when the diagnosis of MTC is secure it may still not be possible to distinguish the sporadic from the familial variety. Because of the close association of phaeochromocytoma and MTC in the MEN 2 familial forms, it is considered mandatory in all patients to exclude this before progressing to any invasive procedure such as surgery. A thyroidectomy performed on a patient with an undiagnosed/untreated phaeochromocytoma is likely to have disastrous clinical consequences.

Preoperative basal calcitonin levels and the response to pentagastrin stimulation tests correlate with the extent of the disease. Patients with levels 10 times over the upper limit of normal are likely to have metastatic disease and will not be cured by surgery. Those with minimal increase in calcitonin levels are likely to have disease limited to the thyroid and local lymph nodes and could be cured by appropriate surgical excision.

Treatment

Total thyroidectomy is the appropriate procedure to adequately treat such patients because many have multicentric and bilateral disease. Due to the embryological origin of C cells, which concentrate in the posterior part of the upper and middle thyroid of the thyroid, many such tumours grow in close proximity to the RLN and its entry point into the larynx. Even when the primary tumour is extensive, the RLN can usually be preserved.

The central and paratracheal lymph nodes are cleared from the level of the thyroid cartilage to the upper mediastinum (level VI–VII), including thymectomy. For tumours larger than 2 cm, a simultaneous ipsilateral modified node dissection should be performed, preserving the internal jugular vein, sternomastoid muscle and spinal accessory nerve.

Because of the multifocal nature of hereditary tumours, a bilateral lymph node clearance is advised. However, when more than one lymph node compartment is involved with metastatic disease there is little chance of normalisation of calcitonin.[59]

Prognosis

The presence or absence of distant metastases and lymph node positivity are major factors in determining the ultimate prognosis. Excellent 10-year survival figures of approximately 90% have recently been reported,[60] but when lymph node metastases are present this survival rate is reduced to 45%. Sporadic disease and MEN 2B tumours are associated with the worst prognosis. A better outlook is seen in patients with non-MEN familial and MEN 2A syndromes.

Follow-up

After surgery, regular clinical and biochemical follow-up is carried out with measurement of calcitonin and CEA concentrations. When increased concentrations of these tumour markers persist after thyroidectomy or develop subsequently, this may signify persistent or recurrent disease.

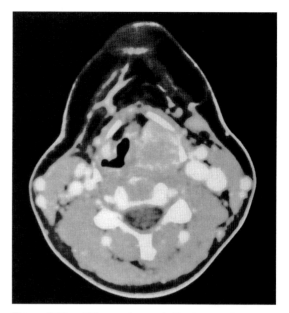

Figure 2.17 • CT scan demonstrating laryngeal metastatic deposit from medullary thyroid carcinoma. Patient treated by hemilaryngectomy.

Ultrasonography, CT, MRI and scanning with MIBG, octreotide or DMSA can be utilised to detect this disease (**Fig. 2.17**). For occult disease, selective venous catheterisation and sampling for calcitonin concentration have been used.[61] Laparoscopic assessment of the liver may detect small metastases not visible by conventional scanning. A proportion of these patients can be helped by re-operative surgery, but the benefits of radical re-operative surgery remain controversial. External irradiation can occasionally produce some benefit, but chemotherapy with doxorubicin is both toxic and response rates disappointing. Results of randomised controlled trials using new tyrosine kinase inhibitors are expected soon.

Anaplastic carcinoma

This tumour has a peak incidence between 60 and 70 years of age, occurs slightly more often in women and has a higher incidence in endemic goitrous areas. The tumour rapidly infiltrates local structures and metastasises via the bloodstream and lymphatics. The frequent finding of foci of papillary or follicular carcinoma in anaplastic tumours gives rise to the view that this disease originates in an unrecognised or untreated differentiated tumour.[62] The clinical findings are typically those of an elderly woman, often with a long history of goitre that suddenly starts to grow rapidly. Involvement of adjacent structures results in hoarseness, dysphonia, dysphagia and a compromised airway.

Although the clinical findings are virtually diagnostic, confirmation can be obtained by FNAC, the aspirate showing bizarre giant, multinucleated and pleomorphic tumour cells. Resection of the thyroid is rarely possible because of the local extent of disease. Incision biopsy for diagnostic purposes should be avoided for fear of initiating uncontrollable local spread of the disease. If surgery is possible, it should relieve an obstructed airway by excision of the isthmus. Radiotherapy and doxorubicin are the main modalities of treatment, but invariably the tumour rapidly progresses, usually leading to death of the patient within 6 months.

Malignant lymphoma

Thyroid lymphoma, usually of the non-Hodgkin's B-cell type, can develop as part of a generalised lymphomatous process involving other viscera, but the disease is usually confined as a primary tumour to the thyroid (**Fig. 2.18**). The majority of such lymphomas arise in a background of long-standing autoimmune Hashimoto's thyroiditis.[63] It must be emphasised that only a very small number of patients with this relatively common disorder ultimately go on to develop lymphoma.

These tumours infiltrate throughout lymphatics and blood vessels, spreading directly into adjacent tissue and involving cervical nodes.

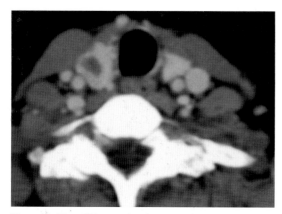

Figure 2.18 • CT scan showing a small lymphoma confined to the right thyroid lobe. No local lymphadenopathy is seen.

As in the case of anaplastic carcinoma, this is primarily a disease of elderly women, a typical patient presenting with a painless firm thyroid mass, rapidly increasing in size. There may be a history of goitre or autoimmune disease, and some patients will be frankly hypothyroid or already receiving T_4. This tumour grows to involve adjacent cervical structures, and lymphadenopathy is invariably present. FNAC usually raises a high degree of suspicion but full characterisation of the lymphoma requires the histological assessment. In most patients this is possible by a needle core biopsy in outpatients. Radiotherapy and chemotherapy are the main treatment modalities. Chemotherapy is of most value for extrathyroidal and disseminated disease. Surgery may be necessary to free the trachea when there is impending obstruction. Although 5-year survival of 85% has been reported,[64] the overall prognosis of the disease is significantly influenced by the histopathological grade of the lesion and the presence of locally extensive or disseminated disease.

Squamous cell carcinoma

This is a rare tumour, distinct from the squamous metaplasia often seen in papillary carcinomas. It is an aggressive disease with a clinical course similar to that of anaplastic carcinoma. Most squamous cell tumours are unresectable.

Metastatic carcinoma of the thyroid

The thyroid gland can be the site of metastatic spread from tumours such as breast and kidney. Careful clinical assessment may suggest the correct diagnosis but confirmation is usually obtained by FNAC. In some instances resection of the thyroid gland is indicated if the primary disease is otherwise well controlled.

Hyperthyroidism

Hyperthyroidism has a prevalence in the UK of approximately 27 per 1000 women and 2.3 per 1000 men.[65] Although Graves' disease is the most common cause of hyperthyroidism, there is an extensive list of other causes which require consideration (**Box 2.2**).

Box 2.2 • Causes of thyrotoxicosis

Common

- Diffuse toxic goitre (Graves' disease)
- Toxic multinodular goitre (Plummer's disease)
- Toxic solitary nodule
- Toxic multinodular goitre with internodular hyperplasia
- Nodular goitre with hyperthyroidism due to exogenous iodine
- Exogenous thyroid hormone excess (factitious)
- Thyroiditis (subacute and autoimmune) – transient

Rare

- Diffuse thyroid autonomy
- Metastatic thyroid carcinoma
- Struma ovarii
- Pituitary tumour secreting thyroid-stimulating hormone
- Choriocarcinoma and hydatidiform mole
- Neonatal thyrotoxicosis
- Postpartum hyperthyroidism
- After ^{131}I therapy

Box 2.3 • Clinical features of thyrotoxicosis (see also Fig. 2.19)

- Palpitations, tachycardia, cardiac arrhythmias, cardiac failure
- Sweating
- Tremor
- Hyperkinetic movements
- Nervousness
- Myopathy
- Tiredness and lethargy
- Weight loss (occasional weight gain due to increased appetite)
- Heat intolerance
- Diarrhoea
- Vomiting
- Irritability
- Emotional disturbance
- Behavioural abnormalities
- Ophthalmic signs
- Irregular menstruation and amenorrhoea
- Pretibial myxoedema
- Thyroid acropathy
- Vitiligo
- Alopecia

Graves' disease (diffuse toxic goitre) is an immunological disorder in which thyroid-stimulating antibodies (TsAbs) of the IgG type bind to the TSH receptor and stimulate the thyroid cell to produce and secrete an excess of thyroid hormones. Human leucocyte antigen (HLA) studies demonstrate that patients positive for HLA B8 and HLA DR3 have an increased susceptibility to the disease. The thyroid gland hypertrophies, producing diffuse enlargement, although nodular varieties of the condition are recognised. An important subgroup is that of internodular hyperplasia in a background of multinodular goitre. Histologically there is acinar hyperplasia, high columnar epithelium, increased vascularity and often lymphoid infiltration.

Clinical features

Most of the symptoms and signs of thyrotoxicosis (**Box 2.3**) result from excess thyroid hormones stimulating metabolism, heat production and oxygen consumption. Cardiac features are caused by beta-adrenergic sympathetic activity. Although Graves' disease can occur at any age, it is especially common in young women between 20 and 40 years of age (**Fig. 2.19**). The onset may be gradual or abrupt, with an extremely variable subsequent course often characterised by exacerbations and remissions. Clinical features due to hypermetabolism tend to predominate, although in elderly people the cardiovascular and neurological features usually dominate. Hyperthyroidism may be severe and even fatal. In children the condition often causes growth abnormalities.

The immunological changes in Graves' disease are complex and undoubtedly cause many of the ophthalmic symptoms and signs.

Ophthalmopathy has two major components:

1. **Non-infiltrative ophthalmopathy,** resulting from increased sympathetic activity leading to upper lid retraction, a stare and infrequent blinking.
2. **Infiltrative ophthalmopathy,** causing oedema of the orbital contents, lids and periorbital

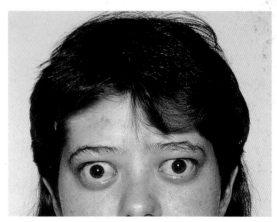

Figure 2.19 • A patient with Graves' disease.

tissues, cellular infiltration and deposition of mucopolysaccharide material within the orbit.

Although the ophthalmopathy is usually bilateral, it may affect only one eye. Diplopia, particularly on upward outward gaze, results from weakening and paralysis of the external ocular muscles. The cornea is vulnerable to damage, and in extreme cases ulceration may occur. Papilloedema, retinal haemorrhage and optic nerve damage (malignant exophthalmos) can progress to blindness (**Fig. 2.20**).

Investigation

Measurement of free T_4, T_3 and TSH concentrations will confirm the diagnosis (in T_3 toxicosis, T_4 concentrations will be normal whereas concentrations of T_3 will be increased and TSH suppressed). A radioactive iodine or technetium scan is not essential in the diagnosis of Graves' disease, although is necessary in the assessment of toxic solitary and multinodular goitre to determine the site of nodular overactivity. Radioactive iodine uptake studies are particularly appropriate when a diagnosis of thyroiditis or factitious hyperthyroidism is being considered.

In Graves' disease there are three treatment options that can be used either alone or in combination to restore the euthyroid state:

- antithyroid drugs;
- radioactive iodine;
- surgery.

Each of these treatments has an important role, but for each patient all factors, medical, personal and social, are carefully considered to produce a treatment plan individualised for each patient.

Medical treatment

Antithyroid drugs (propylthiouracil, carbimazole and methimazole)

These drugs interfere with the incorporation of iodine into tyrosine residues and prevent the coupling of iodotyrosines into iodothyronines. Carbimazole may also have some immunosuppressive action on TsAb production. Medical treatment with thionamides has two principal roles:

1. Treatment of patients with a new diagnosis of Graves' disease in the hope of inducing a permanent remission.
2. To render the toxic patient euthyroid in preparation for surgery.

Although most patients can be rendered euthyroid with antithyroid drugs there is a less than optimum remission rate after an 'adequate' course of medication. A relapse rate of approximately 43% is seen in the first year after stopping drugs, and approximately 20% of the remaining patients relapse in each of the subsequent 5 years.[66] Antithyroid drugs are therefore not a satisfactory long-term solution to the problems of hyperthyroidism for most patients. Carbimazole is prescribed in a dose of 10–15 mg 8-hourly, reducing to 5 mg 8-hourly once the euthyroid state has been achieved. Iatrogenic hypothyroidism may be prevented by the administration of a small dose of T_4 in a so-called blocking/replacement regimen. Patients must be followed up carefully, with regular clinical assessment and measurement of thyroid function tests. All patients should be warned concerning side-effects, particularly those relating to effects on the bone marrow resulting in leucopenia, agranulocytosis and aplastic anaemia. Instructions are given to discontinue carbimazole and seek medical advice immediately should buccal ulceration or a sore throat develop. Other side-effects include rashes, pruritus, arthritis and nausea.

Propylthiouracil is more widely used in the USA than elsewhere and can be used effectively if *mild* side-effects have occurred with carbimazole. The other major indication for administration of antithyroid drugs is to render the patient euthyroid once a decision has been made to proceed with surgery.

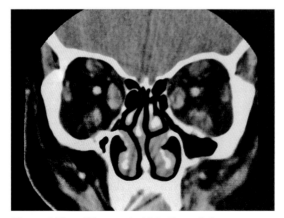

Figure 2.20 • CT scan of orbit in Graves' disease ophthalmopathy demonstrating marked infiltration of the extraocular muscles.

Beta-adrenergic blockers

Many of the manifestations of hyperthyroidism, particularly those relating to the cardiovascular system, can be ameliorated by the administration of beta-blockers such as propranolol. This agent also reduces peripheral conversion of T_4 to T_3. Beta-blockers are usually used in combination with one of the thionamides, particularly in patients who are severely toxic and in those being prepared for surgery. The usual dose of propranolol is 20–40 mg 8-hourly. New long-acting beta-blockers can be administered once daily. Beta-blockers are absolutely contraindicated in patients with asthma. When used as preoperative preparation, propranolol must not be omitted on the morning of surgery and must be continued for at least 5 days postoperatively because of the 8-day half-life of circulating T_4.

Radioactive iodine

^{131}I can be used to control thyrotoxicosis by destruction of overactive thyroid tissue. There would seem to be no adverse effects of ^{131}I treatment with respect to leukaemia, thyroid carcinoma, fetal damage or genetic mutation, and in the USA the therapy is even given to children. ^{131}I (555 MBq) is administered as an ablative dose and the patient covered with carbimazole 10 mg t.d.s. started 3 days after the administration and continued for approximately 1 month to counter the effects of thyroid hormone release, which might precipitate a thyroid crisis.

Although some patients require additional doses of ^{131}I as a result of an inadequate initial response, most patients will be cured of toxicity. An ablative dose (555 MBq) renders more than 60% of patients hypothyroid in 1 year.[67] Regular long-term surveillance is required and T4 replacement given as necessary. Thyroid eye disease may worsen after radioactive iodine treatment. Steroids should be given to reduce this risk.

Surgery

Thyroidectomy in patients with Graves' disease is safe and rapidly renders the patient euthyroid. The principal indications for surgery are:

1. Relapse after an adequate course of antithyroid drugs.
2. Severe thyrotoxicosis with a large goitre.

3. Difficulty in controlling toxicity with antithyroid drugs (including poor compliance).
4. High T_4 concentrations (>70 pmol/L).

Surgery would be offered to most patients under 40 years of age fulfilling the above criteria.

Operative strategy

Details of thyroidectomy are covered in the section dealing specifically with surgical technique, Essentially two surgical options are available, bilateral subtotal thyroidectomy (leaving a 3–4 g posterior remnant of thyroid tissue on each side of the trachea) or total thyroidectomy. Increasingly many endocrine surgeons seem to favour total thyroidectomy as a treatment for Graves' disease. This approach removes the possibility of recurrent disease and appears to improve the outlook for patients with significant eye disease.

Special circumstances in Graves' disease

Reaction to antithyroid drugs

Toxic patients who have demonstrated reaction to antithyroid drugs may be prepared for surgery by the use of beta-blockers. However, in patients who have asthma or where antithyroid drugs have not rendered the patient completely euthyroid, Lugol's iodine or potassium iodide tablets (60 mg t.d.s.) is an extremely useful alternative.

Children

Treatment should be started with antithyroid drugs and continued for no more than 12–18 months. When treatment is discontinued, relapse may follow in up to 50% of patients. These children are usually candidates for surgery, and the resection must be more radical than in adults because remnant growth and recurrent hyperthyroidism are more likely.

Pregnancy

Hyperthyroidism occurring in pregnancy poses a difficult management problem.[68] Radioactive iodine is absolutely contraindicated. Antithyroid drugs are used, propylthiouracil being the drug of choice as it crosses the placenta less readily than carbimazole. Furthermore, there is a risk of congenital malformations after carbimazole (e.g. imperforated anus).

Once control of thyrotoxicosis has been achieved, the dose of antithyroid drugs should be reduced as far as possible and the thyroid status of the mother carefully measured. A blocking/replacement regimen must not be used, as T_4 does not cross the placenta in sufficient amounts to avoid fetal hypothyroidism. In a patient still requiring high doses of antithyroid drugs or in whom hyperthyroidism is difficult to control, surgery may be safely performed in the second trimester.

Recurrent hyperthyroidism after surgery

Further surgery is not indicated as it is likely to be unsuccessful and carries a significant risk of damage to recurrent laryngeal nerves and parathyroid glands. Over the age of 40, ^{131}I is the treatment of choice, whereas under 40 years of age, antithyroid drugs are prescribed in the hope of achieving lasting remission.

Neonatal hyperthyroidism

TsAbs crossing the placenta may stimulate the fetal thyroid, to produce transient hyperthyroidism.[69] Active supportive treatment with antithyroid drugs is necessary and the whole process is usually self-limiting within a period of 1–2 months.

Ophthalmic Graves' disease

The effect of surgery on this condition is somewhat unpredictable, although in the past total thyroidectomy has been advocated in an attempt to arrest the progress of the eye disease. Patients must be warned that effective treatment of the thyrotoxicosis is not a guarantee that ophthalmopathy will regress. Mild symptoms can be treated by the administration of methylcellulose eye drops, but more severe disease may require steroids, lateral tarsorrhaphy or even orbital decompression.

Toxic multinodular goitre

Antithyroid drugs are of no value as a long-term treatment in the younger patient because toxicity is due to autonomy and will recur once any medication is discontinued. However, in the older patient who is unsuitable for surgery, long-term treatment with carbimazole may be appropriate. [131]I can be used for small goitres, but usually a total thyroidectomy is most appropriate after achievement of the euthyroid state with antithyroid drugs.

Toxic solitary nodule

This condition is caused by a single autonomous thyroid nodule. Patients with a nodule greater than 3–4 cm are more commonly treated by thyroid lobectomy; tumours below this size can successfully be managed by [131]I (the normal thyroid gland being protected from iodine uptake as it is suppressed).

Follow-up

Because of the risk of developing postoperative hypothyroidism, patients who have undergone any form of treatment for hyperthyroidism must be followed up on a long-term basis, with regular clinical and biochemical assessment.

Thyroiditis

The thyroid gland may be subject to inflammatory change in a variety of conditions, which may be focal or diffuse and often associated with thyroid dysfunction.

Subacute thyroiditis

This condition, often called granulomatous thyroiditis or de Quervain's thyroiditis, is probably of viral origin. It is characterised by painful swelling of one or both thyroid lobes, with associated malaise and fever. Often there is a preceding history of sore throat or viral infection a week or two before the onset of thyroid symptoms. Approximately one-third of patients are asymptomatic apart from enlargement of the thyroid gland, but 10–15% have a more acute illness with symptoms and signs of hyperthyroidism resulting from the outpouring of thyroid hormones into the circulation from the damaged inflamed thyroid. Thyroid hormone concentrations are increased but in contrast to Graves' disease there is low uptake of radioactive iodine on scintigraphy. The erythrocyte sedimentation rate is invariably raised. The disease process is usually self-limiting, with resolution of local symptoms and thyroid dysfunction. A few patients, however, pass through a mild hypothyroid phase. Local symptoms can be controlled with aspirin but, if severe and prolonged, a course of steroids can be helpful. The transient hyperthyroidism does not require treatment with antithyroid drugs.

Autoimmune thyroiditis (Hashimoto's thyroiditis)

Focal thyroiditis is often seen in association with other thyroid disease, particularly Graves' hyperthyroidism, and is a common finding in autopsy studies. A condition of lymphomatous thyroiditis was described by Hashimoto and occurs as a diffuse process throughout the gland, which usually enlarges to several times normal size. Although classically the gland enlargement is diffuse, there may be nodularity and lobulation, making the distinction from simple multinodular goitre or even malignant disease difficult.

Histologically there is infiltration of the thyroid by lymphocytes and plasma cells, frequently secondary lymphoid nodules and adjacent stromal fibrosis. The condition is due to an immunological disorder characterised by thyroid antibodies (antithyroglobulin and antimicrosomal (TPO)) in the serum. A positive family history of other autoimmune disease such as pernicious anaemia, gastritis, vitiligo, diabetes mellitus, Addison's disease, autoimmune liver disease and thyrotoxicosis is often obtained.[70] As a result of destructive changes within the infiltrated thyroid, hypothyroidism usually ensues and when present requires treatment with T_4. This medication suppresses TSH and leads to shrinkage of the thyroid gland with relief of any local symptoms. Pressure symptoms and involvement of adjacent structures are rare and surgery is usually not required. The risk of developing lymphoma of the thyroid, although small, is increased several times in the presence of Hashimoto's thyroiditis.[55] When a gland that is involved with autoimmune disease is seen to enlarge rapidly or develop a firm asymmetrical nodular area, exclusion of lymphoma by FNAC or core biopsy is required.

Riedel's thyroiditis

This condition, sometimes called invasive fibrous thyroiditis, is characterised by a dense fibrous inflammatory infiltrate throughout the gland, sometimes extending through the capsule to involve adjacent structures. The condition is rare but is important because the clinical picture mimics thyroid malignancy. Sclerosing cholangitis and retroperitoneal, mediastinal and retro-orbital fibrosis may coexist.

Needle biopsy is likely to be uninformative, and often an open incision biopsy is required to establish a precise diagnosis. Surgical resection of the isthmus will be required to free a compromised airway.

Acute suppurative thyroiditis

The thyroid gland can be affected by a variety of bacterial or fungal agents, producing clinical features of an acute painfully inflamed organ. Confirmation of diagnosis and bacteriology is obtained by needle aspiration and appropriate antibiotics administered. The condition is rare in Western practice.

Postpartum thyroiditis

Postpartum thyroiditis is now recognised more often and is characterised by an early thyrotoxic phase, usually with mild symptoms and transient dysfunction.[71,72] There is a later hypothyroid phase, sometimes requiring treatment with T_4, long-term hypothyroidism occurring in up to 25% of patients.

Hypothyroidism

Hypothyroidism is a clinical state resulting from insufficient thyroid hormone or more rarely a resistance of the tissues to T_4. Causes can be classified as congenital (cretinism) or acquired (adult type). Retardation of growth and mental development are the serious features of hypothyroidism in the infant. The child fails to thrive, is constipated and displays the classic physical signs of a puffy face, large tongue and protuberant abdomen. In adults the extreme presentation is that of myxoedema, characterised by weight gain, facial puffiness and pallor, dry skin, hair loss, hoarseness of the voice, declining intellect and, in extreme cases, psychiatric disturbance and even coma. The causes of hypothyroidism are listed in **Box 2.4**.

Hypothyroidism is confirmed by measurement of TSH, which is raised. Free T_4 and T_3 concentrations will be low in primary hypothyroidism. Treatment is with thyroxine. Caution must be exercised in myxoedematous and elderly patients (who may already be suffering from heart disease). Initially a low dose of thyroxine is administered (0.025 mg), increasing gradually to full replacement level.

Box 2.4 • Causes of hypothyroidism

Primary hypothyroidism

- Thyroid agenesis

Disorders of thyroid hormone synthesis

- Iodine deficiency
- Dyshormonogenesis
- Antithyroid drugs

Thyroid gland damage

- Hashimoto's thyroiditis
- Surgical resection of the thyroid
- Radioactive iodine ablation
- Post-subacute thyroiditis

Secondary hypothyroidism (pituitary)

- Pituitary tumour
- Autoimmune hypophysitis

Tertiary hypothyroidism (hypothalamic)

- Hypothalamic tumour
- Generalised or peripheral thyroid hormone resistance

Thyroidectomy

The term 'thyroidectomy' embraces a variety of surgical procedures but the precise procedure should be tailored to the existing pathology (**Table 2.3**).

Unilateral total thyroid lobectomy

Informed consent should be obtained from all patients. Preoperative examination of the vocal cords (by indirect laryngoscopy) needs to be considered. This procedure will exclude an unsuspected, pre-existing unilateral nerve palsy; this is particularly important if the patient has undergone previous thyroid surgery.

General anaesthesia, with endotracheal intubation and muscle relaxation, is used. Bilateral superficial cervical blocks are beneficial for intra- and post-operative pain control.

The patient is placed supine on an operating table tilted 15° upwards at the head end to reduce venous engorgement. A small degree of neck extension aids access to the thyroid but care must be taken not to extend the neck too much (this may result in cervical trauma, particularly in the elderly patient).

A skin incision should be marked out to lie in a suitable skin crease above the sternal notch. The length of the incision will depend on the degree of thyroid enlargement and whether further procedures (such as modified neck dissection) are contemplated.

The incision is deepened through the platysma, and upper and lower skin flaps are raised by a combination of sharp and blunt dissection in the plane anterior to the anterior jugular vessels. The upper flap is freed to the level of the thyroid notch and the lower flap to the suprasternal notch. These skin flaps are held apart with a suitable self-retaining retractor and a midline incision made through the fascia over the thyroid. It is the length of this vertical incision that determines access to the thyroid. The strap muscles will be separated, dissected from the thyroid and retracted laterally. These muscles need not be routinely divided, but if greater exposure is required to gain safe access to a large or vascular goitre, then they may be.

The thyroid lobe is dislocated and delivered forward by the insertion of the index finger between the thyroid lobe and strap muscles. The middle thyroid veins, if apparent at this stage, should be ligated and divided. Any adhesions lateral to the thyroid lobe are divided by a combination of sharp and blunt dissection and

Table 2.3 • Thyroid surgery

Procedures	Indications
Unilateral total lobectomy, including pyramidal lobe and isthmus	Solitary nodules
	Unilateral multinodular disease
Bilateral subtotal thyroidectomy (unilateral lobectomy and contralateral resection)	Diffuse toxic goitre of Graves' disease
	Bilateral non-toxic and toxic multinodular goitre
	Hashimoto's disease
Total thyroidectomy	Most cases of papillary, follicular and medullary carcinoma
Excision of isthmus	May be only procedure possible in anaplastic carcinoma or lymphoma to free airway
	Riedel's thyroiditis

the thyroid lobe retracted further medially, usually with a gauze swab between the operator's thumb and the gland. Tissue forceps must not be placed on the thyroid when performing surgery for a solitary nodule, in case the lesion should prove to be malignant and cell spillage occur.

Full mobilisation of the thyroid lobe is achieved by ligation and division of the superior thyroid vessels at the upper pole. To gain access to these vessels it is often helpful to pass a finger upwards in the plane behind the vessels, breaking down adhesions and then with gentle downward traction on the thyroid the vessels come clearly into view. The space medial to the superior thyroid artery is carefully opened with a pledget or artery forceps to expose the external branch of the superior laryngeal nerve (ESLN). This may be identified on the inferior pharyngeal constrictor before entering the cricothyroid muscle. A non-toothed forceps is then passed under the vascular pedicle to lift the vessels forward. The branches of the superior thyroid artery and vein must be individually tied close to the thyroid gland to avoid damage to the ESLN. In approximately 20% of patients, this nerve may pass between the branches of the vessels and is in great danger if mass ligation is carried out (**Fig. 2.21**). In a further 20% of patients the nerve runs its distal course through the inferior pharyngeal constrictor muscle, is not visible at surgery and is at no risk of damage.

The RLN should now be identified before continuing with dissection of the thyroid lobe. The nerve may run close to the tracheo-oesophageal groove but there is enormous variability of its position, course and relationship to key anatomical structures in the neck. If damage is to be avoided, an accurate knowledge of the normal anatomy and these variations is of paramount importance. Palpation of the RLN as a cord-like structure against the trachea is often a useful initial guide to the nerve's location. The nerve can then be exposed by gentle dissection of the overlying fascial layers with a small artery clip. The nerve often has a small blood vessel running on its surface. Vulnerability is somewhat greater on the right than on the left because of the obliquity of the nerve's course in the lower third of the wound. The nerve usually lies deep to the inferior thyroid artery but can be rendered vulnerable by anterior fixation in a fork formed by the glandular branches of this artery (**Fig. 2.22**). Precise definition of the nerve/artery relationship is most important. A potential pitfall for the unwary exists when the RLN passes superficial to the inferior thyroid artery, appears to pulsate and may therefore be mistaken for a vessel and ligated.

The RLN can be displaced from its usual position by nodules, particularly in the posterior part of the thyroid lobe, and occasionally is displaced

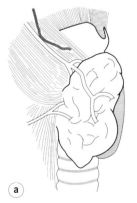 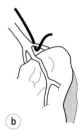

a b

Figure 2.21 • (a) The external superior laryngeal nerve (ESLN) passing medial to the superior thyroid artery before entering the cricothyroid muscle. **(b)** The ESLN is in a vulnerable position when passing between branches of the superior thyroid artery.

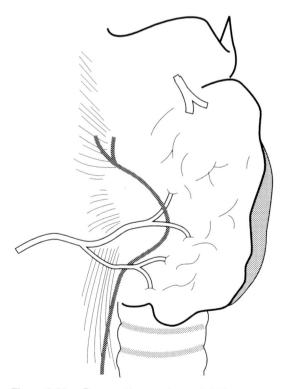

Figure 2.22 • Recurrent laryngeal nerve held in a vulnerable anterior position by fork of inferior thyroid artery branches.

anteriorly, close to the lower pole of the thyroid into a dangerous position where it may be ligated and divided with the inferior thyroid veins. Clearly these veins must not be clipped until the nerve has been identified in its lower third. During unilateral lobectomy, the small arterial branches to the thyroid must all be individually clipped and tied close to the gland, staying on the thyroid capsule. The trunk of the inferior thyroid artery is not ligated.

The nerve is perhaps in most danger close to its point of entry into the larynx as it passes through Berry's ligament, often adopting a curving, looping course before entering the larynx. To identify the nerve in this region the suspensory fascia must be carefully divided. This manoeuvre is most safely accomplished by staying close to the thyroid and picking up superficial layers one at a time with fine haemostats, being absolutely certain that at each stage only fascia and small arterial branches are included. The nerve is soon seen at a deeper level, glistening, with its fine accompanying arterial blood vessel aiding identification. The inferior cornu of the thyroid cartilage is a most dependable landmark for the point of entry of the RLN into the larynx.

In approximately 1% of patients the nerve on the right is non-recurrent, arising from the vagus and passing medially close to the inferior thyroid artery before turning to ascend and enter the larynx (**Fig. 2.23**). Ligation of the main trunk of the inferior thyroid artery in these circumstances could result in permanent damage to the nerve. It is well recognised that the RLN can divide into several branches before entering the larynx and therefore clear identification of all divisions is necessary for their preservation.

The parathyroid glands should also be identified. When they are in their usual positions, the inferior gland can be located close to the lower pole of the thyroid anterior to the RLN. The superior gland is usually seen just above the inferior thyroid artery; in more than 90% of patients it is within a 1-cm radius of the junction of the inferior thyroid artery and the RLN. The dissection of the thyroid should continue close to the capsule of the gland, with ligation and division of the individual branches of the inferior thyroid artery, preserving those branches that supply the parathyroid glands. It is possible to tease the parathyroid glands away from the thyroid with their blood supply intact, leaving them free but perfectly viable. It must be

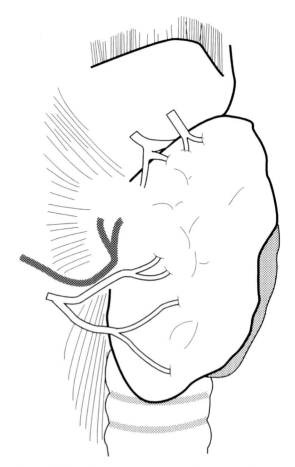

Figure 2.23 • Non-recurrent laryngeal nerve passing in close proximity to the inferior thyroid artery before ascending to the larynx.

remembered that enlargement of the thyroid can carry the parathyroid glands far forward onto the anterolateral surface of the thyroid when they may be devascularised or inadvertently excised. In these circumstances they should be diced into 1-mm cubes and autotransplanted into several pockets in the sternomastoid muscle.

It is important to keep diathermy usage to a minimum as heat conduction may damage the RLN, the blood supply to the parathyroids or the delicate joints within the larynx.

The thyroid lobe is now almost completely free and is dissected further medially by dividing the vascular fascia binding it to the trachea and larynx. The division of Berry's ligament is completed, taking care to re-identify the RLN. Small vessels close to the nerve at this point require careful clipping and ligation otherwise troublesome bleeding may obscure the nerve's entry point to the larynx. Indeed, safe thyroidectomy is utterly dependent on careful haemostasis as it is only by this discipline that the RLN and parathyroid glands can be identified and left undamaged.

Mobilisation of the thyroid lobe is now complete, and the resection must include the isthmus and pyramidal lobe. The cut surface of the contralateral thyroid lobe is usually sutured to the trachea with Vicryl® to obtain haemostasis. The wound is closed in layers with absorbable material to the muscle layers, and the skin is closed with a subcuticular prolene suture or skin clips, which can be removed at 3 days.

Total thyroidectomy

Total thyroidectomy is usually performed for cancer but occasionally for gross multinodular disease. The opposite lobe is mobilised in a similar manner to that described for unilateral lobectomy. If the procedure is for cancer an appropriate lymph node clearance will also be necessary.

Subtotal thyroidectomy

When subtotal thyroidectomy is performed, perhaps for Graves' disease, the principles of identification of the vital structures are the same as those employed in a unilateral total lobectomy. In Graves' disease a small remnant, usually 3–4 g, of tissue is left in situ on each side of the trachea and haemostasis secured by suturing the lateral edge of each remnant, without tension, to the anterior surface of the trachea with Vicryl®. As in unilateral lobectomy, the main trunk of the inferior thyroid artery is not ligated, but individual small bleeding vessels on the surface of the remnant may require ligation. Unilateral total lobectomy and a contralateral resection leaving a larger single remnant may be an acceptable alternative strategy.

Recently minimally access and endoscopic techniques have been adapted to permit thyroidectomy, usually by performing a unilateral lobectomy for benign disease. The precise role and relevance of this technique in the management of thyroid disease remains to be defined. The use of high-frequency vibrating shears to cut and secure blood vessels in place of ties or clips has facilitated minimally invasive techniques and made the open operation easier and quicker.

Retrosternal goitre

Retrosternal goitres derive their blood supply from the superior and inferior thyroid arteries, and these are usually accessible in the neck. Ligation and division of the superior pole vessels is an essential, preliminary step before mobilisation of the gland is attempted. The retrosternal portion can then be delivered from behind the sternum by gentle traction aided by the introduction of a finger alongside the gland. Placement of traction sutures in the thyroid or the gentle introduction of a dessert spoon alongside the gland may also facilitate delivery. Median sternotomy is rarely necessary to remove a retrosternal thyroid.

Recurrent goitre

Surgery for recurrent thyroid disease is particularly hazardous with respect to damage to the RLN and parathyroid gland, as identification of these structures is likely to be impeded by the presence of scar tissue. A lateral approach to the thyroid lobe can be gained by dissecting in the plane between the strap muscles and the anterior border of the sternomastoid (where there may be fewer adhesions).

Complications of thyroidectomy

The most important complications of thyroidectomy are shown in **Box 2.5**. Complications relating to damaged individual structures can be kept to a minimum by operating in a bloodless field and performing a meticulous anatomical dissection.

RLN

Damage to the RLN should be extremely rare after routine thyroidectomy, although the risk of damage is increased when performing re-operative thyroid

Box 2.5 • Complications of thyroid surgery

- Recurrent laryngeal nerve injury
- External superior laryngeal nerve injury
- Hypoparathyroidism
- Laryngeal oedema – airway obstruction
- Bleeding – haematoma
- Hypothyroidism
- Hyperthyroidism
- Wound infection
- Keloid
- Suture granuloma

surgery.[73,74] Identification of the RLN at surgery is the fundamental step to avoiding damage. When this policy is employed, any nerve damage is likely to be a transient neuropraxia and recovery will be expected, usually after a period of a few weeks or months. If the nerve has not been identified, then paralysis will be permanent in up to one-third of patients whose nerves have been injured. Extremely low nerve injury rates have been reported, even when performing extensive surgery for thyroid cancer.[75]

ESLN

Assessment of damage to the ESLN is difficult, as the changes may be subtle and easily overlooked. Disability results in changes of voice pitch, range and projection. Damage to the ESLN is particularly devastating in singers. The nerve is most likely to be damaged at the time of ligation and division of the superior thyroid vessels.[76] To avoid this complication the arterial branches should be individually ligated close to the thyroid and the nerve identified whenever possible.

Hypoparathyroidism

Careful identification of the parathyroid glands and preservation of their delicate arterial blood supply can avoid this complication. In bilateral subtotal resection for Graves' disease, the incidence of hypoparathyroidism should be no more than 0.5%. The complication is more common after total thyroidectomy for cancer, but even in these circumstances the incidence has been reported within the range of only 1–3%.[72]

Hypothyroidism

This sequel of thyroidectomy is most likely to occur after surgery for Graves' disease, with an incidence as high as 50%. This is not a true complication but an acceptable feature of the treatment of hyperthyroidism and is easily managed by the administration of T_4.

Recurrent hyperthyroidism

If this occurs after surgery for Graves' disease, it represents a failure of the operation. The incidence is approximately 5% and varies depending on the size of the thyroid remnants left in situ, the complex immunological processes taking place in primary hyperthyroidism and iodine intake.

Thyroid crisis

This potentially life-threatening condition is rarely seen but classically occurs in the postoperative period. It is usually encountered in patients who have undergone surgery for thyrotoxicosis without adequate preoperative preparation or where a diagnosis of thyrotoxicosis has not been established prior to emergency or elective surgery. Hormones released by gland manipulation result in an acute postoperative thyrotoxicosis. The condition may also result from stress or infection. The clinical picture includes extreme distress, dyspnoea, tachycardia, hyperpyrexia, vomiting, diarrhoea, confusion and/or delirium.

Propylthiouracil (200–250 mg) is given every 4 hours, by nasogastric tube if necessary, and Lugol's or potassium iodide should be given. Adrenergic effects are treated by careful administration of propranolol under ECG-monitored control. General supportive measures consist of rehydration with intravenous fluids, cooling with ice packs, the administration of oxygen, digoxin (if there is evidence of cardiac failure), appropriate sedation and corticosteroids.

Haemorrhage

Bleeding into the wound is a serious complication of thyroidectomy. When the bleeding and haematoma occur deep to the strap muscles, the situation can rapidly develop into a life-threatening emergency because of associated airway obstruction resulting from laryngeal and subglottic oedema.

Airway obstruction

Although mortality from thyroidectomy is extremely rare, airway obstruction remains the most potentially dangerous complication. It was once thought that airway obstruction caused by postoperative bleeding was due to compression of the trachea by the expanding haematoma. This is unlikely to be the case except in the rare condition of tracheomalacia. It is subglottic and laryngeal mucosal oedema consequent upon venous and lymphatic obstruction that occludes the airway. It must be appreciated that airway obstruction can occur by this mechanism as a result of operative manipulation of the trachea without any postoperative bleeding or haematoma deep to the strap muscles. It is crucial that early signs of airway obstruction (patient distress and stridor) should be recognised and the immediate action of suture removal taken.

If symptoms are mild and there is no haematoma, conservative measures of humidified oxygen or heliox (a combination of helium and oxygen) and intravenous steroids may suffice. A senior anaesthetist must be consulted immediately. Intubation may prove necessary to restore an occluding airway. If a skilled anaesthetist is not immediately available, the situation can be retrieved by insertion of two or three white needles directly into the trachea. Any obvious haematoma should be evacuated, and this should ideally be performed under general anaes-thesia with endotracheal intubation in the operating room. Rarely is it necessary to remove sutures on the ward.

Wound complications

The use of absorbable suture material has virtually abolished the complication of suture granuloma after thyroidectomy. Keloid scars may still occur in susceptible individuals.

Key points

- Family history is important in thyroid disease.
- Clinical examination and FNAC are essential in evaluating the thyroid nodule.
- Thyroid nodules in children are more likely to be cancers.
- Smaller intrathyroidal papillary, micropapillary and minimally invasive follicular cancers may be adequately treated by total thyroid lobectomy and TSH suppression.
- Larger intrathyroidal, extrathyroidal and widely invasive follicular cancers should be treated by total thyroidectomy and radioiodine ablation.
- Prophylactic lymph node dissection is not necessary in differentiated thyroid cancer.
- Overall prognosis in differentiated thyroid cancer is very good.
- Medullary thyroid cancer requires a more aggressive surgical approach than differentiated thyroid cancer. Genetic testing should be considered.
- Treatment options in thyrotoxicosis should be tailored to individual patient needs.
- Patients should be fully counselled with regards to the complications of thyroid surgery prior to operation.

References

1. Beever K, Bradbury J, Phillips D et al. Highly sensitive assays of autoantibodies to thyroglobulin and to thyroid peroxidase. Clin Chem 1989; 35:1949–54.

2. Van Herle AJ, Uller RP. Elevated serum thyroglobulin: a marker of metastases in differentiated thyroid carcinoma. J Clin Invest 1975; 56:270–7.

3. Doullay F, Ruf J, Codaccioni JL et al. Prevalence of autoantibodies to thyroperoxidase in patients with various thyroid and autoimmune diseases. Autoimmunity 1991; 9:237–44.

4. Rees-Smith B, McLachlan SM, Furmaniak J. Autoantibodies to the thyrotropin receptor. Endocr Rev 1988; 9:106–21.

5. Melvin KEW, Tashjian AH. The syndrome of excessive thyrocalcitonin produced by medullary carcinoma of the thyroid. Proc Natl Acad Sci USA 1968; 59:1216–22.

6. Mulligan LM, Kwok JBJ, Healey CS et al. Germ-line mutations of the RET proto oncogene in multiple endocrine neoplasia type IIA. Nature 1993; 363:458–60.

7. Turner JW, Spencer RB. Thyroid carcinoma presenting as a pertechnetate hot nodule without 131I uptake. Case report. J Nucl Med 1976; 17:22–3.

8. Ochi H, Yamamoto K, Endo K et al. A new imaging agent for medullary carcinoma of the thyroid. J Nucl Med 1984; 25:323–5.

9. Hoefnagal CA, Delprat CC, Marcuse HR et al. Role of thallium-201 total-body scintigraphy in follow up of thyroid carcinoma. J Nucl Med 1986; 27:1854–7.

10. Clarke SEM, Lazarus CR, Wraight P et al. Pentavalent (^{99m}Tc) DMSA, ^{131}I MIBG, and (^{99m}Tc) MDP. An evaluation of three imaging techniques in patients with medullary carcinoma of the thyroid. J Nucl Med 1988; 29:33–8.

11. Rosen IB, Walfish PG, Miskin M. The ultrasound of thyroid masses. Surg Clin North Am 1979; 59:19–33.

12. Rosen IB, Wallace D, Strawbridge HG et al. Re-evaluation of needle aspiration cytology in detection of thyroid cancer. Surgery 1981; 90:747–56.

13. Soderstrom N. Aspiration biopsy punctures of goitres for aspiration and biopsy. Acta Med Scand 1952; 144:237–44.

14. Lowhagen T, Granberg PO, Lundell G et al. Aspiration biopsy cytology (ABC) in nodules of the thyroid gland suspected to be malignant. Surg Clin North Am 1979; 59:3–18.

15. Grant CS, Hay ID, Gough IR et al. Long term follow up of patients with benign thyroid FNA cytologic diagnosis. Surgery 1989; 106:980–91.

16. Stephenson BM, Wheeler MH. Carcinoma of the thyroglossal duct. Aust NZ J Surg 1994; 64:212.

17. Gaitin E, Nelson NC, Poole GV. Endemic goitre and endemic thyroid disorders. World J Surg 1991; 15:205–15.

18. Gaitin E. Aetiology of benign thyroid disease-environmental aspects. In: Wheeler MH, Lazarus JH (eds) Diseases of the thyroid. Pathophysiology and management. London: Chapman & Hall Medical, 1994; pp. 73–84.

19. Vander JB, Gaston EA, Dawber TR. The significance of non toxic thyroid nodules: final report of a 15 year study of the incidence of thyroid malignancy. Ann Intern Med 1968; 69:537–40.

20. Hellwig CA. Thyroid gland in Kansas. Am J Clin Pathol 1935; 5:103–11.

21. Hayles AB, Johnson LM, Beahrs OH et al. Carcinoma of the thyroid in children. Am J Surg 1963; 106:735–43.

22. Harness JK, Thompson NW, Nishiyama RH. Childhood thyroid carcinoma. Arch Surg 1971; 102:278–84.

23. Cuello C, Correa P, Eisenberg H. Geographic pathology of thyroid carcinoma. Cancer 1969; 23:230–9.

24. Williams ED, Doniach I, Bjarnason O et al. Thyroid cancer in an iodine rich area: a histopathological study. Cancer 1977; 39:215–22.

25. Duffy BJ, Fitzgerald PJ. Cancer of the thyroid in children: a report of 28 cases. J Clin Endocrinol Metab 1950; 10:1296–308.

26. DeGroot LJ, Paloyan E. Thyroid carcinoma and radiation: a Chicago endemic. JAMA 1973; 225:487–91.

27. Naunheim KS, Kaplan EL, Straus FH et al. High dose external radiation to the neck and subsequent thyroid carcinoma. In: Kaplan EL (ed.) Surgery of the thyroid and parathyroid glands. Edinburgh: Churchill Livingstone, 1983; pp. 51–62.

28. Henry JF, Denizot A, Porcelli A et al. Thyroperoxidase immunodetection for the diagnosis of malignancy on fine-needle aspiration of thyroid nodules. World J Surg 1994; 18:529–34.

29. Delbridge L, Lean CL, Russell P et al. Proton magnetic resonance and human thyroid neoplasia II: potential avoidance of surgery for benign follicular neoplasms. World J Surg 1994; 18:512–17.

30. Monzani F, Caraccio N, Iacconi P et al. Prevalence of cancer in follicular thyroid nodules: is there still a role for intraoperative frozen section analysis? Thyroid 2003; 13(4):389–94.

31. Reeve TS, Delbridge L, Cohen A. Total thyroidectomy: the preferred option for multinodular goitre. Ann Surg 1987; 206:782–6.

This treatment option has become increasingly popular amongst surgeons in recent years; it removes the need for dangerous re-operative surgery and the increased risk of damage to the RLN.

32. Thompson NW, Nishiyama RH, Harness JK. Thyroid carcinoma. Current controversies. Curr Probl Surg 1978; 15:1–67.

33. Thompson NW. In: Johnston IDA, Thompson NW (eds). The thyroid nodule: surgical management in endocrine surgery. London: Butterworths, 1983; pp. 14–24.

34. Reeve TS. Operations for non medullary cancer of the thyroid gland. In: Kaplan EL (ed.) Surgery of the thyroid and parathyroid glands. Edinburgh: Churchill Livingstone, 1983; pp. 63–74.

35. Wynford Thomas D. Molecular basis of epithelial tumorigenesis: the thyroid model. Crit Rev Oncogen 1993; 4:1–23.

36. Lemoine NR, Mayall ES, Wyllie FS et al. High frequency of Ras oncogene activation in all stages of human thyroid tumorigenesis. Oncogene 1989; 4:159–64.

37. Lemoine NR, Hughes CM, Gullick WJ et al. Abnormalities of the EGF receptor system in human thyroid neoplasia. Int J Cancer 1991; 49:558–61.

38. Fagin JA, Matsuo K, Karmakar A et al. High prevalence of mutations of the p53 gene in poorly differentiated human thyroid carcinomas. J Clin Invest 1993; 91:179–84.

39. Garcia-Rostan G, Zhao H, Camp RL et al. Ras mutations are associated with aggressive tumor phenotypes and poor prognosis in thyroid cancer. J Clin Oncol 2003; 21(17):3226–35.

40. Lote K, Anderson K, Nordal E et al. Familial occurrence of papillary thyroid carcinoma. Cancer 1980; 46:1291–7.

41. McConahey WM, Hay ID, Woolner LB et al. Papillary thyroid cancer treated at the Mayo Clinic, 1946 through 1970: initial manifestations, pathologic findings, therapy and outcome. Mayo Clin Proc 1986; 61:978–96.

42. Noguchi S, Yamashita H, Murakami N et al. Small carcinomas of the thyroid – long term follow up of 867 patients. Arch Surg 1996; 131:187–91.

A comprehensive study showing that the vast majority of minimal papillary cancers are treated adequately by surgery alone and that the likelihood of death from this tumour is small.

43. Thompson NW. Differentiated thyroid carcinoma. In: Wheeler MH, Lazarus JH (eds) Diseases of

the thyroid, pathophysiology and management. London: Chapman & Hall Medical, 1994; pp. 367–77.

44. Ozaki O, Ito K, Kobayashi K et al. Familial occurrence of differentiated non medullary thyroid carcinoma. World J Surg 1988; 12:565–71.

45. Thompson NW. Total thyroidectomy in the treatment of thyroid carcinoma. In: Thompson NW, Vinik AI (eds) Endocrine surgical update. New York: Grune & Stratton, 1983; pp. 71–84.

46. Stephenson BM, Wheeler MH, Clark OH. The role of total thyroidectomy in the management of differentiated thyroid cancer. In: Daly JM (ed.) Current opinion in general surgery. Philadelphia: Current Science, 1994; pp. 53–9.

47. Phillips AW, Fenwick JD, Mallick UK et al. The impact of clinical guidelines on surgical management in patients with thyroid cancer. Clin Oncol (R Coll Radiol) 2003; 15(8):485–9.

48. Hay ID, Grant CS, Taylor WF et al. Ipsilateral lobectomy versus bilateral lobe resection in papillary thyroid carcinoma: a retrospective analysis of surgical outcome using a novel prognostic scoring system. Surgery 1987; 102:1088–95.

49. Mazzaferri EL, Young RL. Papillary thyroid carcinoma: a 10 year follow up report of the impact of therapy in 576 patients. Am J Med 1981; 70:511–18.

Keystone study detailing the long-term outcome from using different treatment modalities in papillary thyroid cancer. It forms the basis for TSH suppression in treating thyroid cancer.

50. Spencer CA, Takeuchi M, Kazarosyan M et al. Serum thyroglobulin autoantibodies: prevalence, influence on serum thyroglobulin measurement and prognostic significance in patients with differentiated thyroid carcinoma. J Clin Endocrinol Metab 1998; 83:1121–7.

51. Vassilopoulou-Sellin R, Kline MJ, Smith TH et al. Pulmonary metastases in children and young adults with differentiated thyroid cancer. Cancer 1993; 71:1348–52.

52. Kouvaraki MA, Shapiro SE, Fornage BD et al. Role of preoperative ultrasonography in the surgical management of patients with thyroid cancer. Surgery 2003; 134(6):946–54; discussion 954–5.

53. Khan N, Oriuchi N, Higuchi T et al. PET in the follow-up of differentiated thyroid cancer. Br J Radiol 2003; 76(910):690–5.

54. Kebebew E, Clark OH. Locally advanced differentiated thyroid cancer. Surg Oncol 2003; 12(2):91–9.

55. Haugen BR, Larson LL, Pugazhenthi U et al. Retinoic acid and retinoid X receptors are differentially expressed in thyroid cancer and thyroid carcinoma cell lines and predict response to treatment with retinoids. J Clin Endocrinol Metab 2004; 89(1):272–80.

56. Hazard JB, Hawk WA, Crile G. Medullary (solid) carcinoma of the thyroid. A clinico-pathologic entity. J Clin Endocrinol Metab 1959; 19:152–61.

57. Williams ED. Histogenesis of medullary carcinoma of the thyroid. J Clin Pathol 1966; 19:114–18.

58. Tashjian AH, Howland BG, Melvin KEW et al. Immunoassay of human calcitonin: clinical measurement, relation to serum calcium and studies in patients with medullary carcinoma. N Engl J Med 1970; 283:890–5.

59. Machens A, Gimm O, Ukkat J et al. Improved prediction of calcitonin normalization in medullary thyroid carcinoma patients by quantitative lymph node analysis. Cancer 2000; 88(8):1909–15.

60. Pyke CM, Hay ID, Goellner JR et al. Prognostic significance of calcitonin immunoreactivity, amyloid staining and flow cytometric DNA measurements in medullary thyroid carcinoma. Surgery 1991; 110:967–71.

61. Sizemore GW. Medullary carcinoma of the thyroid. Semin Oncol 1987; 14:306–14.

62. Backdahl M, Hamberger B, Lowhagen T et al. Anaplastic giant cell thyroid carcinoma. In: Wheeler MH, Lazarus JH (eds) Diseases of the thyroid. Pathophysiology and management. London: Chapman & Hall Medical, 1994; pp. 379–85.

63. Sirota DK, Segal RL. Primary lymphomas of the thyroid gland. JAMA 1979; 242:1743–6.

64. Devine RM, Edis AJ, Banks PM. Primary lymphoma of the thyroid: a review of the Mayo Clinic experience through 1978. World J Surg 1981; 5:33.

65. Tunbridge WMG, Evered DC, Hall R et al. The spectrum of thyroid disease in a community: the Wickham survey. Clin Endocrinol 1977; 7:481–93.

66. Sheldon J, Reid DJ. Thyrotoxicosis: changing trends in treatment. Ann R Coll Surg Engl 1986; 68:283–5.

67. Kendall-Taylor P, Keir MJ, Ross WM. Ablative radioiodine therapy for hyperthyroidism: long term follow up study. Br Med J 1984; 289:361–3.

68. Masiukiewicz US, Burrow GN. Hyperthyroidism in pregnancy: diagnosis and treatment. Thyroid 1999; 9:647–52.

69. Zimmerman D. Foetal and neonatal hyperthyroidism. Thyroid 1999; 9:727–33.

70. Furmaniak J, Rees-Smith B. Diagnostic tests of thyroid function and structure – thyroid antibodies. In: Wheeler MH, Lazarus JH (eds) Diseases of the thyroid. Pathophysiology and management. London: Chapman & Hall Medical, 1994; pp. 117–30.

71. Lazarus JH, Othman S. Thyroid disease in relation to pregnancy. Clin Endocrinol 1991; 34:91–8.

72. Amino N, Miyai K, Onishi T et al. Transient hypothyroidism after delivery in autoimmune thyroiditis. J Clin Endocrinol Metab 1976; 2:296–301.

73. Wade JSH. Vulnerability of the recurrent laryngeal nerves at thyroidectomy. Br J Surg 1955; 43:164–80.

74. Beahrs OH, Vandertoll DJ. Complications of secondary thyroidectomy. Surg Gynaecol Obstet 1963; 117:535–9.

75. Clark OH. Total thyroidectomy: the treatment of choice for patients with differentiated thyroid cancer. Ann Surg 1982; 196:361–70.

76. Lennquist S, Cahlin C, Smeds S. The superior laryngeal nerve in thyroid surgery. Surgery 1987; 102:999–1008.

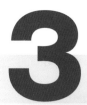

The adrenal glands

Richard D. Bliss
Tom W.J. Lennard

Anatomy

The two adrenal glands have a characteristic golden colour due to the cholesterol in the cortex and are both retroperitoneal structures, weighing approximately 5–7 g in the adult male. Their positions and shapes are slightly different from each other. The right gland is pyramidal in shape and lies at the upper pole of the right kidney, between the right crus of the diaphragm and the inferior vena cava. The left adrenal gland is crescentic and lies on the upper part of the medial aspect of the left kidney. The tail of the pancreas may lie over the inferior part of the left adrenal and the left crus of the diaphragm lies behind this gland. Each gland consists of two distinct parts, which have different structures and functions – the outer cortex and the inner medulla.

Blood supply

The blood supply is similar for both glands, although there are a few differences due to the embryology of the major vessels. Classically, there are three arteries and a single vein for each gland. The arteries include branches from the inferior phrenic arteries, the renal arteries and direct branches from the aorta. In practice, the major vessels often divide before entering the glands to enter as a leach of vessels.

The adrenal vein is most commonly a single vessel that drains into the left renal vein on the left and directly into the inferior vena cava on the right.

The right vein is therefore extremely short and is a major landmark for the surgeon. The veins drain from the medulla and therefore the venous return from the cortex flows through the medulla. This is relevant in that an enzyme involved in the synthesis of catecholamines (phenylethanolamine N-methyltransferase) is influenced by the levels of glucocorticoid hormones secreted by the cortex.

Lymph drainage

There are two lymphatic plexuses, one in the medulla and one under the capsule of the gland. As expected, the lymphatics follow the arterial supply to the pre-aortic nodes, then to the para-aortic and paracaval nodes and on to the thoracic duct.

Nerve supply

The gland has a rich nerve supply, primarily to the adrenal medulla. The cortex has a few vasomotor nerve fibres but the rest supply the medulla and are derived from the splanchnic nerves (T5–9). The medulla itself should be regarded as a collection of modified postganglionic nerve fibres where the axon has degenerated and been replaced with innumerable granules containing either adrenaline or noradrenaline. The preganglionic sympathetic nerve fibres pass through the hilum of the adrenal to synapse with the phaeochromocytes in the medulla.

Microscopic anatomy

As mentioned above, the adrenal gland should be considered as two separate glands with distinct macroscopic and microscopic appearances. The medulla accounts for only 15% of the volume of the adrenal gland and consists of eosinophilic cells known as phaeochromocytes. They have a variable size and shape to their nuclei and hence the diagnosis of malignancy is difficult for the pathologist without the presence of invasion. They possess multiple granules in the cytoplasm attached to the membrane of the cell. These are characterised histologically by their reaction to various salts and typically stain brown to dichromate salts, hence they are referred to as chromaffin cells. There are large vascular spaces within the medulla.

The cortex of the adrenal gland is divided into three layers: the outer zona glomerulosa, the zona fasciculata and the innermost zona reticularis. There is a noticeable border between the zona reticularis and the medulla.

The zona glomerulosa produces mineralocorticoids, particularly aldosterone. It consists of an arrangement of columnar cells organised into clusters. There is relatively little cytoplasm compared with the nucleus. The zona fasciculata is the largest of the cortical zones. It occupies approximately 75% of the adrenal cortex and the cells are poorly staining, polyhedral and organised in columns running radially through the zone. It is primarily responsible for the production of glucocorticoids. The zona reticularis is characterised by large clusters of cells and is easily differentiated from both the zona fasciculata and the medulla. It produces the sex hormones, particularly dehydroepiandrosterone (DHEA).

Embryology

The embryological origins of the two layers of the adrenal are completely different. The cortex starts to appear at approximately the fifth week of gestation as two clefts, either side of the embryonic dorsal mesentery. This is mesodermal in origin. It enlarges to form the primitive (or fetal) cortex by the seventh week. At this stage, the developing adrenal gland is invaded by cells migrating from the neural crest (ectodermal in origin) to form the adrenal medulla. At the seventh week, the mesodermal layer produces another group of cells known as the secondary cortex, which becomes the mature adult adrenal cortex. The primary cortex produces large amounts of DHEA, which is made available for conversion to oestrogens by the placenta. The fetal adrenal does not produce cortisol itself until just before delivery.

At birth, the adrenal gland is large and is approximately one-third the size of the kidney. The primary cortex shrinks rapidly after delivery of the baby until it has disappeared after a year or so. It takes until puberty for the adrenal gland to regain the size it had at birth. Prior to delivery, the zona glomerulosa starts to appear, followed after delivery by the inner zona fasciculata and finally the zona reticularis emerges a few months after birth.

Accessory cortical adrenal tissue is often found (up to 50% of neonates) in the tissue around the adrenals or more rarely in relation to structures from the urogenital ridge. This usually disappears but may persist or even enlarge if the adrenals are stimulated. Ectopic medullary tissue is often found in masses around the aorta or the sympathetic plexus (organ of Zuckerkandl). Phaeochromocytomas may arise in any tissue derived from the neural crest.

Physiology

Adrenal medulla

The adrenal medulla produces adrenaline (epinephrine), noradrenaline (norepinephrine) and dopamine. It is basically a modified sympathetic ganglion, whereby the postganglionic cells have lost their axons and developed secretory functions.

The catecholamines are synthesised from tyrosine via a series of steps, outlined in **Fig. 3.1**. It should be noted that tyrosine hydroxylase controls the rate-limiting step. Cortisol (produced in the cortex) is necessary for the induction of phenylethanolamine N-methyltransferase (PNMT), which converts adrenaline to noradrenaline.

The catecholamines are released after stimulation of the medulla as the secretory granules fuse with the cell membrane (exocytosis) in a calcium-dependent process.

The majority of the released catecholamines are taken back up into the presynaptic terminals of the chromaffin cells, the rest being transported away from the adrenal into the systemic circulation. The catecholamines taken up by neural tissue are

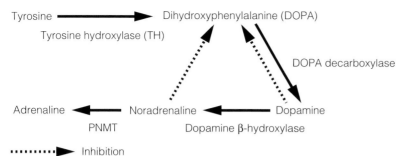

Figure 3.1 • Synthesis of catecholamines.

broken down by monoamine oxidase, into hydroxy-methoxy mandelate (HMMA) and homovanillic acid (HVA) (from dopamine). Carboxy-O-methyl-transferase produces the deactivation of adrenaline and noradrenaline taken up by extraneural tissue, via metadrenaline and normetadrenaline to vanyl-lmandelic acid (VMA).

Physiological effects

Catecholamines affect most tissues in the body but particularly the cardiovascular system and they have several metabolic effects. Basal secretion is quite low and substantial release of preformed catecholamines requires a marked stimulus during special conditions.

The actions are mediated via characteristic cell-membrane-bound receptors, the α- and β-adrenergic receptors, each with their own subclasses. The physiological effects are typified as the flight or fight response, i.e. preparing the organism for opti-mal performance in times of threat. An increase in heart rate, blood pressure and cardiac output, excitation of the central nervous system, contrac-tion of iris, changes in tone of arterioles depend-ing upon the organ affected – increased blood flow to muscles, decreased to the splanchnic circulation – and a breakdown of lipid, glycogen and protein to provide metabolic substrate for action all occur.

Adrenal cortex

Each of the three zones of the cortex produces differ-ent hormones. The outer zona glomerulosa produces the salt-retaining hormone aldosterone, the zona fasciculata produces cortisol, and the innermost zona reticularis produces the sex hormones. All are derivatives of cholesterol and have a characteristic molecular shape.

Mineralocorticoids

Aldosterone is the main mineralocorticoid hormone and causes an increase in resorption of sodium. This leads to an increase in the volume of the extracel-lular fluid by acting on the epithelium of the distal tubule and collecting duct of the kidney. Aldosterone therefore causes a fall in potassium and hydrogen ions in exchange for sodium. It is produced under the control of renin via angiotensin. A fall in the circulating volume or blood pressure, or an increase in sympathetic output, stimulates the secretion of renin from the juxtaglomerular apparatus of the kidney. Renin has a half-life in the circulation of 80 minutes and splits angiotensin I from circulating angiotensinogen. Angiotensin-converting enzyme (ACE) then converts angiotensin I to angiotensin II, mostly in the lungs. This stimulates the secretion of aldosterone from the adrenal cortex. Numerous other stimuli are known to initiate aldosterone secretion, including adrenocorticotropic hormone (ACTH) from the pituitary and a direct stimulatory effect of an elevated plasma potassium.

Glucocorticoids

Cortisol is the major glucocorticoid along with corticosterone. Synthesis is via a series of steps as outlined in **Fig. 3.2**. The major effects of glucocor-ticoids are upon glucose and protein metabolism. They are necessary for maintaining hepatic glyco-gen stores, they stimulate protein catabolism and lipolysis and cause hyperglycaemia. They also have a weak mineralocorticoid effect. In supraphysi-ological doses (therapeutic or pathological), skele-tal weakening is caused by a decrease in intestinal absorption and increasing urinary excretion of calcium.

Cortisol is secreted under the direct control of ACTH. The cortisol level is continually regulated via a negative-feedback mechanism on both the

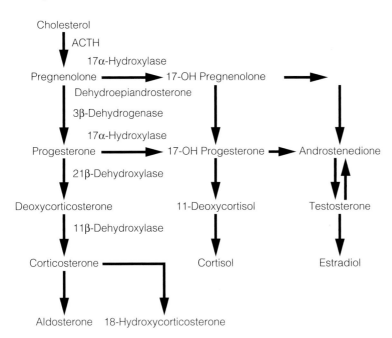

Figure 3.2 • Synthesis of steroids.

hypothalamus and pituitary. The hypothalamus secretes corticotropin-releasing hormone (CRH) to stimulate the secretion of ACTH from the anterior pituitary. Serum levels of cortisol show a diurnal rhythm, with the highest levels in the early morning; this is also controlled by the hypothalamus.

Steroids are fat-soluble and enter cells to bind to a receptor. The ligand–receptor complex then diffuses into the nucleus of the cell and there binds to DNA to affect protein synthesis over a relatively long period of time (hours to days).

Sex steroids

Dehydroepiandrosterone (DHEA) and androstenedione are weakly androgenic sex steroids. They are converted in peripheral tissues to testosterone and oestrogens, via the aromatase enzyme system. Corticotropin stimulates the secretion of the adrenal androgens. Tumours producing DHEA, androstenedione and DHEA precursors cause virilisation in women.

Congenital adrenal hyperplasia and adrenogenital syndromes

Congenital adrenal hyperplasia (CAH) includes a group of conditions that are usually inherited as an autosomal recessive disorder. They are charac-

terised by a block in the synthesis of cortisol. This can occur anywhere on the synthetic pathway from cholesterol, and the clinical effects depend upon the level of the block. Due to failure of the negative-feedback loop, there is an increase in the levels of ACTH secreted by the pituitary and this leads to hyperplasia of the adrenal glands. The adrenogenital syndrome is a subcategory of CAH characterised by abnormalities in the external genitalia.

In all of these syndromes there is a deficiency of the end steroid and overproduction of the steroid intermediary at the level of the enzyme deficiency. The most common enzyme block is a deficiency of 21-hydroxylase, which accounts for 90% of cases, causing a deficiency of glucocorticoid and mineralocorticoid. Due to the high concentrations of the intermediary prior to 21-hydroxylase, there are high levels of androgens. This deficiency causes ambiguous genitalia in females as the child is masculinised in utero. There is also salt loss and hyperkalaemia, which requires the administration of mineralocorticoid and salt to correct it. All of the CAH deficiencies are treatable by replacement of glucocorticoid, mineralocorticoid or both. Some also require sex hormone treatment from puberty.

Management

The standard treatment for CAH and adrenogenital syndrome includes the replacement of the steroid beyond the enzyme block. This results in restoration of the feedback loop, a subsequent reduction of ACTH and a reduction of the androgens causing the virilisation. The genital effects of androgen excess may require surgical intervention prior to and after puberty.[1]

Treatment may be difficult in some patients as there may be inadequately treated hyperandrogenism and iatrogenic hypercortisolism. Recently, more evidence has emerged indicating that patients with CAH who are proving difficult to manage medically may benefit from bilateral adrenalectomy. This can lead to a further decrease of androgens, and improved control of the signs and symptoms of hypercortisolism (particularly obesity), as the dose of exogenous steroids may be reduced.[2,3] The adrenal gland can become significantly enlarged in these syndromes and may need to be removed for this reason (**Fig. 3.3**).

- Congenital adrenal hyperplasia is due to an inherited enzyme deficiency occurring at a variety of places in the steroid synthetic pathway.

- The deficiency causes a build-up of steroid precursor and stimulation of the negative-feedback loop to increase ACTH, thus making the adrenal gland large and hyperplastic.

- Build-up of precursor steroids can produce ambiguous gender at birth, and deficiencies of steroid will need to be replaced.

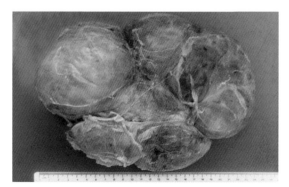

Figure 3.3 • Excised adrenal gland from patient with congenital adrenal hyperplasia. Note nodular appearance caused by high circulating ACTH and large overall size (scale in cm).

Cushing's syndrome

Cushing's syndrome is characterised by increased levels of circulating glucocorticoids. It is conveniently divided into two types: ACTH-dependent, due to either pituitary or ectopic origin; and ACTH-independent, due to adrenal origin. The most common cause of hypercortisolism is iatrogenic administration of steroids for the treatment of other diseases. The characteristics of the syndrome, however, are identical regardless of the cause.

Features of Cushing's syndrome (Figs 3.4 and 3.5)

Cushing's syndrome is a rare disorder but may be responsible for many symptoms and therefore frequently enters a list of differential diagnoses. It has a prevalence of 10 cases per million per year. The majority of these patients have ACTH-dependent Cushing's syndrome.

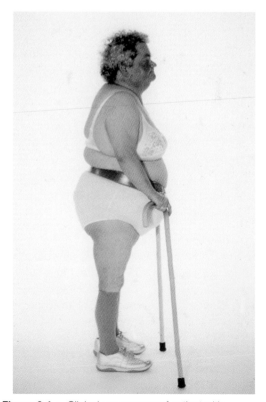

Figure 3.4 • Clinical appearance of patient with Cushing's syndrome. Note body habitus.

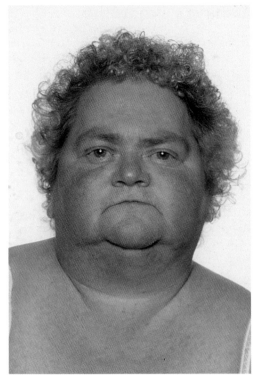

Figure 3.5 • Cushing's syndrome. Note facial plethora and moon face.

Table 3.1 • The symptoms and signs of Cushing's syndrome

Signs and symptoms	Occurrence (%)
Obesity	95
Facial plethora	80
Hirsutism	80
Menstrual disorders	80
Hypertension	75
Muscular weakness	60
Striae	50
Acne	40
Psychological symptoms	40
Congestive heart failure	20
Oedema	20
Headache	10
Hyperpigmentation	10
Back pain	60
Buffalo hump	55
Diabetes	15
Fractures	20
Bruising	40

The clinical presentation of Cushing's syndrome has numerous and variable features, as outlined in Table 3.1.[4,5]

Aetiology

ACTH-dependent Cushing's

There are two main causes of ACTH-dependent Cushing's syndrome: pituitary adenoma that secretes ACTH or ectopic ACTH secretion.

ACTH-secreting pituitary adenoma

This was the form of Cushing's syndrome described by Harvey Cushing in 1932,[6] and is often referred to as Cushing's disease. These tumours are usually microadenomas (<1 cm), so pituitary magnetic resonance imaging (MRI) is the imaging modality of choice. Nevertheless, very small tumours may not always be detected. Moreover, MRI cannot distinguish between corticotropin adenomas and non-functioning pituitary incidentalomas. Therefore, biochemical confirmation is also required to achieve a confident diagnosis.

Ectopic secretion of ACTH

This is usually secondary to small-cell lung cancer and accounts for 10–15% of ACTH-dependent Cushing's syndrome.[7] Clinical examination and/or abnormal chest X-ray (CXR) appearance usually make the diagnosis obvious, without the need to perform specialised imaging. ACTH levels are usually higher than in pituitary disease, resulting in relatively greater prevalence of pigmentation, muscle weakness and hypokalaemia. Most of the remainder of ectopic ACTH cases are caused by carcinoid tumours, usually of bronchial origin.[8,9] Such tumours may be so small and slow growing that even high-resolution MRI or spiral computed tomography (CT) are not always able to identify them reliably.

ACTH-independent Cushing's syndrome

Causes of ACTH-independent Cushing's syndrome fall into one of three categories.

Adrenal adenoma and carcinoma

ACTH is usually suppressed by negative feedback, and levels are therefore low. Carcinomas are most reliably identified preoperatively as a result of their size or concomitant hypersecretion of androgens. Postoperative histology can be difficult to interpret as distinguishing between adrenocortical adenomas and carcinomas is rarely possible on histological grounds alone.

Bilateral adrenal hyperplasia

This is a rare condition and may be associated with other symptoms of Carney's syndrome (see Chapter 4) such as myxomas, blue naevi and pigmented lentigines.[10] Note that Cushing's disease can cause nodular hyperplasia of the adrenals secondary to stimulation by high circulating levels of ACTH.[11]

Iatrogenic

Symptoms are usually mild and only after long-term administration of steroids are the gross symptoms and signs of Cushing's syndrome evident.

Diagnosis

Once the diagnosis has been considered and drugs excluded, blood and urine tests are employed to confirm Cushing's syndrome.[12]

1. **Twenty-four-hour urinary cortisol.** This reflects the average plasma cortisol level. It is reliable, and sensitivities of up to 95% have been recorded, although the investigation may need repeating two or three times.[13] Note that in alcoholics, if alcohol is withdrawn, then the cortisol may well fall to give a false-negative result. Stress may increase the levels of cortisol and give a false-positive result.
2. **Cortisol diurnal rhythm.** An elevated (>50 nmol/L) sleeping midnight cortisol level is said to have 100% sensitivity and specificity in the investigation of Cushing's syndrome. However, this investigation is best performed in a dedicated inpatient investigation unit. Level of noise, disturbance and general patient stress on the average acute medical or surgical ward might be expected to result in loss of cortisol diurnal rhythm even in normal individuals! Loss of diurnal rhythm is also a feature of chronic alcohol abuse and severe depression.
3. **Low-dose dexamethasone suppression test.** A dose of dexamethasone is given to exploit the loss of negative feedback. After administration of dexamethasone (1–2 mg) the night before,

the 09.00 cortisol level should be suppressed (<50 nmol/L) in normal people, but it fails to do so in those with Cushing's syndrome. False-positive results may be obtained if the patient is taking drugs that speed up the metabolism of dexamethasone such as phenytoin, carbamazepine and rifampicin.[14]

Once the diagnosis has been established, the cause of the Cushing's syndrome must be established, i.e. is the elevated cortisol ACTH-dependent or not?

- **ACTH measurement.** If the elevated cortisol is ACTH-dependent, then the ACTH will be elevated; if it is ACTH-independent, then the measured ACTH will be low or undetectable. ACTH is measured with a two-site immunometric assay and should be measured on two or three separate occasions to minimise any variability.

ACTH-independent Cushing's syndrome

As mentioned above, if Cushing's is ACTH-independent, then it is due to adrenal disease. Imaging of the adrenals is therefore required to localise the site of the adrenal disease.

CT scan (**Figs 3.6 and 3.7**)

A CT scan will reveal an adrenal adenoma or carcinoma. It is impossible to distinguish between the two accurately by CT scan alone, although a size

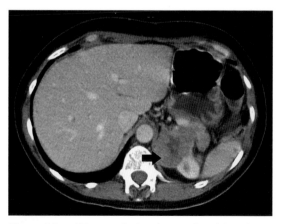

Figure 3.6 • CT scan of adrenal mass. Suspicion of carcinoma is raised by the irregular outline and non-homogeneous nature suggestive of central necrosis. Carcinoma was later confirmed histologically.

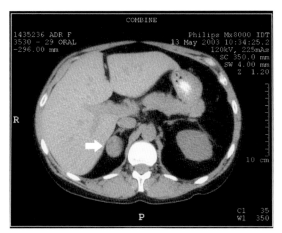

Figure 3.7 • CT scan of adrenal adenoma (arrowed) in contrast to Fig. 3.6.

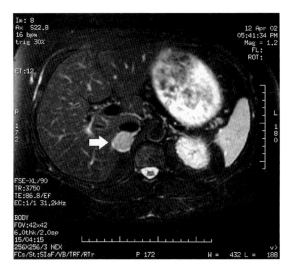

Figure 3.9 • MRI scan of right adrenal adenoma. Fast spin echo T2-weighted to highlight water. Note bright appearance of adrenal indicating high water content and likelihood of the mass being a benign adenoma. This was subsequently confirmed histologically.

>3.5 cm increases the risk of malignancy. Local invasion or heterogeneity of the tumour all point towards a malignant lesion.[15,16] This risk is also raised if the tumour is secreting multiple hormones, particularly virilising hormones (measure testosterone and DHEA). Note that after prolonged stimulation of the adrenals with high levels of ACTH (ACTH-dependent Cushing's), nodular changes may occur in the adrenals and this may be mistaken for a true adrenal mass.

MRI scan (**Figs 3.8 and 3.9**)

This may help to distinguish between an adenoma and carcinoma because an adenoma has a higher water content than a carcinoma. T2-weighted, both unenhanced and gadolinium-enhanced T1-weighted scans and chemical shift studies can be performed. With all of these images, sensitivities of 95% for distinguishing adenoma from carcinoma have been reported.[17]

ACTH-dependent Cushing's syndrome

To make the diagnosis in ACTH-dependent Cushing's syndrome, both blood work and imaging will be required.

High-dose dexamethasone suppression test

This is based on the fact that pituitary tumours usually retain some negative feedback control, but this is lost in patients with an ectopic source of ACTH. Dexamethasone is a synthetic glucocorticoid that binds to the cortisol receptors in the pituitary and so would prevent the normal secretion of ACTH. A dose of 2 mg dexamethasone is given 6-hourly for 2 days. A reduction in serum cortisol to <50% of the baseline value points towards Cushing's being due to pituitary secretion of ACTH. In ACTH-independent Cushing's or ectopic ACTH-dependent Cushing's, then no significant drop in cortisol will be seen.[18]

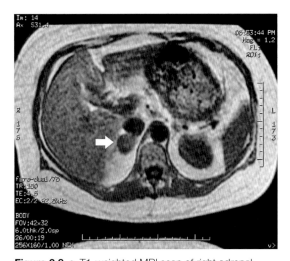

Figure 3.8 • T1-weighted MRI scan of right adrenal adenoma.

Overnight high-dose dexamethasone suppression test

This involves giving 8 mg dexamethasone, and measuring serum cortisol at 09.00 the next morning and again the morning following this. If plasma cortisol is reduced to less than 32% of baseline, then the sensitivity is 71% and specificity is 100%.[19]

Inferior petrosal sinus catheterisation

This directly measures the ACTH produced from the pituitary gland as the pituitary secretions drain into the petrosal sinus via the cavernous sinus.[20] Peripheral blood levels of ACTH must also be measured to detect any concentration gradient. Both sinuses should be sampled as ACTH may only be secreted into a single sinus, and corticotropin-releasing factor (CRF) should be infused to avoid the possibility that the ACTH is being produced in an episodic fashion.[21]

Imaging

Once the pituitary gland has been identified as the source of the ACTH, it should be imaged. This is achieved by MRI or CT scan, but note that the offending lesion is often a pituitary microadenoma. This means that the pituitary may often appear normal and an adenoma is detected in only 50–60% of patients.[22] CT or MRI of the chest should be used if ectopic ACTH-dependent Cushing's is diagnosed.

Treatment

Surgery is the mainstay of treatment for Cushing's syndrome of both pituitary and adrenal origin. Pituitary surgery will not be dealt with in detail in this book, suffice to say that this is usually performed through the trans-sphenoidal route. Surgery to the adrenal will be discussed in detail at the end of this chapter.

If primary surgery to the pituitary to excise the microadenoma is unsuccessful (which it may be in up to 40%), or if a treatable ectopic source of ACTH is not found, then bilateral adrenalectomy may be indicated to excise the target organs. Other options to treat the pituitary directly include external beam irradiation or complete surgical ablation of the pituitary, which results in the other hormones of the anterior pituitary becoming deficient. If bilateral adrenalectomy is performed, the patient will be left with permanent adrenal failure and will have to take both glucocorticoid and mineralocorticoid replacement to avoid Addisonian crises. The patient should always wear an alert badge and carry a shock pack of glucocorticoids for rapid treatment of stress, such as infection and trauma. The results of bilateral adrenalectomy for the treatment of pituitary ACTH-dependent Cushing's syndrome are encouraging, with a remission rate of 95%. Quality-of-life questionnaires show a less favourable outcome, with several symptoms remaining, and there may be long-term recurrence if adrenal remnants are left.[23,24] A complication of bilateral adrenalectomy after previous pituitary surgery is Nelson's syndrome, which results in marked hyperpigmentation and possible mass effects on the pituitary as the ACTH-secreting tumour enlarges and secretes large quantities of ACTH (with melanocyte-stimulating hormone) due to the lack of negative feedback. The incidence of Nelson's syndrome may be reduced, or at least delayed, by prior radiotherapy to the pituitary.[25]

If the cause of the Cushing's syndrome is localised to a unilateral lesion in the adrenal, then adrenalectomy is indicated. Treatment for these patients needs to be particularly careful, as they are prone to postoperative infections, skin injury, fractures and hypoglycaemia, as complications of the Cushing's syndrome. Prophylactic antibiotics should be given preoperatively, and it is also important to bear in mind that the remaining adrenal gland will be suppressed; therefore steroid replacement will be required until it recovers. This should be confirmed with a Synacthen test before complete withdrawal of steroid supplements (this may take over a year). There is no role for subtotal adrenalectomy or adrenal autotransplantation.[26]

If the cause of the Cushing's is ectopic ACTH production, treatment of the primary tumour is indicated if possible. But this is often impossible,[27] and so controlling the symptoms becomes paramount. This may be achieved medically by the use of ketoconazole, metyrapone, aminoglutethimide or mitotane, which inhibit cortisol production or secretion. However, even in patients with limited life expectancies, bilateral adrenalectomy may still be the best way to achieve good palliation, particularly if this can be achieved laparoscopically.

- Cortisol excess can be driven by ACTH or independent of that (adrenal).
- Clinical suspicion of the classical syndrome is confirmed by biochemistry and then appropriate imaging.
- There is a time in the natural history of the disease where the autonomous cortisol production will not be clinically evident (subclinical Cushing's). The patient is particularly vulnerable at this time from missed diagnosis.
- Laparoscopic adrenalectomy is the procedure of choice for adrenal causes or when pituitary surgery has failed to cure ACTH-driven cases.
- Postoperatively patients need careful steroid replacement regimens delivered through a multidisciplinary team.

Adrenocortical carcinoma

Adrenocortical carcinoma is fortunately a rare tumour and has an incidence of 2 per million per year. It is, however, one of the most lethal endocrine tumours, with overall survival rates of only 20–35% at 5 years.

There is a slight gender bias, with a female:male ratio of 4:3, and it presents at two peak incidences of age, namely the first and fifth decades. Most of the tumours are hormonally functional and commonly present by producing more than one hormone – in particular virilising tumours in women (this may account for the slight sex distribution bias).[28] Approximately one-third of adrenocortical carcinomas are biochemically silent, however, and this obviously is highly relevant to the investigation of incidental adrenal masses (see below).

Inherited susceptibility (see also Chapter 4)

Adrenocortical carcinoma is associated with three named syndromes:

- Multiple endocrine neoplasia type 1 (MEN 1) – pituitary, parathyroid, pancreatic and foregut carcinoid tumours. This has a known mutation on chromosome 11.
- Beckwith–Wiedemann syndrome – affects children and is associated with exophthalmos, macroglossia and nephromegaly. This involves two mutations on chromosome 11: IGF-2 and H19.
- Li–Fraumeni syndrome – affects children and young adults and is characterised by breast carcinomas, osteosarcomas and brain tumours. It is caused by inactivation of the tumour suppressor gene *p53*.

Diagnosis

Diagnosis of adrenocortical carcinoma is usually only made histologically and this can be difficult, with the only absolute criterion being the presence of metastases. Like many endocrine tumours, it is impossible to distinguish cytologically between an adrenal adenoma or carcinoma and therefore percutaneous biopsy is not helpful as this may be falsely reassuring and has a relatively high morbidity rate. In addition, seeding of tumour cells in the biopsy track has also been reported, which should increase the concern about requesting this procedure.[29]

Functioning tumours may, as previously mentioned, present by the clinical effects of multiple hormones. If only a single hormone is produced, this is most commonly a virilising tumour, but feminising, cortisol-secreting or, rarely, aldosterone-secreting carcinomas can occur.

In assessing resectability, evidence of invasion of local structures should be sought on CT or MRI scans, and on the right side a venogram may assist in evaluating caval involvement (**Fig. 3.10**).

Suspicion of malignancy may be raised on imaging of the adrenal glands. The likelihood of malignancy increases with increasing size of the adrenal mass: the larger the adrenal tumour, the greater the risk of malignancy.[16] Malignancy in adrenal tumours smaller than 5 cm is rare, but has been reported in masses smaller than 2.5 cm.[30] Logic would suggest that all malignant tumours must at some stage have been small. Evidence of malignancy in small adrenal masses should therefore be carefully sought for. This may be provided by CT appearances: non-homogeneous tumours, those with irregular edges and marked enhancement after the administration of intravenous contrast all support the diagnosis of malignancy. MRI can be helpful as adrenal carcinomas have a low fat content when compared with adrenal adenomas and, with gadolinium contrast, malignant tumours have a high rate of enhancement with a long washout phase (Figs 3.8 and 3.9). None of these features,

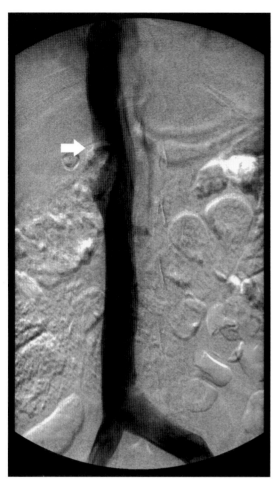

Figure 3.10 • Venogram indicating invasion of inferior vena cava from a malignant phaeochromocytoma in the right adrenal gland.

however, are diagnostic of malignancy. MRI is particularly useful if invasion of the inferior vena cava is suspected. Scintigraphy with iodocholesterol or 6-β-iodomethylnorcholesterol (NP-59) has been used for further imaging of the adrenals, as uptake of the isotope is decreased or absent in adrenal carcinomas.[31] However, availability of these radiopharmaceuticals is severely restricted and thus the regular use of these imaging tests is diminishing. Adrenal adenomas and nodular hyperplasia usually produce images in which the gland takes up tracer. With scintigraphy the patient is exposed to significant doses of radiation and the scan takes 3 days to complete as it requires the adrenal to metabolise the cholesterol. The cost, availability and duration mean that many medical physics departments may have difficulty and/or reluctance in providing these scans.

Treatment

Surgery

If a likely diagnosis of malignancy has been made preoperatively, the surgeon should be prepared to deal with a locally advanced tumour and laparoscopic surgery should not be performed electively. Direct access to the major vessels should be easily attainable and radical resection is the best chance of achieving a cure.

A transabdominal approach is the method of choice and this can be extended to include a thoraco-abdominal approach if necessary, particularly on the right side to gain control of the inferior vena cava if needed. The role of laparoscopic surgery in adrenal carcinoma is unknown, due in part to few reports of its use and because port-site recurrences have been reported. Laparoscopic surgery for benign adrenal tumours is the gold standard (see below) but many carcinomas are only diagnosed as malignant on postoperative histology. Reassuringly, when this happens after laparoscopic removal the prognosis does not appear to be unduly worsened. Surgery may also be needed to treat recurrent disease.

Medical

The first-line medical therapy is mitotane (o,p-DDD). This compound was first used as a pesticide and causes adrenal necrosis. Mitotane also inhibits cortisol synthesis as well as being cytotoxic, but is still effective in non-functioning adrenal carcinomas. The role of mitotane as adjuvant treatment is unclear but as first-line therapy for adrenal carcinoma a response rate of 30% is reported, with recent reports suggesting improved survival with adjuvant use.[32] Suramin, a polysulphonated naphthylurea, has been used with some effect as a single agent. Standard cytotoxic chemotherapy and radiotherapy have a very limited role. Single-agent use is disappointing and multiple-agent chemotherapy only has a response rate in the region of 30%.[33]

Prognosis

The overall outcome of treatment for adrenocortical carcinoma is poor. Most series report 5-year survival rates between 20% and 35% for those who have undergone potentially curative surgery.[15] Median survival is 20–25 months but depends upon the stage at diagnosis. Non-curative surgery has a median survival of 9 months.[34] Endocrine function of the tumour makes no difference to the survival,[35] although those presenting as an acute Cushing's syndrome have an even poorer mean survival of 3 months.

- Adrenal carcinoma is rare and can be sporadic or part of inherited predisposition.
- The tumours are rapidly growing and can produce a variety of active hormones.
- Biopsy is not advised for risk of disseminating the tumour.
- Open surgery based on suspicion (clinical, biochemical or radiological) is the treatment of choice.
- The overall prognosis is poor but adjuvant treatment with mitotane may improve outcome.

Phaeochromocytoma

Phaeochromocytoma is the term given to a functioning tumour of the adrenal medulla producing excessive amounts of catecholamines or their derivatives. Most commonly these tumours are benign; they arise within the adrenal gland and are unilateral. However, approximately 10% can be malignant, some occur in both adrenal glands (10%), and they can occur in ectopic sites where there is any embryological chromaffin tissue derived from the neural crest (10%).[36] A diagram of the extra-adrenal chromaffin tissue is shown in **Fig. 3.11**. Phaeochromocytomas are most commonly sporadic, but rarely they can be associated with multiple endocrine neoplasia syndrome or in association with von Recklinghausen's disease (**Fig. 3.12**), von Hippel–Lindau syndrome and occasionally as familial inherited autosomal dominant tumours (see Chapter 4). Of the extra-adrenal tumours approximately 2% are situated in the neck and the thorax, and they can even be in the myocardium (**Figs 3.13 and 3.14**). Multiple, bilateral and extra-adrenal tumours are more common in children, and malignancy is also more common in extra-adrenal tumours.[37] Phaeochromocytomas can also occur in association with Sturge–Weber syndrome and tuberosclerosis. Autopsy studies suggest 0.3% of all autopsies have an undiagnosed phaeochromocytoma, and the estimated incidence of phaeochromocytoma is 1–2 per 100 000 adults per year.[38] It is probable that this rare condition is underdiagnosed and under-recognised in life.

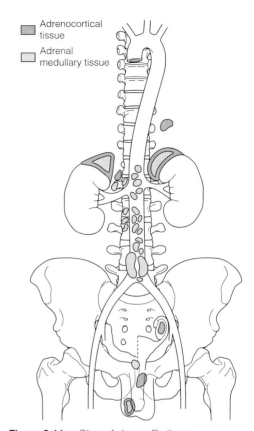

Adrenocortical tissue

Adrenal medullary tissue

Figure 3.11 • Sites of chromaffin tissue.

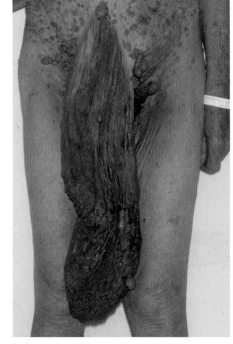

Figure 3.12 • von Recklinghausen's disease.

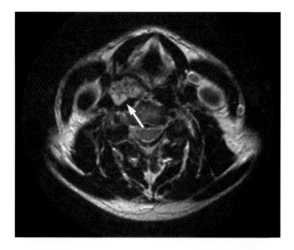

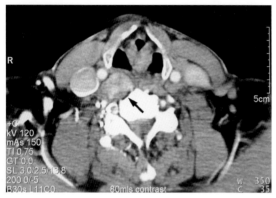

Figure 3.13 • MRI and CT scan of cervical phaeochromocytoma.

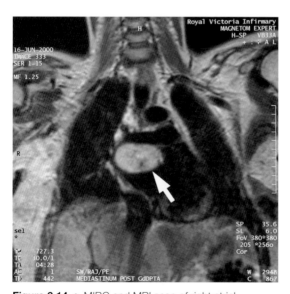

Figure 3.14 • MIBG and MRI scan of right atrial phaeochromocytoma.

Clinical presentation

The diverse hormones produced by these tumours and their widespread effects produce a wide spectrum of clinical presentations. Hypertension and its associated complications is the commonest presentation. The patient may have headaches, dizziness or visual problems secondary to hypertensive retinopathy or, rarely, papilloedema. Secondary effects on the cardiovascular system include palpitations, heart failure, myocardial ischaemia and arrhythmia. The characteristic feature of all presenting symptoms is that they are intermittent or paroxysmal. This reflects the intermittent secretion of catecholamines into the circulation and further makes the diagnosis difficult as the patient may be perfectly well for reasonable periods of time and then have paroxysmal attacks of symptoms that may or may not be witnessed by anybody else. Typically during one of these paroxysms the patient will appear pale, sweaty and tremulous and relatives will describe them as looking 'ghostlike'. During such a paroxysm patients will commonly complain of a desperate and unpleasant sense of doom.

Direct trauma to the tumour or any stress (including anaesthesia and surgery) may precipitate symptoms. Attacks and symptoms may last for minutes or hours. Symptoms in virtually all of the major systems of the body can be caused by phaeochromocytoma, and the diagnosis will only be made if the clinician is alert to the possibility of the disease.

Conditions associated with phaeochromocytoma

Multiple endocrine neoplasia (MEN)

Phaeochromocytoma is a component of MEN types 2A and 2B (see Chapter 4). In these patients screening for the disease annually will often identify the condition before it is clinically evident. Phaeochromocytoma may be the presenting feature of MEN 2A or 2B and therefore a careful family history and history of other endocrine disease within the patient should be sought in everyone presenting with a phaeochromocytoma. In MEN 2B there are other clues to the syndrome, namely multiple mucosal neuromas, a megacolon and a typical marfanoid habitus. Screening for MEN 2A using RET mutation analysis now allows individuals susceptible to developing phaeochromocytoma and other components of the syndrome to be identified and to be monitored on an annual basis with early detection of the disease.[39]

Neurofibromatosis

Phaeochromocytoma is associated with neurofibromatosis (Fig. 3.12). The features of the disease may not be as prominent as those shown in Fig. 3.12, but nevertheless neurofibromas, axillary freckling and a family history of this syndrome should raise the clinician's level of alertness to the diagnosis of phaeochromocytoma.

Von Hippel–Lindau syndrome

This syndrome, which consists of cerebellar haemangiomas, renal tumours and phaeochromocytomas, is rare and can be tested for by analysis of the VHL gene.[40,41]

Very rarely the phaeochromocytoma can appear as a familial autosomal dominant condition in young individuals due to a mitochondrial enzyme defect,[42] caused by a mutation in the gene encoding succinate dehydrogenase complex subunit D (SDHD) or subunit B (SDHB). Recurrence and malignancy are more common in SDHB mutations than SDHD.

Diagnosis and preoperative management

Diagnosis is made on clinical suspicion first and then confirmatory biochemical tests. These will include measurement of excessive catecholamine excretion in the urine. Traditionally this is performed with 24-hour urinary collections, but overnight excretion of urinary catecholamines and their metabolites can be helpful in the detection of phaeochromocytoma and is often more socially acceptable.[43] In addition to confirmation of excess levels of urinary catecholamines, it is traditional also to measure plasma catecholamines, but these are difficult and costly to measure. The patient should be at rest when the blood is drawn, the blood rapidly centrifuged in a chilled centrifuge and then frozen pending batch analysis. Phaeochromocytoma should be actively excluded before operating on the thyroid of any patients with MEN 2 or medullary thyroid carcinoma to ensure that there is not a silent tumour awaiting activation by the anaesthetic and thyroidectomy. Once the biochemical diagnosis is made, immediate blockade with α-adrenergic drugs should be instituted prior to scanning. Uncontrollable hypertension and uncontrollable paroxysmal hypertension are dangerous and take priority over localisation studies. Phenoxybenzamine is the agent most frequently used, in a dose initially of 20 mg twice daily, escalating the dose until postural hypotension occurs and the patient is maximally vasodilated. A safe and satisfactory alternative to phenoxybenzamine is doxazosin.[44] Some units prefer to control blood pressure with drugs such as calcium channel blockers or magnesium. These may result in quicker control of hypertension preoperatively. At all costs the sole use of a beta-blocking drug should be avoided lest a hypertensive crisis be precipitated.[45] Once alpha blockade has been instituted localisation studies can begin; these will include CT scan, which is probably the most sensitive, but should be from at least the diaphragm down to the symphysis with small cuts through the adrenal gland. Ultrasound rarely may add to the value of the CT, as may MRI. Additional localisation with radioisotopes, including [^{131}I]meta-iodobenzylguanidine (MIBG), is helpful (**Fig. 3.15**). MIBG is taken up in areas of catecholamine production within chromaffin tissue and can subsequently

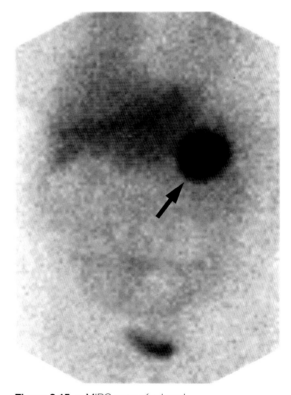

Figure 3.15 • MIBG scan of adrenal phaeochromocytoma.

identify not only the primary lesion but also secondary deposits in cases of malignancy. When labelled with an appropriate radiopharmaceutical it can be used as a therapeutic method of ablating irremovable metastases or recurrences.[46]

The use of positron emission tomography to visualise phaeochromocytomas is gaining in popularity as the technology to exploit the dihydroxyphenylalanine (DOPA) and fluorodeoxyglucose (FDG) receptors on these tumours advances.[47]

Further preoperative preparation will need to take place once localisation has been achieved, and this will include escalation of the dose of alpha-blocking agents being used, and the possible introduction of a beta-blocker if the patient is tachycardic. The period of blockade will depend upon the activity of the tumour and the patient's general cardiovascular condition. During blockade regression of cardiomyopathy is to the advantage of the patient and a sustained improvement in blood pressure allows the heart to recover and the patient to be fitter for surgery. There is no need to rush into surgery for phaeochromocytoma, and although various crash blockade and rapid blockade programmes have been advocated, a cautious approach to getting the patient into the optimal condition for surgery is advised. Typically this is going to take around 2–4 weeks, but in cases of severe cardiomyopathy may take longer.

Surgical removal

The treatment of choice for phaeochromocytoma in the 21st century is laparoscopic adrenalectomy. Most tumours will be amenable to this, but extremely large tumours and malignant tumours may be more easily managed by open operation. Careful liaison between surgeon and anaesthetist during the operation is essential. Undue handling of the tumour can result in secretion of catecholamines and wide dispersions in blood pressure. Once the tumour is devascularised a significant fall in catecholamines will occur and the patient's blood pressure may subsequently fall, requiring significant volume replacement and/or inotropes. Phaeochromocytomas can be diagnosed during a coincidental operation when, in the unblocked patient, characteristic rises in blood pressure and pulse and arrythmias may occur during induction of anaesthesia and in surgery (**Fig. 3.16**). If a surgeon

encounters an undiagnosed phaeochromocytoma at laparotomy no attempt should be made to remove this. The tumour should be handled as little as possible. The primary disease for which the laparotomy was indicated should be treated providing the patient is stable, and immediate blockade, work-up and subsequent elective removal of the phaeochromocytoma should be planned in the postoperative period. Surges in blood pressure during the operation can be controlled by the anaesthetist with agents such as nitroprusside. Full cardiac monitoring including the use of a Swan–Ganz catheter to measure cardiac output and epidural anaesthesia is advised, if an open approach to the phaeochromocytoma has been employed.

In the postoperative period the patient should be returned to a high-dependency or intensive care unit for regular monitoring of blood pressure and cardiovascular status. In addition, regular monitoring of the blood sugar is advised as the metabolic consequences of removing a phaeochromocytoma and a sudden reduction in circulating catecholamines include hypoglycaemia, which can on occasions be severe and profound. This is due to the sudden removal of the lipolytic, glycolytic and glycogenolytic effects of catecholamines that were produced by the phaeochromocytoma.

Phaeochromocytoma in pregnancy and in special circumstances

As mentioned above the removal of an adrenal tumour found coincidentally at laparotomy for some other reason is ill-advised in case it is a phaeochromocytoma. A profound fall in blood pressure and cardiovascular instability can occur in this setting, and it would be advisable to leave the tumour alone, investigate, block and remove it at a later date. Phaeochromocytoma in pregnancy is rare, but dangerous. There is a significant mortality both for the infant and the mother.[48] When the diagnosis is made during pregnancy it is customary to block the tumour with alpha blockade and then in the third trimester carry out a Caesarean section with or without a synchronous adrenalectomy. Vaginal delivery is contraindicated. Early operation after Caesarean section to deal with the phaeochromocytoma once the haemodynamics of pregnancy and raw area of the uterus has healed is another safe approach.

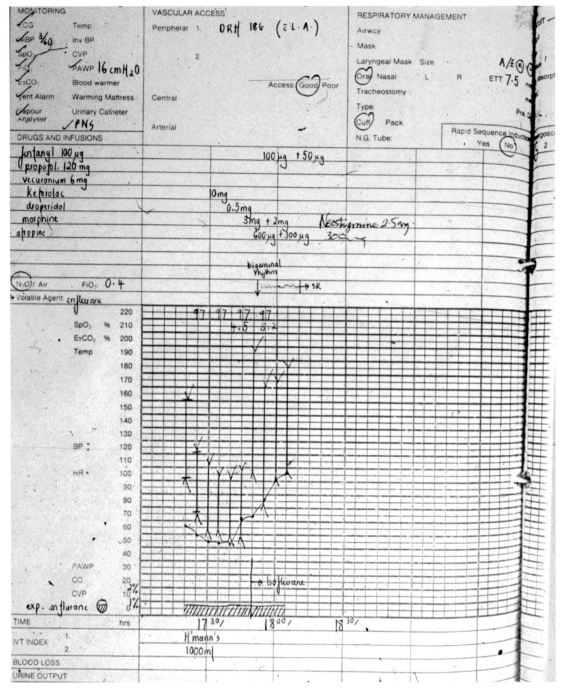

Figure 3.16 • Anaesthetic chart of patient undergoing general anaesthesia and surgery for melanoma, with an undiagnosed phaeochromocytoma.

In children the treatment and diagnosis are similar to the approach in adults, but awareness of inherited syndromes will be higher.[49]

Malignant phaeochromocytomas are difficult to diagnose on the basis of histopathology. All phaeochromocytomas show bizarre cellular arrangements within the tumour. They are highly vascular, and there are multiple mitotic figures – this applies equally to benign and subsequently proven malignant tumours. Frank invasion of local structures will of course increase the likelihood of a tumour being malignant (Fig. 3.10), as will demonstrable metastases. The treatment of distant or non-resectable local metastases is best dealt with by using radiolabelled MIBG.[46] External beam radiotherapy is unproven, but a variety of chemotherapeutic regimens can be tried, though no randomised control trials exist to inform the best choice of medication.

- Hypertension under the age of 40 years should prompt investigation.
- Phaeochromocytomas cause paroxysmal symptoms of catecholamine excess, often induced by stress.
- Overnight urinary and plasma levels of catecholamines and their metabolites wil confirm the diagnosis and are used in follow-up.
- These tumours are mostly benign (90%), sporadic (80%) and solitary (80%).
- Familial syndromes exist in patients with phaeochromocytomas in isolation or combined with other affected organs, endocrine and non-endocrine.
- Early involvement of genetics teams is important in all patients under the age of 45 years with phaeochromocytomas.
- Laparoscopic resection is the operation of choice for adrenal and some extra-adrenal tumours.
- Careful preoperative blockade of catecholamine excess is essential.

Primary aldosteronism (Conn's syndrome)

Primary aldosteronism is due to autonomous adrenal cortical tissue secreting excessive amounts of aldosterone. It presents as a result of investigations for hypertension or hypokalaemia.

Whilst a single benign adenoma of the adrenal cortex is the most common cause of primary hyperaldosteronism (**Fig. 3.17**), rarely the disease can be due to bilateral micronodular or macronodular hyperplasia of the zona glomerulosa of the adrenal gland. Exceptionally rare are aldosterone-secreting carcinomas of the adrenal and the so-called familial glucocorticoid-suppressible hyperaldosteronism

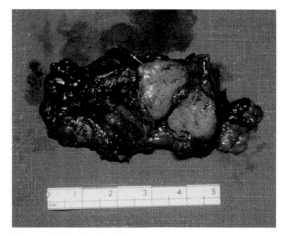

Figure 3.17 • Typical Conn's tumour.

syndrome, which is dominantly inherited. The anatomy and physiology of the adrenal cortex were reviewed at the beginning of the chapter, and it can be seen that aldosterone is the final common product of the pathway of hydroxylase enzymes converting pregnenolone into progesterone, corticosterone and ultimately aldosterone. Aldosterone produced by the zona glomerulosa controls the resorption of sodium by the distal renal tubules through the Na^+/K^+ and H^+ pumps. Along with the resorption of sodium (an active transport mechanism) water will follow, thus aldosterone will cause retention of water and an increase in the circulatory volume. The secretion of aldosterone is controlled primarily by angiotensin II, which in turn is generated through the activity of renin and angiotensin-converting enzyme on angiotensinogen. Renin, secreted from the juxtaglomerular apparatus of the kidney, is traditionally measured as well as aldosterone in reaching a diagnosis.[50] Aldosterone will also be increased by an increase in serum potassium concentration, and secondary hyperaldosteronism occurs in the presence of liver disease, cardiac failure and nephrotic syndrome. The feedback loop controlling renin and aldosterone secretion exists to regulate intravascular volume and electrolyte balance. Disturbance in the renin/aldosterone loop can be complex and the factors leading up to the onset of autonomous aldosterone production are varied.[51] In early disease more than half the patients with primary aldosteronism will have a normal circulating potassium level, and hence if this alone is used to diagnose the disease or lead to its investigation, a significant number of cases will be missed.

Indeed Jerome Conn, who first described hypertension caused by a benign adrenal cortical tumour in 1954, recognised that hypokalaemia was not present in all cases.[52] Selective venous sampling is the most accurate way of diagnosing the syndrome, by measuring aldosterone, cortisol and renin from the adrenal gland via a catheter in the inferior vena cava.[53] In cases of bilateral adrenal hyperplasia this will also allow the dominant side to be identified in case unilateral adrenalectomy is indicated. Using these more sensitive but invasive investigative tests, the incidence of Conn's syndrome in the population is approximately 5%. In addition the use of the fludrocortisone suppression test may also be helpful in confirming the diagnosis. In the experimental setting, there is a correlation between the in vitro release of aldosterone and cortisol and the expression of genes responsible for steroid-synthesising enzymes (hydroxylases). This enables confirmation that these tumours not only have the **potential** to secrete aldosterone but do so.[54]

All the hormonal assays described above must be performed without the influence of drugs that may affect the renin–angiotensin–aldosterone axis. Therefore spironolactone, ACE inhibitors and diuretics must be stopped several weeks before the assays are performed. Once the biochemistry is confirmed then localisation with CT scan and/or MRI can be performed. In cases where imaging is inconclusive or confusing, selective venous sampling (see above) may be helpful. Where possible iodocholesterol scanning may be a further imaging modality if there remains doubt, and it has been estimated that this has an 83% positive predictive value for the diagnosis of adenoma.[55] Once the diagnosis is confirmed and the disease localised, blood pressure and potassium where abnormal must be corrected prior to operative intervention. Single adenomas are eminently treated by surgery; nowadays most typically this will be laparoscopic (see below). In bilateral disease selective venous sampling may identify the dominant side, removal of which can significantly reduce medications. Patients with glucocorticoid-remediable hyperaldosteronism should be treated with steroids. A typical postoperative stay after laparoscopic surgery will be 1–3 days.[56] At best two-thirds of patients will be cured of their hypertension, and of those continuing with antihypertensives the vast majority will benefit from reduced medication requirement. The typical appearance of an adenoma is shown in Fig. 3.17.

Neuroblastoma

Neuroblastoma is a malignant tumour of childhood arising in the developing neuroendocrine system. Most (80%) produce abnormal levels of sympathetic amines. The incidence is 8–10 per million per year in children up to 15 years of age. It is the most common solid tumour in childhood and accounts for 10% of all paediatric malignancies, although it is the most frequent malignancy in children aged under 5 and has a median age at diagnosis of 2 years. Generally, the younger the child at presentation, the better the prognosis.[57]

Presentation

Most neuroblastomas present as an asymptomatic abdominal mass and may be very large, with any symptoms attributable to the organ that is being compressed. Twenty percent are in the posterior mediastinum rather than the abdomen, and rarely the tumour may present in the neck or pelvis. The tumour has usually metastasised by the time it is discovered, with the bone and bone marrow being the most commonly affected secondary sites.

Diagnosis

The primary tumour is usually confirmed by imaging – most commonly CT scan and/or MRI. The diagnosis requires histological confirmation, as the differential diagnosis includes other small-cell tumours including lymphoma and Ewing's sarcoma. Urinary catecholamines may be raised and urinary levels of VMA, HVA and dopamine will be elevated in 90% of patients. Infiltration of bone marrow produces classical pseudorosettes in the aspirate, and this may also be diagnostic. Skeletal metastases are detected with MIBG scans or a technetium scan. Various gene abnormalities have been identified with neuroblastomas. Amplification of the *MTCN* oncogene is associated with a poor prognosis. DDX1, NAG and N-cym have also been demonstrated to be co-amplified.[58]

Treatment

Neuroblastoma exists in three clinical patterns: non-metastatic loco-regional disease, metastatic disease, and the spontaneously regressing widespread disease (stage IVs). Treatment must be tailored to the type and stage of the tumour as well as the age of the patient. Surgical resection is most effective in low-stage tumours, but localised, operable tumours account for only 20% of neuroblastomas. In 20–25% the presentation is with disease that has spread beyond the midline, and is therefore inoperable.[59,60] Chemotherapy is the mainstay of treatment for these children, followed by surgery if the tumour has regressed sufficiently. For those children with disseminated disease at presentation, the outcome is poor if they are over 1 year old. Chemotherapy response rates have improved recently with the intensification of doses used. Multifocal disease (stage IVs) is most commonly found in children aged under 1 year and accounts for 5–10% of patients. Bizarrely, this small group of patients have a good long-term survival rate as spontaneous remission of the disease may occur after resection of the primary tumour.[61] Increased understanding of tumour biology should in future allow appropriate selection of therapies.[62]

Incidentaloma

Adrenal masses are found in approximately 1% of patients having cross-sectional imaging of the abdomen for a variety of indications. The incidence of adrenal tumours presenting as clinical problems is approximately 10 per million of the population so it is self-evident that more masses are found in the adrenal gland than produce symptoms, and thus a careful strategy is required to identify those that need intervention and investigation and those that can be safely ignored. Investigation and management of an incidental finding of an adrenal mass requires a thorough understanding of adrenal pathophysiology. Only a small percentage of such incidentally found tumours are found to be malignant (5%) and a further small percentage are metastases from an otherwise occult primary tumour.[63] Nevertheless, a significant number will be metastases from a known primary tumour, roughly one-third will be benign cortical adenomas (either functioning or non-functioning) and a further 5% will be phaeochromocytomas. Box 3.1 summarises the differential diagnosis of adrenal masses incidentally noted while imaging the abdomen. Initial assessment of a patient with an incidentaloma should start with

Box 3.1 • Differential diagnosis of adrenal masses incidentally noted while imaging the abdomen

Functional

Adrenal cortex

- Adenoma
- Nodular hyperplasia
- Carcinoma

Adrenal medulla

- Phaeochromocytoma
- Ganglioneuroma
- Ganglioneuroblastoma

Non-functional

Adrenal masses

- Myelolipoma
- Cyst
- Haematoma
- Hamartoma
- Amyloidosis
- Xanthomatosis
- Neurofibroma
- Teratoma
- Granulomatosis

Metastases

- Breast
- Lung
- Lymphoma
- Leukaemia

Pseudo-adrenal masses

- Lymph nodes
- Renal
- Splenic
- Pancreas
- Vessels

Imaging artefacts

the patient and not by focusing on the X-ray. Reflex biopsy and unconsidered investigation of coincidentally found adrenal masses can lead to disasters, and a careful strategy must be employed to elucidate the cause of the problem. Clinical examination should be carefully undertaken looking for evidence of Cushing's disease, hypertension, diabetes or any other symptoms that could be associated with pituitary–adrenal axis imbalance. A past medical history of malignant disease or a family history of endocrine disease should also be sought. Simple investigations, including a chest X-ray, urea and electrolyte estimation and a full blood count, may lead to a diagnosis, but if there is still no obvious cause for the abnormality then specialist endocrine investigations will be required.[64] These will include exclusion of a phaeochromocytoma by measuring urinary catecholamine excretion,[43] and exclusion of Cushing's syndrome through urinary cortisol levels, plasma cortisol levels and ACTH levels. These can, however, be insensitive tests in the setting of preclinical Cushing's syndrome. The gold standard for a diagnosis of autonomous cortisol production is the overnight dexamethasone suppression test (2 mg). Conn's syndrome may need to be considered (see above) and evidence of androgen secretion by the adrenal gland should be investigated by measuring serum testosterone levels and dehydroepiandrosterone sulphate (DHEA-S). If any of these investigations prove positive then appropriate treatment can be instituted. In a significant number of individuals, however, there will be no endocrine function of the adrenal mass and further investigation is required to elucidate the cause of the enlarged adrenal gland. In a patient with a history of malignant disease in the recent past, guided fine-needle aspiration biopsy may be helpful. Cells retrieved that resemble those of the original primary tumour can be diagnostic and save unnecessary surgery on occasions. In the absence of a history of previous malignant disease then fine-needle aspiration biopsy or core biopsy is generally unhelpful as the interpretation of primary adrenal pathology is difficult if not impossible in such small samples. Dynamic gadolinium-enhanced MRI may be helpful in predicting the status of adrenal masses,[65] but it is likely that a combination of CT scan, MRI and, where appropriate, fine-needle aspiration biopsy will identify the cause of the adrenal mass in the majority of cases[66] (Figs 3.6–3.9). In small (<3 cm), apparently benign non-functioning adrenal tumours a watch policy with serial CT scanning on a yearly basis seems safe.[67] In tumours over 3.5 cm the threshold for surgical removal is less because there appears to be a significant risk of malignancy in larger tumours.[68] Incidentalomas that are growing on serial scanning or in which there is any suspicion of malignancy should be removed surgically and the laparoscopic approach will usually be the preferred option.

The management of incidentalomas should be conducted in the context of a full endocrine work-up and should not be handled by surgeons, anaesthetists or physicians unfamiliar with the routine management of such patients. In this way the inadvertent operation on an unsuspected phaeochromocytoma or removal of an adrenal containing autonomous cortisol-secreting tissue resulting in postoperative Addison's disease can be avoided.

Addison's disease (adrenal insufficiency)

Adrenal insufficiency is most commonly caused by autoimmune adrenalitis or more rarely by pituitary disease resulting in failure of the hypothalamic–pituitary–corticotropic axis. In addition adrenal insufficiency can be caused by removal of overactive adrenal tissue and a failure to recognise hypofunction in a suppressed normal adrenal gland remaining on the contralateral side. The main presenting features of adrenal insufficiency include fatigue, anorexia and weight loss, and in the acute postoperative phase failure to wean off the ventilator, poor healing and hypotension.[69]

Glucocorticoid replacement therapy and mineralocorticoid replacement therapy are life saving, but clearly the disease must be recognised first. In addition to the above causes of adrenal insufficiency, therapeutic glucocorticoid administration will cause secondary adrenal insufficiency if steroid replacement therapy is withdrawn or not increased at times of stress. Adrenal infiltration by a secondary tumour or haemorrhage into the adrenal gland are rare causes of primary adrenal insufficiency, but in the context of disseminated malignancy, shock or other surgical interventions these must be borne in mind. The natural history, evolution and development of primary Addison's disease are lengthy and patients who are stressed by, for example, surgery can be tipped into full acute adrenal insufficiency.

Diagnosis

Concentrations of ACTH and cortisol vary throughout the day due to the diurnal rhythm. Random samples are therefore not generally helpful. Hence, the combined measurement of an early morning serum cortisol and plasma ACTH level is helpful. The short Synacthen test will expose an inability of the adrenal cortex to respond to ACTH. Serum cortisol levels are measured before and 30 or 60 minutes after intravenous or intramuscular injections of ACTH. In healthy individuals this will lead to an increase in serum cortisol to a level of >500 nmol/L. In patients who have primary adrenal failure the exogenous administration of extra ACTH will not normally produce any further increase in serum cortisol. Caution must be taken in interpreting these investigations in critically ill patients in whom the corticotropic axis is greatly activated. In this setting there is reduced sensitivity to dexamethasone and enhanced responses to ACTH and cortisol concentrations after the administration of corticotropin-releasing hormone. In settings where there is doubt about whether or not there has been acute adrenal failure, blood samples should be drawn to estimate ACTH and serum cortisol levels followed by the administration of exogenous glucocorticoid, pending the results of the blood work.

Adrenalectomy

The operation of adrenalectomy should never be commenced without a working diagnosis of the lesion, and in particular an assessment of its function. If an adrenalectomy is performed for an unrecognised phaeochromocytoma, then there is a high mortality rate. If an undiagnosed adenoma producing cortisol is excised, then a postoperative Addisonian crisis may ensue (see above). Preparation of patients prior to adrenalectomy is discussed in each section of this chapter. The operation should nearly always aim for total excision of the affected adrenal gland. Subtotal adrenalectomy in certain defined situations is an acceptable operation, particularly where the need to avoid steroid dependence is paramount (e.g. bilateral disease or when a contralateral adrenalectomy has been performed previously). Laparoscopic adrenalectomy has become accepted as the procedure of choice, and should be regarded as the norm for benign adrenal surgery. Benefits for patients from this approach have been widely reported, although a truly randomised trial has not been published. Most surgeons would choose to perform an open adrenalectomy for tumours with a high degree of suspicion for malignancy as open access to the major blood vessels may be essential but difficult if not impossible laparoscopically. The basic principles of adrenalectomy are the same for both the open and laparoscopic approaches to the glands; in each case the procedure is essentially the same, but with different access.

Open adrenalectomy

Open adrenalectomy has been the main means of access to the adrenal gland for many years. The first reported adrenalectomy was performed in 1889 by Thornton, who utilised a transabdominal approach. The first description of a phaeochromocytoma was in 1886, and the first successful adrenalectomy for phaeochromocytoma was performed in 1927 by Charles Mayo. Traditionally, three approaches have been used – transperitoneal, loin or posterolateral, and posterior. In addition a thoraco-abdominal approach may be needed for large tumours. The approach employed by the surgeon depends upon the size of the tumour, any invasion of surrounding tissues, bilateral disease, previous surgery and coexisting disease.

Anterior approach

This may be achieved with either a subcostal or midline incision – the advantage of the latter being that both glands can be more easily explored. Traditionally, phaeochromocytomas have been approached anteriorly, so that extra-adrenal or bilateral lesions can be excised. This has rather fallen into obsolescence as MIBG scans and better imaging with CT and MRI have improved preoperative detection and rendered this approach unnecessary. The main disadvantage of this approach is the morbidity associated with a major laparotomy. The blood loss, postoperative stay and operative time have all been shown to be higher with an anterior approach when compared with other open approaches (and especially when compared with laparoscopic approaches).

Loin approach

This is generally the most popular open approach to the adrenal gland and is widely accepted as the normal approach to the kidney. The patient is positioned in the lateral decubitus position with the table broken to open the space between the 12th rib and the iliac crest. An incision is made along the line of the 11th or 12th rib, which is then excised. The adrenal is exposed taking care to injure neither the pleura nor the peritoneum. This gives more limited exposure than an anterior approach, but better exposure than the posterior approach to the glands. Only one side can be operated upon, and if bilateral surgery is required the patient needs to be moved after completion of one side and repositioned.

Posterior approach

This gives the most direct access to the adrenals and both are able to be operated upon without moving the patient. This approach was initially described in 1936 by Hugh Young. It involves positioning the patient prone and flexing the back by jack-knifing the table. A near-vertical incision (moving slightly towards the iliac crest) is then made and the neck of the 12th rib divided (or completely excised) to expose the gland. The advantage of the posterior approach is that a bilateral adrenalectomy may be performed without moving the patient by the use of bilateral parallel incisions. Access is limited, however, particularly in the obese, and excision of tumours larger than 5 cm should not be attempted by this approach. This is frustrating as bilateral adrenalectomy is most commonly indicated in Cushing's syndrome, and these are the most obese patients and technically most difficult to approach in this way.

Thoraco-abdominal approach

This is indicated only for large malignant adrenal tumours as it provides the widest exposure to the adrenal and in particular its vessels and adjacent organs.[70]

Laparoscopic adrenalectomy

Laparoscopic adrenalectomy was initially described by Michel Gagner in 1992.[71] It has rapidly become widely accepted by surgeons, anaesthetists and patients, and should now be considered the standard technique for adrenalectomy.[72] It has been demonstrated to have lower blood loss, shorter hospital stay, faster return to normal daily activities and lower postoperative pain than open adrenalectomy, but a slightly longer operative time.[73–75] The intra-abdominal procedure is the same as in the open operation and there are three approaches in laparoscopic surgery as in open surgery: transperitoneal, lateral retroperitoneal and posterior retroperitoneal.

The approach chosen by the surgeon will depend upon his or her experience but certain factors should be taken into account when contemplating surgery. Any surgeon who is going to attempt a laparoscopic adrenalectomy should also be comfortable with the open procedure. The size of the tumour is important both for access by laparoscopic surgery[73] and for the risk of malignancy, which should be regarded as a relative contraindication to laparoscopic surgery.[76] Most surgeons would regard a tumour size of 6–10 cm as the upper limit for laparoscopic surgery, although Gagner will operate laparoscopically on tumours up to 15 cm in diameter.[77] Bear in mind that the duration of surgery is relative to the size of the tumour, and large tumours will require more surgical time and are more difficult dissections. Phaeochromocytoma is not a contraindication to laparoscopic surgery assuming the patient has been adequately prepared preoperatively.[78] Relative contraindications to laparoscopic adrenalectomy include a coagulopathy and previous surgery in the area (particularly nephrectomy and splenectomy). Conversion rates to the open approach are usually quoted as 5–10%.

Transperitoneal approach

This is the most commonly used approach to the adrenal glands laparoscopically. The patient is placed in the lateral decubitus position with the table jack-knifed to open the lumbar space between the ribs and the iliac crest (similar to the open loin approach). The patient is placed slightly head-up so irrigation fluid, the omentum and intra-abdominal contents will tend to fall away from the site of dissection. The operation can also be performed with the patient supine, although access to the adrenal will be more difficult. The advantage of the flank approach is that the organs act as their own retractors and gravity is used to facilitate access to retroperitoneal structures.

Left adrenalectomy

Once the patient has been correctly positioned, a 10- or 12-mm trocar is introduced into the peritoneal cavity under direct vision in the left subcostal space and the pneumoperitoneum is created. Two further subcostal ports are then placed under direct vision (**Fig. 3.18**). The splenic flexure is mobilised and the lienorenal ligament is divided. The spleen retracts forwards under gravity to allow entry into the retroperitoneum behind the lesser sac. The adrenal will be recognised superomedial to the kidney in the perinephric fat by its characteristic colour. The ease with which the adrenal gland is then dissected out of the fat depends upon the vascularity of the gland and density of the periadrenal fat. The dissection can be performed by diathermy or the use of a harmonic scalpel, for example Ace Harmonic (Ethicon J and J) (preferred by the authors). Care must be taken to ensure that the adrenal vein is

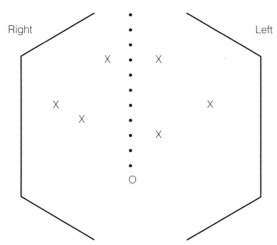

Figure 3.18 • Port sites for left and right laparoscopic adrenalectomy.

identified and is controlled. Adjacent organs must be protected from injury, particularly the spleen and the tail of the pancreas as it lies just in front of the adrenal gland. When freed from blood vessels and surrounding structures the adrenal gland is placed in a bag prior to removal from the abdomen.

Right adrenalectomy

Once the patient has been placed in the correct position, the trocars are introduced in a similar fashion as on the left side. A fourth trocar is more often required on the right to retract the liver. The right triangular ligament of the liver is divided to mobilise the liver, which allows retraction of the liver medially and good exposure of the space between the right adrenal and the inferior vena cava. The peritoneum below the liver and overlying the adrenal gland is then divided above and medial to the right kidney. Once the gland has been identified by its characteristic colour, it is dissected from the surrounding tissue. It is advisable to dissect the superior pole of the adrenal first, so that the gland remains attached to the kidney and does not migrate further away from the dissection point and upwards.

Again, great care must be taken to ensure that the adrenal vein is identified and controlled prior to division from the vena cava.

Retroperitoneal approach

The retroperitoneal approach is similar to the traditional open loin approach to the adrenal gland. It is less widely used than the transperitoneal approach in the UK. The surgeon positions the patient in the same lateral decubitus position as for an open or transperitoneal approach. A port is placed under direct vision through the muscles in the subcostal plane and into the retroperitoneal tissue. A balloon is then inflated to create a space. This balloon may be either passed down the port and then inflated, or some ports are produced with the balloon attached as an integral part of the port itself. This approach is limited as the space provided is smaller, and thus the size of the adrenal that can be removed may be more restricted. Bleeding may be more difficult to control and hypercapnoea and surgical emphysema are more likely to occur. However, it has been claimed that postoperative pain control is better and the duration of hospital stay is shorter.

Posterior retroperitoneal approach

Again, the patient is positioned in the same position as for the open posterior approach, i.e. prone with the table jack-knifed. Three ports are used for each side, in a line in the subcostal plane. This has the same advantages and disadvantages in comparison with the open posterior approach as the laparoscopic loin approach has compared with the open loin approach.[Reference Martin Walz?]

In conclusion, the different techniques that are available all have their supporters.[79] The laparoscopic approach to the adrenal gland is now considered the 'gold standard' technique for benign tumours. Different surgeons use different techniques, but no approach has been demonstrated as yet to have significantly better results in all hands.

Key points

- Adrenal function is essential to sustain normal healthy life.
- Adrenal malfunction is rare.
- Tumours of the adrenal can be functioning or non-functioning, benign or malignant.
- Via the negative-feedback loop cortisol overproduction by one adrenal will suppress the contralateral gland.
- Functioning or familial syndromes must be excluded before removing any adrenal gland.
- Most adrenal pathology can be safely and optimally removed by the laparoscopic route.

References

1. Young MB, Hughes IA. The response to treatment of congenital adrenal hyperplasia in infancy. Arch Dis Child 1990; 65:441–4.

2. Merke DP, Bornstein SR, Avila NA et al. NIH conference. Future directions in the study and management of congenital adrenal hyperplasia due to 21-hydroxylase deficiency. Ann Intern Med 2002; 136:320–4.

3. Van Wyk JJ, Ritzen EM. The role of bilateral adrenalectomy in the treatment of congenital adrenal hyperplasia. J Clin Endocrinol Metab 2003; 88:2993–8.

4. Clutter WE. Cushing's syndrome; hypercortisolism. In: Doherty GM, Skogseid B (eds) Surgical endocrinology. Philadelphia: Lippincott Williams & Wilkins, 2001; p. 237.

5. Ross EJ, Lynch CD. Cushing's syndrome: killing disease. Lancet 1982; ii:64–9.

6. Cushing H. The basophil adenomas of the pituitary body and their clinical manifestations (pituitary basophilism). Bull Johns Hopkins Hosp 1932; 50: 137–95.

7. Wajchenberg BL, Mendonca BB, Liberman B et al. Ectopic ACTH syndrome. Endocr Rev 1994, 15:752–87.

8. Delisle L, Boyer MJ, Warr D et al. Ectopic corticotropin syndrome and small-cell carcinoma of the lung: clinical features, outcome and complications. Arch Intern Med 1993; 153:746–52.

9. Limper AH, Carpenter PC, Scheithauer B et al. The Cushing syndrome induced by bronchial carcinoid tumours. Ann Intern Med 1992; 117:209–14.

10. Young WF, Carney JA, Musa BU et al. Familial Cushing's syndrome due to primary pigmented nodular adrenocortical disease. N Engl J Med 1989; 321:1659–64.

11. Samuels MH, Loriaux DL. Cushing's syndrome and the macronodular adrenal gland. Endocrinol Metab Clin North Am 1994; 23:555–69.

12. Crapo L. Cushing's syndrome: a review of diagnostic tests. Metab Clin Exp 1979; 28:955–77.

13. Orth DN. Cushing's syndrome. N Engl J Med 1995; 332:791–803.

14. Newell-Price J, Trainer P, Besser M et al. The diagnosis and differential diagnosis of Cushing's syndrome and pseudo-Cushing's states. Endocr Rev 1998; 19:647–72.

15. Icard P, Goudet P, Charpenay C et al. Adrenocortical carcinomas: surgical trends and results of a 253-patient series from the French Association of Endocrine Surgeons Study Group. World J Surg 2001; 25:891–7.

16. Copeland PM. The incidentally discovered adrenal mass. Ann Intern Med 1983; 98:940.

17. Prager G, Heinz-Peer G, Passler C et al. Can dynamic gadolinium-enhanced magnetic resonance imaging with chemical shift studies predict the status of adrenal masses? World J Surg 2002; 26:958–64.

18. Katznelson L, Bogan JS, Trob JR et al. Biochemical assessment of Cushing's disease in patients with corticotroph macroadenomas. J Clin Endocrinol Metab 1998; 83:1619–23.

19. Dichek HL, Nieman LK, Oldfield EH et al. A comparison of the standard high-dose dexamethasone suppression test and the overnight 8 mg dexamethasone suppression test for the differential diagnosis of ACTH-dependent Cushing's syndrome. J Clin Endocrinol Metab 1994; 78:418–22.

20. Zovickian J, Oldfield EH, Doppman JL et al. Usefulness of inferior petrosal sinus venous endocrine markers in Cushing's disease. J Neurosurg 1988; 68:205–10.

21. Oldfield EH, Doppman JL, Nieman LK et al. Petrosal sinus sampling with and without corticotropin-releasing hormone for the differential diagnosis of Cushing's syndrome. N Engl J Med 1991; 325:897–905.

22. Findling JW, Doppman JL. Biochemical and radiological diagnosis of Cushing's syndrome. Endocrinol Metab Clin North Am 1994; 23:511–37.

23. Nagesser SK, van Seters AP, Kievit J et al. Long-term results of total adrenalectomy for Cushing's disease. World J Surg 2000; 24:108–13.

24. Sarkar R, Thompson W, McLeod MK. The role of adrenalectomy in Cushing's syndrome. Surgery 1990; 108:1079–84.

25. Moore TJ, Dluhy RG, Williams GH et al. Nelson's syndrome: frequency and effect of prior pituitary irradiation. Ann Intern Med 1976; 85:731.

26. Nagesser SK, Kievit J, Derksen J et al. Autologous adrenal transplantation for Cushing's disease. In: Clark OH, Duh QY (eds) Textbook of endocrine surgery. Philadelphia: WB Saunders, 1997; pp. 506–11.

27. Aniszewski JP, Young WF, Thompson GB et al. Cushing's syndrome due to ectopic adrenocorticotropic hormone secretion. World J Surg 2001; 25:934–40.

28. Wooten MD, King DK. Adrenal cortical carcinoma. Epidemiology and treatment with mitotane and a review of the literature. Cancer 1993; 72: 3145–55.

29. Mighell AJ, High AS. Histological identification of carcinoma in 21-gauge needle tracks after fine-needle aspiration biopsy of head and neck carcinoma. J Clin Pathol 1998; 5:241–3.

30. Lee MJ, Hahn PF, Papanicolau N et al. Benign and malignant adrenal masses: CT distinction with

attenuation coefficients, size and observer analysis. Radiology 1991; 179:415–418.

31. Gross MD, Wilton GP, Shapiro B et al. Functional and scintigraphic evaluation of the silent adrenal mass. J Nucl Med 1987; 28:1401–7.

32. Terzolo M, Angeli A, Fassnacht M et al. Adjuvant Mitotane treatment for adrenocortical carcinoma. N Engl J Med 2007; 356:2372–80.

33. Ahlman H, Khorram-Manesh A, Jansson S et al. Cytotoxic treatment of adrenocortical carcinoma. World J Surg 2001; 25:927–33.

34. Pommier RF, Brennan MF. An eleven-year experience with adrenocortical carcinoma. Surgery 1992; 112:963–71.

35. Venkatesh S, Hickey RC, Sellin RV et al. Adrenal cortical carcinoma. Cancer 1989; 64:765–9.

36. Madani R, Al-Hashmi M, Bliss R et al. Ectopic phaechromocytoma: does the rule of tens apply? World J Surg 2007; 31(4):849–54.

37. Kebebew E, Duh Q-Y. Benign and malignant phaeochromocytoma. Diagnosis, treatment and follow up. Surg Oncol Clin North Am 1998; 7:765–89.

38. St John Sutton MG, Sheps SG, Lie TJ. Prevalence of clinically unsuspected phaeochromocytoma: review of a 50 year autopsy series. Mayo Clin Proc 1981; 56:354–60.

39. Williams DT, Dann S, Wheeler MH. Phaeochromocytoma – views on current management. Eur J Surg Oncol 2003; 29:483–90.

40. Richard D, Beigelman C, Dudas J-M et al. Phaeochromocytoma as the first manifestation of Von Hippel–Lindau disease. Surgery 1994; 116:1076–108.

41. Woodward ER, Eng C, McMahon R et al. Genetic predisposition to phaeochromocytoma: analysis of candidate genes GDNF, RET, and VHL. Hum Molec Genet 1997; 6:1051–6.

42. Astuti D, Douglas F, Lennard TWJ et al. Germline SDHD mutation in familial phaeochromocytoma. Lancet 2001; 357:1181–2.

43. Peaston RT, Lennard TWJ, Lai LC. Overnight excretion of urinary catecholamines and metabolites in the detection of phaeochromocytoma. J Clin Endocrinol Metab 1996; 81:1378–84.

44. Prys-Roberts C, Farndon JR. Efficacy and safety of doxazocin for perioperative management of patients with phaeochromocytoma. World J Surg 2002; 26:1037–42.

45. Sibal L., Jovanovic A, Agarwal SC et al. Phaeochromocytomas presenting as acute crises after beta blockade therapy. Clin Endocrinol (Oxf) 2006; 65(2):186–90.

46. Bouloux PG, Fakeeh M. Phaeochromocytoma. In: Sheaves R, Jenkins PJ, Wass JH (eds) Clinical endocrine oncology. Blackwell Science, 1988; pp. 299–305.

47. Trimmers HJLM, Kozupa A, Chen CC et al. Superiority of FDG PET to other functional imaging techniques in the evaluation of metastatic SDHB associated phaeochromocytoma and paraganglioma. J Clin Oncol 2007; 25(16):2262–9.

48. Dreier DT, Thompson NW. Phaeochromocytoma and pregnancy: the epitome of high risk. Surgery 1993; 114:1148–52.

49. Hume DM. Phaeochromocytoma in the adult and in the child. Am J Surg 1960; 99:458.

50. Hiramatsu K, Yamada T, Yukimura Y et al. A screening test to identify aldosterone producing adenoma by measuring plasma renin activity. Arch Intern Med 1981; 141:1589.

51. Gordon RD, Stowasser M, Rutherford JC. Primary aldosteronism: are we diagnosing and operating on too few patients? World J Surg 2001; 25:941–7.

52. Conn JW. Plasma renin activity in primary aldosteronism: importance in differential diagnosis and in research of essential hypertension. JAMA 1964; 190:222.

53. Melby JL, Spark RF, Dale S et al. Diagnosis and localization of aldosterone producing adenomas by adrenal vein catheterization. N Engl J Med 1967; 277:1050.

54. Enberg U, Farnebo LO, Wedell A et al. In vitro release of aldosterone and cortisol in human adrenal adenomas correlates to mRNA expression of steroidogenic enzymes for genes CYP 11 B2 and CYP 17. World J Surg 2001; 25:957–66.

55. Wheeler MH, Harris DA. Diagnosis and management of primary aldosteronism. World J Surg 2003; 27:627–31.

56. Harris DA, Au-Yong I, Basnyat PS et al. Review of surgical management of aldosterone secreting tumours of the adrenal cortex. Eur J Surg Oncol 2003; 29:467–74.

57. Hayes FA, Smith EI. Neuroblastoma. In: Pizzo PA, Poplack DG (eds) Pediatric oncology, principles and practice. Philadelphia: JB Lippincott, 1989; pp. 607–22.

58. Scott D, Elsden J, Pearson A et al. Genes coamplified with MYCN in neuroblastoma: silent passengers or co-determinants of phenotype? Cancer Lett 2003; 197:81–6.

59. De Bernardi B, Conte M, Mancini A et al. Localised resectable neuroblastoma: results of the second study on the Italian Co-operative Group for neuroblastoma. J Clin Oncol 1995; 13:884–93.

60. Garaventa A, De Bernardi B, Pianca C et al. Localised but unresectable neuroblastoma: treatment and outcome of 145 cases. J Clin Oncol 1993; 11:1770–9.

61. De Bernardi B, Milanaccio C, Occhi M. Neuroblastoma. In: Sheaves R, Jenkins PJ, Wass JAH et al. (eds) Clinical endocrine oncology. Oxford: Blackwell Scientific Publications, 1997; pp. 306–11.

62. Brodeur GM. Neuroblastoma: biological insights into a clinical enigma. Nature Rev 2003; 3:203–16.

63. Lumachi F, Borsato S, Tregnaghi A et al. CT scan, MRI and image guided FNA cytology of incidental adrenal masses. Eur J Surg Oncol 2003; 29:689–92.

64. Ross NS, Aron OC. Hormonal evaluation of the patient with an incidentally discovered adrenal mass. N Engl J Med 1990; 323:1401–5.

65. Prager G, Heinz-Peer G, Passler C et al. Can dynamic gadolinium-enhanced magnetic resonance imaging with chemical shift studies predict the status of adrenal masses? World J Surg 2002; 26:958–64.

66. Patel HRH, Harris AM, Lennard TWJ. Adrenal masses: the investigation and management of adrenal incidentalomas. Ann R Coll Surg Engl 2001; 83:250–2.

67. Siren J, Tervahartiola P, Sirula A et al. Natural course of adrenal incidentalomas: seven year follow up study. World J Surg 2000; 24:579–82.

68. Kjellman M, Larsson C, Backdahl M. Genetic background of adrenocortical tumour development. World J Surg 2001; 25:948–56.

69. Arlt W, Allolio B. Adrenal insufficiency. Lancet 2003; 361:1881–93.

70. Prinz RA, Falimirski. Operative approaches to the adrenal glands. In: Clark OH, Duh QY (eds) Textbook of endocrine surgery. Philadelphia: WB Saunders, 1997; pp. 529–34.

71. Gagner M, Lacroix A, Bolte E. Laparoscopic adrenalectomy in Cushing's syndrome and phaeochromocytoma. N Engl J Med 1992; 327:1003.

72. Gagner M. Laparoscopic adrenalectomy. Surg Clin North Am 1996; 76:523–37.

73. Prinz RA. A comparison of laparoscopic and open adrenalectomies. Arch Surg 1995; 130:489–94.

74. Dudley NE, Harrison BJ. Comparison of open posterior versus transperitoneal laparoscopic adrenalectomy. Br J Surg 1999; 86:656–60.

75. Duh QY, Siperstein AE, Clark OH et al. Laparoscopic adrenalectomy: comparison of the lateral and posterior approaches. Arch Surg 1996; 131:870–5.

76. Henry JF, Sebag F, Iacobone M et al. Result of laparoscopic adrenalectomy for large and potentially malignant tumours. World J Surg 2002; 26:1043–7.

77. Gagner M, Pomp A, Heniford BT et al. Laparoscopic adrenalectomy: lessons learned from 100 consecutive procedures. Ann Surg 1997; 226:238–46.

78. Gagner M, Breton G, Pharand D et al. Is laparoscopic adrenalectomy indicated for phaeochromocytomas? Surgery 1996; 120:1076–80.

79. Lezoche E, Guerrieri M, Feliciotti AM et al. Anterior, lateral and posterior retroperitoneal approaches in endoscopic adrenalectomy. Surg Endosc 2002; 16:96–9.

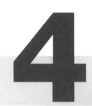

Familial endocrine disease: genetics, clinical presentation and management

Stephen G. Ball
Paul Brennan
Tom W.J. Lennard

Introduction

The diagnosis and management of familial endocrine syndromes epitomises the complex and changing interface between surgery, medicine and molecular genetics. The last decade has seen an explosion in our understanding of the molecular basis of these rare syndromes, and the rapid translation of research-based findings into clinical practice. As a result, we are already witnessing genetic testing leading to highly effective, targeted intervention. The next decade is likely to see continued progress, with expansion and refinement of molecular diagnostics and further integration of these developments into clinical practice.

This chapter will cover the genetics, presentation and management of a range of conditions relevant to endocrine surgical practice. This is a complex clinical area, one that encompasses several professional boundaries and the interface between paediatric and adult medicine. A coordinated and integrated approach is essential.

Multiple endocrine neoplasia type 1 (MEN 1)

MEN 1 is an autosomal dominant familial syndrome characterised by the development of multiple and metachronous endocrine and non-endocrine tumours (Table 4.1). Approximately 10% of cases arise de novo, without a prior family history of the syndrome.[1] The precise prevalence of MEN 1 is unclear. This in part reflects variability in disease expression, even though penetrance may be high. The hallmark features of MEN 1 are endocrine tumours of the pituitary, pancreas and parathyroid.

Genetics

MEN 1 is associated with heterozygous germline loss of function mutations in the *MEN1* gene located on chromsome 11q13.[2] Endocrine tumours from patients with MEN 1 demonstrate loss of heterozygosity for the MEN 1 locus, indicating that tumour formation is dependent on the development of a second somatic mutation in the wild-type allele. *MEN1* therefore acts as a tumour suppressor gene. Heterozygous *MEN1* mutant mice develop tumours mimicking the human phenotype.[3] The *MEN1* gene encodes a 67-kDa protein – menin – which has multiple functional domains (**Fig. 4.1**).

The functions of menin

Menin can influence a number of key cellular processes including transcription, DNA repair and cytoskeletal function. Menin is known to bind several signalling proteins including JunD and Smad3. Recent data have highlighted menin's role in the

Table 4.1 • Clinical features of multiple endocrine neoplasia type 1 (MEN 1)

Tumour/site*	Hormonal/ other characteristics*
Parathyroid adenoma (90%)	
Enteropancreatic islet tumour (30–80%)	NF (80%) Gastrinoma (40%) Pancreatic polypeptidoma (20%) Insulinoma (10%) Glucagonoma VIPoma Somatostatinoma ACTHoma (rare) GRFoma (rare)
Anterior pituitary tumour (10–60%)	Prolactinoma (20%) NF (6%) GHoma (5%) ACTHoma (2%)
Foregut carcinoid	Gastric ECL tumour (10%) Thymic carcinoid (2–8%) Bronchial carcinoid (2%)
Adrenocortical tumour	Non-functioning adenoma (25%) Adrenocortical carcinoma (rare) Hyperaldosteronism (rare)
Cutaneous manifestations	Lipoma (30%) Angiofibroma (85%) Collagenoma (70%)

*Values in parentheses are estimates of penetrance of given characteristic at age 40.
ACTH, adrenocorticotropin; ECL, enterochromaffin-like; GH, growth hormone; GRF, growth hormone-releasing factor; NF, non-functioning; VIP, vasoactive intestinal peptide.

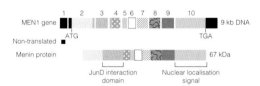

Figure 4.1 • Schematic representation of *MEN1* gene and menin protein, indicating functional domains of menin protein.

regulation of key developmental genes through influences on histone methylation.[4,5]

Some patients and families manifest MEN 1 but do not have demonstrable mutations in the *MEN1* gene on gene sequencing. There are several potential explanations for this phenomenon:

- Mutation in a non-coding region of the *MEN1* gene regulating gene expression (e.g. promoter).
- Presence of a whole exon deletion or duplication. Most mutation searching strategies now include an exon dosage assay.
- Disease mediated though an alternative MEN 1 locus.
- Phenocopy – this refers to the chance co-occurrence of two or more features of MEN 1, one of which is usually primary hyperparathyroidism.

A normal *MEN1* gene sequence analysis should therefore not be taken as excluding the disease. Gene dosage studies will help to clarify how many cases of apparently mutation-negative MEN 1 are due to germ-line hemizygosity for the *MEN1* gene.

MEN 1 exhibits two classical characteristics of genetic disease: variable penetrance (not all mutation carriers develop the disease) and variable expressivity (those who do develop the disease can manifest in different ways). Not all features of MEN 1 will occur in a single patient or indeed a single family. Some families exhibit only hyperparathyroidism.[1] There is considerable variation in age-related tumour penetrance and no clear genotype–phenotype correlation. It is therefore difficult to predict with any degree of accuracy the natural history of MEN 1 in an individual or and within a family.[6]

Presentation

Presentation is dependent upon the herald lesion. More than one component may be apparent at presentation.

Primary hyperparathyroidism

Primary hyperparathyroidism (PHP) is the most common endocrinopathy in MEN 1, and is thought to be present in at least 90% of cases aged 50 years or over. It is also the most common initial clinical expression of MEN 1, with typical detection or presentation in the third decade of life, significantly earlier than that found in sporadic PHP. Patients with MEN 1 generally have asymmetric, independent parathyroid adenomas in three to four glands. PHP often recurs following subtotal parathyroidectomy. PHP can exacerbate coexistent hypergastrinaemia from gastrinoma.

Enteropancreatic islet tumours

The prevalence of enteropancreatic islet tumours in patients with MEN 1 may be as high as 80%, although the majority of such tumours are clinically silent and non-functional. Functional tumours can present in the second decade of life. Many asymptomatic patients have radiologically detectable tumours by the third decade. Tumours can arise throughout the pancreas and the duodenal submucosa. They are commonly multicentric, metachronous, and range in size and characteristics from micro- and macroadenomas to invasive and metastatic carcinoma. The prognosis of these tumours may relate to specific somatic molecular changes.[7]

Up to 40% of patients with MEN 1 develop gastrinoma, and current data suggest that up to 25% of all patients with gastrinoma have MEN 1. Though presentation with invasive or metastatic disease is unusual before 30 years of age, metastatic disease (possibly occult) can be present in up to 50% of MEN 1-associated gastrinoma at diagnosis. The presence of multiple, discrete gastrinomas can be mistaken for local disseminated disease. Tumours secreting pancreatic polypeptide are manifest biochemically and radiologically, but are generally clinically silent.[8]

Pituitary tumours

The prevalence of pituitary tumours in MEN 1 is uncertain, due to the range of patients and methods employed in the majority of studies to date. A large European multicentre study of 324 patients with MEN 1 found pituitary tumours in 42% of cases.[9] The most common pituitary lesion is prolactinoma. There are few prospective data on age-related penetrance of pituitary disease. However, MEN 1-associated pituitary macroadenoma has occurred as early as 5 years of age.[10]

Foregut carcinoids

MEN 1-associated foregut carcinoid tumours are found in the thymus, stomach and bronchi. They are not generally hormonally active, and do not present with carcinoid syndrome. Their true prevalence is unclear. Gastric enterochromaffin-like (ECL) tumours are generally discovered at endoscopy. They exhibit loss of heterozygosity at the *MEN1* gene locus and are promoted by hypergastrinaemia. Thus, they generally arise in MEN 1 patients with gastrinoma. They can regress with normalisation of gastrin levels after surgical excision of gastrinoma.[11] Thymic carcinoid disease has been highlighted as a major cause of mortality in MEN 1. However, relatively little is known about its natural history.

A prospective study of 85 patients with MEN 1 found an incidence of 8% over a mean follow-up period of 8 years.[12] Patients were all male, and most had no symptoms of the tumour at the time of detection. Interestingly, 4 of 7 of the tumours did not show somatic loss of heterozygosity at the *MEN1* locus, raising questions as to the mechanism of tumour development. Serum chromogranin A was elevated in 6 of 7 tumours. Mean time interval between diagnosis of MEN 1 and development of thymic carcinoid was 19 years. It may be that as early mortality reduces in MEN 1 due to improved surgical and medical treatment, this relatively late expression of the disease increases in prevalence and impact.

Adrenocortical tumours

Adrenocortical disease occurs in 20–40% of patients with MEN 1. It is unusual in patients who do not have pancreatic disease. Pathology may include diffuse hyperplasia, solitary adenoma and carcinoma.[13] Disease can be bilateral. Excess hormone secretion is rare, and the majority of lesions are detected on routine radiological monitoring.[14]

Cutaneous manifestations

A variety of cutaneous pathologies are now firmly established as components of MEN 1. Cutaneous lipomas are often nodular and multicentric. Visceral lipomas have also been described. Cutaneous manifestations of MEN 1 are useful clinically in the presymptomatic diagnosis of MEN 1 in affected families.[15]

Diagnosis

A diagnosis of MEN 1 is considered in any patient presenting with two synchronous or metachronous tumours in the three characteristic sites (pituitary, pancreas and parathyroid). If there is a first-degree relative with a lesion typical of MEN 1, the diagnosis should be considered in the presence of a single lesion. Patients with recurrent PHP, especially multiglandular disease, should have the diagnosis excluded.

The application of diagnostic DNA analysis has altered the phenotypic spectrum of MEN 1, revealing both asymptomatic individuals and those with atypical phenotypes. DNA analysis does not always provide answers, however, as illustrated by phenocopies: the association of an endocrine tumour that has a low population prevalence – such as growth hormone (GH)-secreting pituitary tumour – with PHP could represent MEN 1 or MEN 1 phenocopy. Recent data suggest that mutations in the *MEN1* coding region are infrequent in those patients without a family history of MEN 1 who develop this combination of endocrinopathies.[16] Absence of a *MEN1* mutation may therefore be difficult to interpret, particularly if the patient is young and there is no supportive family history.

Management

MEN 1 is associated with premature death, most commonly (30%) through metastatic islet cell tumours.[17] Advances in the medical management of gastrinoma and hyperparathyroidism may result in a paradoxical increase in cumulative morbidity from other facets of the condition in the coming decade. The principal organs involved in MEN 1 are difficult to screen for early tumours, and prophylactic surgery is either not appropriate or has not been shown to prevent the development of tumour (cervical thymectomy).[12] The challenge is therefore to improve morbidity and mortality through targeted surgical and medical interventions as directed by surveillance and molecular screening programmes that aim to detect disease expression at an early stage in an inclusive manner.[18]

Primary hyperparathyroidism

PHP in MEN 1 is characterised by asynchronous involvement of all parathyroid glands. However, there remains debate as to the optimum type and timing of parathyroid surgery. Subtotal parathyroidectomy for PHP in MEN 1 is associated with a surgical cure rate (as defined by the number of patients not hypercalcaemic) of 60% at 10 years and 51% at 15 years.[19] The alternative, total parathyroidectomy with or without autograft, is associated with postoperative hypoparathyroidism and lifelong treatment with vitamin D analogues. Preoperative imaging and minimally invasive approaches may be difficult because of the need to examine all four glands. Transcervical thymectomy is recommended at the time of parathyroidectomy.

Enteropancreatic islet tumours

Enteropancreatic tumours in MEN 1 are often multiple, recurrent and heterogeneous in behaviour. Correct management requires the correlation of symptoms, hormonal and imaging studies (which may be discordant) and experience in the natural history of the pathology. This can pose a significant challenge to the clinician.

Surgery is the main treatment for patients with insulinoma in MEN 1 (**Figs 4.2 and 4.3**). All other syndromes of hormone excess due to enteropancreatic tumours respond well to medical therapy with proton-pump inhibitors (gastrinoma) or somatostatin analogues (VIPoma). The timing of surgery in the management of these conditions is debated.

Gastrinomas in MEN 1 are often multifocal and small, and can be situated in the duodenum. Extensive pancreato-duodenal surgery can be associated with significant morbidity. Surgery for gastrinoma in MEN 1 is frequently not curative, in part due to the multifocal nature of the problem.[20] Furthermore, metastatic disease is found at surgery in a substantial number of patients in whom it is not apparent preoperatively.[21] Nevertheless, the outcome of patients treated surgically for locally

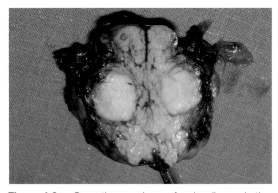

Figure 4.2 • Operative specimen of an insulinoma in the tall of the pancreas, bisected.

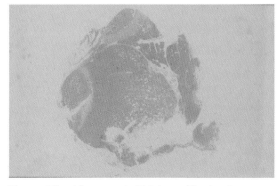

Figure 4.3 • Macroscopic histology of the insulinoma in Fig. 4.2.

advanced disease can be the same as those with limited disease. Indeed, there are data that demonstrate that surgery is beneficial in increasing disease-related survival and decreasing advanced disease in Zollinger–Ellison syndrome.[22]

A subset of MEN 1 patients with gastrinoma has aggressive disease and decreased survival.[23] Features associated with aggressive tumour behaviour include:

- diagnosis of MEN 1 before 35 years of age;
- onset of gastrinoma at 27 years or younger;
- markedly elevated gastrin levels at presentation;
- tumour size greater than 3 cm.

Aggressive antitumour treatment in this group needs to be considered.

Non-functioning enteropancreatic islet cell tumours and those secreting pancreatic polypeptide are generally clinically silent. There is no consensus as to best treatment in this situation. Some advocate surgical removal if the lesion is greater than 3 cm or growing on serial radiological monitoring, while others suggest excision as a preventive measure in the absence of data suggestive of aggressive behaviour.

The standard surgical approach other than for gastrinoma is spleen-preserving distal pancreatectomy (**Fig. 4.4**) and intraoperative bidigital palpation, coupled with intraoperative ultrasound and enucleation of any tumour found in the pancreatic

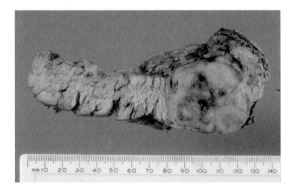

Figure 4.4 • Spleen-preserving distal pancreatectomy specimen, showing a large neuroendocrine tumour in the body of the pancreas.

head and duodenal submucosa. Surgery for gastrinoma should include duodenotomy.[24] A Whipple procedure may be considered for tumours at the pancreatic head. Preoperative localisation of the target lesion with corroborative intraoperative ultrasound is useful in planning the appropriate approach. This can be important in the management of functional tumours as the pancreas and duodenum may contain multiple abnormalities, leading to uncertainty as to which of several lesions is the source of excess hormone production. Surgery prompted by abnormal biochemistry but in the absence of any scan-detected lesion should be considered to prevent malignant transformation of microadenomas. Distal 80% subtotal pancreatectomy should be considered for risk modification in any patient undergoing surgery for localised islet-cell tumour in MEN 1.[25]

Pituitary tumours

Pituitary tumours should be managed in the same manner as in isolated pituitary disease. Prolactinomas should be treated with dopamine agonists, with biochemical and radiological confirmation of response. Normalisation of prolactin levels without tumour shrinkage suggests misdiagnosis of a non-functioning pituitary adenoma with secondary hyperprolactinaemia. Non-functioning tumours should be treated with surgery. GH-secreting adenomas are best treated with primary surgery followed by consideration of external beam radiotherapy and somatostatin analogue therapy for persistent disease.[15]

Foregut carcinoids

The optimum management of this generally late expression of MEN 1 is unclear. Resection of bronchial carcinoid is usually required to make the diagnosis. Long-term follow-up is then required to check for recurrence. The natural history and malignant potential of ECL-like gastric carcinoids is unclear. Thymic carcinoid tumours are generally asymptomatic when detected through radiological screening, and can behave aggressively. Relapse is common after surgery, and the optimum adjuvant medical and radiotherapeutic approaches are not yet established.[12]

Screening

The multiple and metachronous nature of endocrine tumours associated with MEN 1 requires lifelong clinical, biochemical and radiological surveillance to detect MEN 1-associated tumour expression as soon as possible, minimising morbidity and optimising outcome. Genetic testing supports this process, facilitating the identification of both individuals within a kindred who will benefit from such long-term surveillance and those who do not require it.

Genetic

MEN1 gene analysis, involving sequencing of all coding exons of the *MEN1* gene, should be offered to patients with MEN 1 to help in determining biochemical and radiological screening strategies for their relatives. Analysis may also be helpful in those patients with atypical presentations, but only if an MEN 1-defining mutation is found. Identification of an *MEN1* mutation in an index case should lead to a screening cascade for the same mutation within the family, beginning with first-degree relatives. Given that 25% of all patients with gastrinoma have MEN 1, genetic testing should be considered in patients presenting with gastrinoma, even in the absence of other features.

 Absence of *MEN1* coding region mutations does not necessarily exclude MEN 1, and should trigger promoter and exon dosage studies if the index of suspicion of MEN 1 is sufficient. If these prove negative in a family with suspected MEN 1, linkage studies may be appropriate.

Biochemical and radiological

Biochemical and radiological screening should be offered to all patients with a diagnosis of MEN 1, to asymptomatic relatives found to harbour an MEN 1-defining *MEN1* mutation on genetic testing, and to those found to be at risk through haplotype and linkage studies (Table 4.2). First-degree relatives of those patients with MEN 1 in whom an *MEN1* mutation has not been found should also be offered screening pending the outcome of promoter and exon dosage analyses. Biochemical and radiological screening should commence in early childhood, balancing age-dependent penetration, sensitivity of specific studies in specific age groups and the inconvenience caused by the process. Screening should be lifelong for those patients with MEN 1, those known to harbour MEN 1-defining *MEN1* mutations, and those defined as 'at risk' by haplotype and linkage studies. It should continue to the age of 50 in those kindreds in whom no genetic risk stratification is possible.

Gastrin levels are elevated in primary (atrophic) and secondary (drug-induced) achlorhydria, which can lead to false-positive screening tests for the disease. Ideally, treatment with H_2 antagonists and proton-pump inhibitors should be stopped for 2 and 4 weeks respectively before assessment of gastrin levels. However, gastrin levels in the normal range do not exclude gastrinoma, and there should be a low threshold for complementary corroborative gastric acid studies.

Table 4.2 • Outline programme for biochemical and radiological screening for MEN 1

Tumour type	Investigation	Age commencing (years)	Frequency
Parathyroid adenoma	ICa²⁺, PTH	8	Annual
Enteropancreatic islet cell	Gastrin	20	Annual
	Glucose, insulin	5	Annual
	VIP, PP	20	Annual
	Glucagon	20	Annual
	Somatostatin	20	Annual
	MRI	20	3- to 5-yearly
Anterior pituitary	Prolactin	5	Annual
	IGF-1		Annual
	MRI		5-yearly
Foregut carcinoid	Chromogranin A	20	Annual
	MRI	20	3- to 5-yearly

Choice of radiological imaging modality may vary with local resources and expertise.

ICa^{2+}, ionised Ca^{2+}; IGF-1, insulin-like growth factor 1; PP, pancreatic polypeptide; PTH, parathyroid hormone; VIP, vasoactive intestinal polypeptide.

Multiple endocrine neoplasia type 2 (MEN 2)

MEN 2 is an autosomal dominant familial cancer syndrome characterised by the metachronous development of medullary thyroid cancer (MTC), phaeochromocytoma and PHP. Overall penetrance of the disease is high in gene carriers although that of individual characteristics is varied. MEN 2 is subclassified into several discrete forms with clinical, pathological and molecular correlates:

- MEN 2A – MTC (90%), phaeochromocytoma (50%) and PHP (20–30%).
- MEN 2A with cutaneous lichen amyloidosis.
- MEN 2A with Hirschsprung's disease (HD).
- Familial medullary thyroid cancer (FMTC) – at least 10 or more carriers or affected cases of MTC in a kindred over the age of 50 with no clinical or detectable evidence of other features of MEN 2.
- FMTC with HD.
- MEN 2B – MTC, phaeochromocytoma, decreased upper/lower body ratio, marfanoid habitus, gastrointestinal and mucosal ganglioneuromatosis.

MEN 2B is the most aggressive form, MTC presenting at a younger age and often with more advanced disease. Historically, the majority of MEN 2B cases represent de novo mutations without a family history of the condition. Earlier diagnosis and improved management strategies may result in a change in this picture over the next 20 years.

MEN 2A shows variable penetrance. Approximately 40% of gene carriers develop clinical manifestations by age 50 and 60% by age 70. Biochemical screening can lead to earlier identification of gene carriers: approximately 90% of individuals with MEN 2A have biochemical abnormality by age 30 even if there are no overt signs of MEN 2A.

Genetics

MEN 2 is associated with heterozygous gain of function mutations in the *RET* gene found on Ch10q11.2. The *RET* gene codes for a membrane-associated tyrosine kinase with two extracellular cadherin-like domains (EC) and two, independent intracellular tyrosine kinase (TK) domains (**Fig. 4.5**). RET protein is expressed by a range of neuroendocrine cell types including the adrenal medulla, thyroid C-cells and parathyroid. In normal physiology, extracellualr signals lead to RET dimerisation triggering TK domain phosphorylation and a downstream signal transduction cascade leading to cell growth and differentiation. Gain of function mutations found in MEN 2 produce constitutive activation of the RET signal transduction cascade outwith normal control processes.[26,27]

In contrast to MEN 1, there is a partial genotype–phenotype correlation in MEN 2. For the majority of families with MEN 2A and FMTC the mutations in *RET* affect cysteine residues in the extracellular domain of the RET protein. The exact position of the cysteine residue involved by any particular mutation affects the likelihood of the phenotype being either MEN 2A or FMTC. Virtually all mutations in MEN 2A are found in exons 10 and 11 of the *RET* gene. For FMTC, mutations may be found in exons 13–15 as well as some in exons 10 and 11. For MEN 2B, 95% have a mutation in exon 16 (codon 918), at a site that is prone to somatic mutation in sporadic MTC (**Fig. 4.6**).[8] There are data to suggest that there may be additional modifying factors, such as key *RET* single nucleotide polymorphisms (SNPs), that impact on disease expression within a given

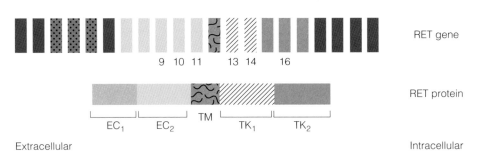

Figure 4.5 • Schematic representation of *MEN2* gene and RET protein, highlighting domain structure of RET protein.

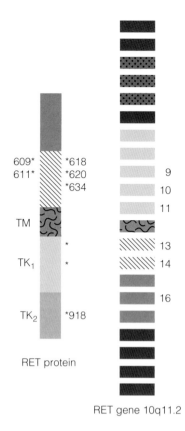

609* *618
611* *620
      *634

TM

TK₁

TK₂ *918

RET protein

9
10
11

13
14

16

RET gene 10q11.2

- MEN2A: RET mutation 95%
  exon 10 c609, 611, 618, 620
  exon 11 c634 (80–90% MEN2A)

- MEN2B: RET mutation 95–98%
  exon 16 c609
  exon 15 c883

- FMTC: RET mutation 85%
  MEN2A mutations
  exon 13 c768
  exon 14 c804

Figure 4.6 • Schematic representation of RET protein, highlighting mapping of common mutation hotspots in MEN 2 to functional domains.

a genotype. These may be particularly relevant in the situation of *RET* mutations that result in relatively weak constitutive activation.[28,29]

Loss of function mutations in *RET* have been demonstrated in some kindreds with familial Hirschsprung's disease. In contrast to the mutation hotspots noted in MEN 2, these mutations are distributed throughout the gene.

Because MEN 2 can manifest in childhood it is important to undertake predictive testing at an early age to help management decisions. Genetic testing should be offered to patients presenting with apparently sporadic medullary carcinoma of thyroid. It is possible to test for specific *RET* mutations in the tumour itself. Somatic *RET* codon 918 mutations are found at moderate frequency in sporadic tumours. Confirmation of this mutation in tumour tissue and its absence in germ-line DNA (consistent with a somatic event) may help in establishing a case of MTC as sporadic. If DNA testing is to be offered, it is important that issues of consent are addressed carefully in view of the potential consequences of identifying germ-line *RET* mutations for both the individual and other family members.

Presentation

Presentation of MEN 2A can be with any specific feature of the condition. MEN 2B can present with additional signs or complications of ganglioneuromatosis (mucosal or gastrointestinal) prior to the development or recognition of an endocrinopathy. Some families present only with MTC.

Medullary thyroid cancer

MTC has been the first manifestation of MEN 2 in most kindreds. It can present in the first decade of life with intrathyroidal, locally advanced or disseminated disease. Historically, MTC has been the major cause of morbidity and mortality in MEN 2. Current management approaches will alter this natural history (see later). MTC in MEN 2 is preceded by C-cell hyperplasia. Recent data have highlighted a 6.6-year window between development of MTC and progression to nodal metastases in MEN 2A patients harbouring the most common (codon 634) *RET* mutation.[30]

Phaeochromocytoma

Phaeochromocytoma can be unilateral or bilateral. Presentation can be with symptoms as in sporadic disease or as the result of positive surveillance studies. Phaeochromocytoma in MEN 2 can present in the first decade of life.

Primary hyperparathyroidism

PHP occurs in 20–30% of patients with MEN 2A, and is more common in those with RET_{634} mutations. Most patients are asymptomatic. PHP associated with MEN 2 is often less severe than that encountered in MEN 1, and synchronous involvement of all four glands is less common.

Management

Medullary thyroid cancer

New cases of MEN 2 presenting with MTC should be treated by thyroidectomy with central or more widespread node dissection depending on pre- and perioperative staging. Thyroidectomy for MEN 2B should include central node dissection. However, the aim of surgical management encompasses and is focused increasingly on prevention of MTC. Surgery for MTC in MEN 2 should be performed before the age at which malignant progression occurs.[31] Historically this decision was based on basal and stimulated levels of the hormone calcitonin, produced by C-cells of the thyroid and a valuable tumour marker for MTC. However, this approach has an unacceptable sensitivity and specificity. Decisions on the timing of thyroidectomy in new cases of MEN 2 without apparent MTC at presentation (such as those cases detected through genetic screening) should follow a stratified approach based on the genotype–phenotype relationships linking specific *RET* mutations with a specific natural history of MTC. Such an approach balances the earliest age at which MTC can present in association with a given *RET* genotype against the potential surgical morbidity of thyroidectomy at a young age (**Fig. 4.7**).

Patients are assigned to one of three risk bands:

- **Risk level 1** – all patients with MEN 2B; patients with *RET* mutations involving codons 883, 918 and 922.
- **Risk level 2** – patients with *RET* mutations involving codons 611, 618, 620 and 634.
- **Risk level 3** – patients with *RET* mutations involving codons 609, 768, 790, 791, 804 and 891.

Patients in risk level 1 should undergo thyroidectomy in the first year of life, and preferably in the first 6 months of life. Those in risk level 2 should undergo thyroidectomy before the age of 5 years. There is no consensus on the optimum approach to patients in risk level 3. MTC presents at an older age in this group, and is commonly less aggressive. Recent data suggest that thyroidectomy need not take place before the age of 10 years, and that central node dissection is unnecessary before 20 years. The cumulative experience on which such recommendations are based remains limited.[30,32]

Accumulating experience suggests that a relatively conservative approach, involving serial monitoring, may be appropriate for some families harbouring 'milder' *RET* mutations.[33] Some have proposed that this approach can be supported by using serial pentagastrin stimulation tests to assist decision-making on the timing of surgery.[34]

Persistence of elevated calcitonin levels following primary surgery should trigger radiological staging with computed tomography (CT) or magnetic resonance imaging (MRI). [111]In pentetreotide scanning can detect somatostatin receptor-positive disease. Fluorodopamine positron emission tomography (PET) is an additional sensitive modality for detection of occult recurrent MTC.[35] Local recurrent or residual disease is the most common cause of persistently elevated tumour markers following primary treatment. In the absence of widespread distant disease, re-operation should be considered. If more distant metastatic disease is found, repeat surgery for tumour debulking should be considered for control of local pressure symptoms or those due to humoral factors secreted by the tumour.

Standard chemotherapy regimens are not particularly effective in the management of systemic metastatic disease. Novel agents targeting angiogenesis and components of the RET signalling pathway

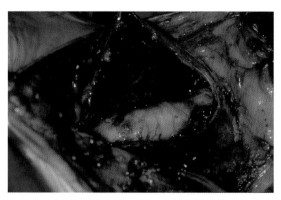

Figure 4.7 • Operative view at the conclusion of a prophylactic thyroidectomy for MEN 2B in a child aged 18 months.

may prove to be beneficial in patients with disseminated disease.[36] External beam radiotherapy can be used for the palliative treatment of bone metastases. However, metastatic MTC can remain asymptomatic, and conservative approaches to management coupled with regular biochemical surveillance of tumour load can result in good quality of life for many years.

Phaeochromocytoma

The principles of diagnosis and intervention should be similar to those applied to sporadic disease (see Chapter 3). However, it is important to exclude active phaeochromocytoma in any patient with suspected or established disease prior to surgical intervention for a separate or linked condition, in early pregnancy and prior to labour.

 Analysis of timed overnight urine metanephrines, together with plasma metanephrines, provides the highest degree of sensitivity and specificity in biochemical diagnostic and surveillance programmes.[37] Plasma metanephrines alone may generate significant false-positive screening data. Positive biochemistry should trigger appropriate imaging studies with MRI, supported by radionuclear imaging if necessary.

Primary hyperparathyroidism

The principles of diagnosis and indications for intervention should be similar to those in sporadic PHP; although all four glands may not be enlarged, the approaches to surgery should be similar too. If enlarged parathyroid glands are encountered at the time of thyroidectomy in a patient who is eucalcaemic, the approach should be the same as if the patient were known to have mild PHP.

Screening

Genetic

 Germ-line RET mutation analysis is accurate, effective and widely available. Routine testing should include analysis of exons 10, 11, 13, 14, 15 and 16. Testing should be offered to the following groups:

- new patients presenting with two synchronous or metachronous features of MEN 2;
- patients presenting with a single manifestation of MEN 2 who have a first-degree relative with an endocrine feature of MEN 2;
- infants presenting with gastrointestinal or mucosal features of MEN 2B;
- patients presenting with MTC;
- infants presenting with Hirschsprung's disease and a family history suggestive of MTC.

First-degree relatives of those patients diagnosed with RET mutations should be offered predictive genetic testing. In a family in which the clinical suspicion of MEN 2 is high and in which no RET mutation is identified, more detailed genetic studies may be helpful in confirming association of the disease with the RET locus and in risk assessment. Such situations are unusual in MEN 2A. Absence of RET mutations have been described in up to 16% of families with apparent FMTC. Though patients presenting with apparent sporadic phaeochromocytoma should be considered for genetic screening, pick-up of RET mutations is very low.[15,38] Failure to detect an RET mutation in cases of apparently sporadic MTC leaves a small possibility that the patient has MEN 2, placing their offspring at risk. This can be defined using Bayes' theorem and the prevalence of germ-line RET mutations in apparent sporadic isolated MTC found in cohort studies (taken as the prevalence of MEN 2 in such cohorts). If there is only one case of MEN 2-associated disease in a kindred of moderate size, the chance of missing a diagnosis of RET mutation-negative familial disease is low.

Biochemical

All patients with MEN 2 or those identified as RET mutation carriers but yet to express the disease should have annual biochemical screening for endocrine components of the syndrome to detect new or recurrent disease:

- MTC – plasma calcitonin, carcinoembryonic antigen.
- Phaeochromocytoma – timed overnight urine metanephrines, plasma metanephrines.
- PHP – ionised Ca^{2+}, parathyroid hormone.

In the high-risk groups (risk levels 1 and 2) biochemical screening should commence at the time of planning thyroidectomy. In remaining patients it should commence between the ages of 5 and 7 years. Catecholamine screening can be difficult in young children. Phaeochromocytoma has not been found in association with certain RET mutations involving codons 609, 768, 804 and 891. It is premature to omit catecholamine screening in these groups, though reduced surveillance frequency can be considered. Positive screening data should trigger appropriate imaging studies and intervention.

Familial hyperparathyroidism (FHP) syndromes

FHP without other features of endocrinopathy has been described extensively. However, advances in our understanding of the calcium receptor and its physiology, the recognition of additional phenotypes found in association with FHP, and the increased application of molecular diagnostics have led to the recognition that many cases may be manifestations of wider syndromes.[39,40]

Presentation

Familial hypocalciuric hypercalcaemia (FHH) and neonatal severe hyperparathyroidism (NSHP)

FHH is inherited as an autosomal dominant condition, and is characterised by lifelong mild to moderate hypercalcaemia that is generally asymptomatic, and normal-range values of parathyroid hormone (PTH). FHH generally presents following detection of hypercalcaemia on routine testing, or on family screening of individuals with a family history. Calcium concentrations are consistent within a kindred. Although pancreatitis has been described as a complication of FHH, most patients in whom it has occurred have had additional risk factors. Renal excretion of calcium and magnesium are characteristically reduced, and the urine calcium:creatinine ratio is less than 0.01 in 80% of cases. The diagnostic value of the urine calcium:creatinine ratio is reduced in patients taking lithium and thiazide diuretics, both of which can reduce calcium excretion, and in mild PHP with concurrent vitamin D deficiency.

NSHP presents in the first week of life with anorexia, constipation, hypotonia and respiratory distress. There is severe hypercalcaemia (total calcium concentration 3.5–7.7 mmol/L), often with hypermagnesaemia. PTH can be significantly elevated. Skeletal radiology shows demineralisation and typical features of severe hyperparathyroidism. As NSHP can result from homozygous or compound heterozygous inheritance of FHH alleles, there may be a history or biochemical evidence of FHH in one or both parents. However, NSHP can arise as a result of a de novo germ-line mutation in a child with normal parents.

Familial hyperparathyroidism–jaw tumour syndrome (FHP-JT)

FHP-JT describes the association of autosomal dominant familial hyperparathyroidism with ossifying tumours (fibromas) of the mandible and maxilla.[41] Polycystic kidney disease has also been described in families with this condition. Hyperparathyroidism presents as in sporadic cases. Jaw and maxillary tumours can be occult, and may only be apparent on screening by orthopantogram. The gene responsible for this condition (*HRPT2*) has been mapped to chromosome 1q21–31, and parathyroid tumours from patients with this condition show loss of heterozygosity at this locus. Increased awareness of this condition has led to its recognition as the underlying problem in kindreds previously thought to have isolated familial hyperparathyroidism.[42] Both somatic and germ-line mutations in *HRPT2* have been identified in patients with apparently sporadic parathyroid carcinoma, suggesting that some patients with this unusual tumour may represent a phenotypic variant of hyperparathyroidism–jaw tumour syndrome (HPT-JT).[43]

Familial isolated hyperparathyroidism (FIHP)

FIHP is an autosomal dominant disorder characterised by uniglandular or multiglandular hyperparathyroidism in the absence of other endocrine disease and without evidence of jaw tumours. Recent data suggest that at least 20% of kindreds thought to have FIHP have inactivating mutations in *MEN1*, suggesting that a significant proportion of FIHP may represent a distinct variant of MEN 1.[1] Further analysis of the *MEN1* promoter (to exclude promoter region mutations) and exon dosage may increase this proportion. Whether more intensive surveillance will detect other features of MEN 1 in these kindreds over time remains unclear.[15] FIHP in some kindreds may thus be a prelude to MEN 1, a distinct variant of MEN 1, or the result of a mutation in a different gene.

Management

Parathyroid surgery should be avoided in FHH, as the hypercalcaemia persists after parathyroidectomy. Efforts should therefore be made to exclude this diagnosis in all patients presenting with hypercalcaemia. Once FHH is diagnosed, it should be treated conservatively without intervention. Appropriate counselling as to the risk of NSHP in offspring should be given. Genetic testing for specific calcium receptor mutations may be useful in certain situations.

NSHP is managed by rigorous rehydration, inhibition of bone resorption with bisphosphonates, and respiratory support in the initial phase. Failure to respond should lead to total parathyroidectomy in the first month of life. Milder forms of the disease may stabilise with medical therapy alone, with progression to a phase resembling FHH after several months.

Hyperparathyroidism in patients with FHP-JT syndrome and FIHP should be managed surgically in the same manner as sporadic disease. Family members should be offered biochemical screening for hyperparathyroidism and radiological screening for mandibular and maxillary tumours. Hypercalcaemic patients with a family history of multiglandular hyperparathyroidism should be offered total parathyroidectomy. Affected members of apparent FIHP kindreds should be offered genetic testing for *MEN1* gene mutations and an orthopantogram. Additional studies of other members of affected kindreds can be considered if a positive diagnosis of an alternative syndrome (MEN 1 or FHP-JT) is found in an index case.

Familial non-medullary thyroid cancer syndromes

Cowden's syndrome and Bannayan–Zonana syndrome

Cowden's syndrome (CS) is an autosomal dominant inherited cancer syndrome characterised by the development of multiple hamartomas (benign tumours comprised of disorganised elements of a particular organ) in multiple systems derived from all three germ-cell layers, together with a predisposition to breast and non-medullary thyroid cancer. Other features are macrocephaly, mild to moderate learning difficulties and occasionally Lhermitte–Duclos disease (LDD), which is an unusual condition of cerebellar ganglion cell hypertrophy, causing ataxia and seizures. Gene carriers may suffer from a variety of thyroid disorders: adenomatous goitre, hypothyroidism or hyperthyroidism and thyroid cancer.[44] Females with CS can also suffer from benign breast disease, and the incidence of breast cancer is high – approximately 25–30%. Most cases of CS are likely to be sporadic, with estimates of familial cases ranging from 10% to 50%.

The International Cowden Syndrome Consortium has defined operational criteria for the diagnosis of CS (Box 4.1). In the absence of a family history of CS, a diagnosis can be made on mucocutaneous findings alone if any of the following criteria are met:

- six or more facial papules of which at least three are trichilemmoma;
- facial papules and oral mucosal papillomatosis;
- oral mucosal papillomatosis and acral keratoses;
- the presence of at least six palmoplantar keratoses.

In the absence of a family history and mucocutaneous signs, a diagnosis of CS can be made if two major criteria (at least one of which is macrocephaly or LDD) or one major together with three minor

Box 4.1 • International Cowden Syndrome Consortium operational criteria for the diagnosis of Cowden syndrome, 1996

Pathognomonic criteria (mucocutaneous lesions)
- Facial trichilemmomas
- Acral keratoses
- Papillomatous papules
- Mucosal lesions

Major criteria
- Breast carcinoma
- Thyroid carcinoma
- Macrocephaly greater than 97th centile
- Lhermitte–Duclos disease (LDD)

Minor criteria
- Thyroid adenoma or multinodular goitre
- Mental retardation
- GI hamartomas
- Fibrocystic disease of the breast
- Lipomas
- Hamartomas
- Reproductive tract tumours or malformation (e.g. uterine fibroadenomas)

criteria are present. If there is a family history of CS, the diagnosis can be made if the pathognomonic mucocutaneous criteria are present; a single major criterion is present; or two minor criteria are present.

Expression of CS is varied. Penetrance is age-dependent, increasing from less than 10% under the age of 20 years to nearly 100% for cutaneous stigmata by the third decade. Thyroid abnormalities occur in 50–67% of CS patients, with 3–10% of patients developing thyroid cancer (generally follicular).

Bannayan–Zonana syndrome (also called Ruvalcaba–Mhyre–Smith or Bannayan–Riley–Ruvalcaba syndrome) is an autosomal dominant condition characterised by intestinal polyps, haemangiomas and lipomas, café-au-lait patches on the penis and macrocephaly.[45] Other features are breast cancer, lipid storage disorder, protein-losing enteropathy and thyroid disease including thyroid cancer. CS and Bannayan–Zonana syndrome have both been shown to be caused by mutations in *PTEN*. There are some reports of both occurring in the same family and presumably due to the same mutation.[46] It is not understood why penetrance and expression of mutations in *PTEN* can be so variable.

Function of *PTEN*

The *PTEN* gene codes for a protein tyrosine phosphatase. *PTEN* expression blocks cell cycle progression in the G1 phase.[47] *PTEN* mutation testing remains an area of research and the usefulness of testing in the clinical setting remains uncertain. Currently, for the vast majority of families, diagnosis of both CS and Bannayan–Zonana syndrome is based on clinical findings.

Presentation

A diagnosis of CS may be made in a patient presenting with thyroid disease (in the presence of other stigmata or relevant history), or may develop in a patient known to have CS who is under endocrine surveillance.

Management

Patients presenting with a thyroid abnormality (goitre or nodule) should be investigated and managed along standard lines. Once a diagnosis of CS has been made, individuals and affected relatives should have endocrine screening with thyroid palpation as part of an annual medical review. The value of routine ultrasound surveillance of the thyroid has not been established. If a family-specific mutation has been identified, screening of other family members for that mutation is of value. If such a mutation cannot be identified and the family fit the criteria established for the diagnosis of CS, predictive testing based on analysis of the *PTEN* gene is not possible. If the family in question is sufficiently large, linkage studies can be considered. The prevalence of germ-line mutations in *PTEN* in kindreds with a high incidence of thyroid cancer but without other criteria for the diagnosis of CS is less than 2%.

Familial papillary thyroid cancer

Between 3% and 13% of patients with papillary thyroid cancer (PTC) have a relative affected by the disease. A small proportion of these patients are members of a kindred in which the PTC is inherited in an autosmal dominant pattern. While somatic rearrangements of RET are a consistent finding in these tumours, the genetic basis for familial clustering and autosomal dominant inheritance is unclear. In keeping with other tumour predisposition syndromes, the disease can be multifocal.

Management

It has been suggested that when two or more family members are identified with PTC, first- and second-degree relatives should be screened clinically for the disease. The onset, frequency, optimum duration, role of ultrasound screening and ultimate cost-effectiveness of this approach remain to be established. Because the disease can be multifocal, total thyroidectomy rather than hemithyroidectomy is recommended when PTC is suspected in this context.

Familial adenomatous polyposis

Genetics

Familial adenomatous polyposis (FAP; also sometimes referred to as Gardner's syndrome) is an autosomal dominant disorder characterised by the occurrence of multiple gastrointestinal adenomatous polyps in association with osteomas, epidermoid cysts, desmoid tumours and retinal pigmentation. Hepatoblastomas and adenomas of the upper gastrointestinal tract and pancreas are more unusual components of the syndrome. Expression is variable, though the disease is usually penetrant in the third decade. FAP is associated with an increased risk of thyroid neoplasia, particularly for women. However, the risk is sufficiently low (affecting approximately 1% of those with FAP) that apart from an awareness of the risk it is unnecessary to organise a screening programme of the thyroid gland.[15] There is some evidence of familial aggregation of thyroid cancer in FAP. For rare families who demonstrate such aggregation it is important to raise awareness and consider screening. FAP is caused by mutations in the *APC* gene.

Presentation

As with CS, a diagnosis of FAP may be made in a patient presenting with thyroid disease or be made in a patient known to have FAP who is undergoing endocrine surveillance.

Management

The role of clinical and/or ultrasound surveillance remains to be established.[48] As disease can be multicentric, total thyroidectomy should be considered as an option for primary surgery in those FAP patients who develop thyroid disease.

Familial non-MEN 2 phaeochromocytoma

Patients presenting with apparent sporadic phaeochromocytoma and functional paraganglioma have a 15–28% prevalence of germ-line mutations in genes predisposing to the disease.[38] These data have informed a change in the management of phaeochromocytoma/functional paraganglioma. Clinical genetics should now be an integral part of the multidisciplinary process.

von Hippel–Lindau (VHL) disease

VHL disease is an autosomal dominant familial syndrome characterised by the metachronous development of multiple benign and malignant tumours. It may occur in an individual as the result of a new mutation. Incidence is of the order of 1 in 40 000 and there is variable penetrance and expression.[49] Key features are central nervous system haemangioblastoma, renal cell carcinoma and phaeochromocytoma. A number of additional lesions are recognised (Table 4.3).

Genetics

VHL disease results from a germ-line mutation in the *VHL* tumour suppressor gene situated at the chromosomal locus 3p25–26 (**Fig. 4.8**) The products of the *VHL* gene (a 213-amino-acid, 18-kDa protein; and a truncated 160-amino-acid, 18-kDa protein arising from an alternative translational start site) are important components in the pathway targeting intracellular proteins for degradation via proteasomes as part of the integrated cellular response to hypoxia. The tumours seen in VHL disease are vascular with pronounced angiogenesis. Their cells exhibit over-expression of vascular endothelial growth factor (VEGF). Production of VEGF is mediated by

Table 4.3 • Clinical characteristics of von Hippel–Lindau (VHL) disease: age at presentation and frequency of expression

Tumour	Age at presentation (years)	Frequency of expression (%)
Retinal haemangioblastoma	1–67	25–60
Cerebellar haemangioblastoma	9–78	44–72
Brainstem haemangioblastoma	12–46	10–25
Spinal cord haemangioblastoma	12–66	13–50
CNS haemangioblastoma (miscellaneous)		<1
Renal cell carcinoma or cysts	16–67	25–60
Phaeochromocytoma	5–58	10–20
Pancreatic tumour or cysts	5–70	35–70
Endolymphatic sac tumours	12–50	10
Epididymal cystadenoma	Unknown	25–60
Broad ligament cystadenoma	Unknown	Unknown

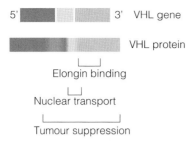

Elongin binding

Nuclear transport

Tumour suppression

Figure 4.8 • Schematic representation of *VHL* gene and VHL protein, highlighting functional domains of the protein.

a pathway of hypoxia detection involving the VHL protein and the elongin complex. Many hypoxia-inducible genes are controlled by hypoxia-inducible factor (HIF). HIF is composed of an α subunit and a β subunit. The HIF α subunit is degraded if oxygen is present; this requires functioning VHL protein.

VHL disease has been divided into four subtypes on the basis of clinical presentation, as depicted in Box 4.2. To date, endolymphatic sac tumours and cystadenomas of the epididymis and broad ligament have not been assigned to a specific disease subtype. Within this classification there is evidence of genotype–phenotype correlation. Patients with type 1 VHL disease are most likely to have deletions or premature termination mutations. Those with type 2 VHL disease are more likely to have missense mutations.[50] Expression of subtype phenotype tends

Box 4.2 • Subtypes of von Hippel–Lindau disease according to clinical presentation

Type 1
- Retinal haemangioblastoma
- CNS haemangioblastoma
- Renal cell carcinoma
- Pancreatic tumours and pancreatic cysts

Type 2a
- Phaeochromocytoma
- Retinal haemangioblastoma
- CNS haemangioblastoma

Type 2b
- Phaeochromocytoma
- Retinal haemangioblastoma
- CNS haemangioblastoma
- Renal cell carcinoma
- Pancreatic tumours and pancreatic cysts

Type 2c
- Phaeochromocytoma only

to be consistent within a given family. Mutations in *VHL* are found in the majority of families with VHL disease.

Presentation

VHL disease has two major endocrine manifestations: phaeochromocytoma and pancreatic islet-cell tumours.[51]

Phaeochromocytoma associated with VHL disease is pathologically distinct from that occurring as part of MEN 2. Tumours have a thick vascular capsule, and contain small to medium-sized tumour cells interspersed with multiple small blood vessels. There is no evidence of adrenomedullary hyperplasia outwith the tumour, as can be found in MEN 2.[52] Clinical presentation of phaeochromocytoma is similar to that in sporadic and other familial forms. However, compared with tumours associated with MEN 2, patients presenting with phaeochromocytoma as part of VHL disease have fewer symptoms. This clinical observation correlates with lower tumour catecholamine content and reduced expression of tyrosine hydroxylase.[53] Increasingly, presentation is with asymptomatic disease detected through routine biochemical and radiological screening. Tumours can be multiple and extra-adrenal.

Diagnosis

Diagnosis of phaeochromocytoma in VHL disease follows the principles established in sporadic and other forms of familial disease: clinical suspicion, biochemical testing and radiological localisation. Phaeochromocytoma associated with VHL disease has a predominantly noradrenergic phenotype. Urine catecholamine excretion can be normal, as can plasma metanephrines. A combination of elevated plasma normetanephrines together with normal plasma metanephrines is highly suggestive of VHL-associated phaeochromocytoma.[53] Localisation of biochemical disease can employ MRI, CT and radioisotope scanning.[37] Adrenal and extra-adrenal masses detected on routine radiological surveillance for renal cell carcinoma should trigger appropriate testing to exclude phaeochromocytoma, with initial biochemical testing followed by further complementary radiological or radioisotope studies.

Treatment

Surgical and non-surgical treatments for phaeochromocytoma in VHL disease follow the same principles as outlined in sporadic and other forms of the tumour (see Chapter 3).

Surveillance and screening

Patients with VHL disease type 2 require annual biochemical screening for phaeochromocytoma with a combination of urine and plasma meta-nephrines and normetanephrines. Elevated screening tests should trigger verification of the result, and then appropriate localisation studies with MRI followed by radioisotope scanning if data are equivocal. Use of MRI in this context reduces lifetime radiation exposure in the context of regular screening for renal and pancreatic disease.

Index cases should be offered genetic testing. These data may help to guide subtype classification and will enable cascade of predictive genetic testing within the wider family. *VHL* gene analysis should form part of the assessment of patients with apparent sporadic phaeochromocytoma,[38] although the genotype–phenotype correlation is not robust enough to enable the broader phenotype to be predicted with accuracy in those patients found to have *VHL* mutations. Comparisons of the relative effectiveness of molecular and clinical approaches in this situation are required.

Pancreatic neuroendocrine tumours in VHL disease

Pancreatic neuroendocrine tumours associated with VHL disease are usually detected during radiological surveillance (CT and MRI). Though they may demonstrate immunopositivity for a variety of pancreatic hormones and neuroendocrine markers, they are clinically silent. Endoscopic ultrasound and ^{111}In-labelled somatostatin scintigraphy can be helpful in differentiating neuroendocrine tumours from pancreatic cysts and cystadenomas, which also occur in VHL disease. Surgical excision has been recommended on the following bases:

1. absence of metastatic disease;
2. tumour larger than 3 cm in the body or tail of the pancreas;
3. tumour larger than 2 cm in the head of the pancreas;
4. independent of tumour size if the patient is undergoing laparotomy for other reasons.

Those tumours below the threshold for surgery should be monitored radiologically at regular (initially annual) intervals.

Familial paraganglioma syndromes

Familial paraganglioma syndromes are autosomal dominant disorders characterised by the development of multiple and metachronous paragangliomas. Parent-of-origin influences may appear to distort the autosomal dominant picture. Familial paraganglioma should be considered in any patient presenting with phaeochromocytoma or paraganglioma in which there is a family history of a similar tumour. Because the spectrum of tumours includes carotid body and glomus jugulare tumours, patients and their affected relatives may present to a wide range of clinical specialties including neurosurgery and head and neck surgery.

Age at presentation varies from childhood to old age and expression is variable. Genetic anticipation may be apparent: the age at presentation seems to be younger in successive generations.

Genetics

Although unusual, familial paraganglioma syndromes have recently gained increased interest because of developments in understanding their genetic basis. Hereditary paragangliomatosis (HP) is caused by mutations in succinate dehydrogenase genes: *SDHB*, *SDHC* and *SDHD*.[54] The protein products of these genes form a complex with SDHA that is a key component of the mitochondrial respiratory chain. The link between this function and the predisposition to paraganglioma formation has not been established in full. As with VHL disease, hypoxia-sensing pathways are likely to be involved. Somatic mutations in *SDHB* can be the underlying molecular pathology in true sporadic phaeochromocytoma.[55] SDH gene analysis should form part of the assessment of patients presenting with apparent sporadic phaeochromocytoma.

Heterozygous loss of function germ-line mutations in *SDHB*, *SDHC* and *SDHD* have also been identified in patients with the diad of paraganglioma and gastrointestinal stromal tumour (the Carney–Stratakis syndrome). This is an autosomal dominant condition with incomplete penetrance. Why some patients express this diad while others only paraganglioma remains to be determined.[56]

Presentation

Familial paraganglioma syndromes can present with tumour in the head and neck, chest or abdomen.

Not all paragangliomas are secretory. Only 5% of those occurring in the head and neck (such as those arising from the carotid body) are thought to secrete catecholamines and thus present with local symptoms. Functional paragangliomas and phaeochromocytomas present in the same manner as in sporadic disease, though the development of effective screening programmes in affected families is likely to lead to increasing detection in the asymptomatic phase.

Patients with familial paraganglioma due to mutations in the genes encoding succinate dehydrogenase subunits B, C and D (SDHB, SDHC, SDHD) can develop both phaeochromocytoma and paraganglioma.[57] Paraganglioma in SDHB-related disease is intrathoracic or intra-abdominal. Malignant behaviour is relatively common. Familial paraganglioma due to mutations in the gene encoding SDHC present with non-functioning head and neck tumours. Recent data have highlighted that these kindreds too can develop phaeochromocytoma.[58] Penetrance of SDHD mutations is dependent upon parent of origin. The disease is not expressed if the mutation is inherited from the mother.[59]

Management

Functional tumours should be removed if possible. Partially excised locally aggressive and metastatic disease may benefit from treatment with [131I]meta-iodobenzylguanidine (MIBG).[60] Excision of non-functional tumours should be considered if there are significant local symptoms, or radiological evidence of growth on serial monitoring. The metachronous nature of the condition means that recurrences and the development of additional tumours are common.

Patients with SDHB, SDHC and SDHD mutations should undergo annual biochemical screening for functional tumours with urine or plasma metanephrines and plasma chromogranin A. At-risk relatives should also be offered biochemical surveillance unless the disease-causing mutation is known in the family and they have had a negative predictive test result. Non-functional tumours are only detectable through clinical and radiological assessment. Optimum strategies for imaging these patients are not yet established.

Index cases should be offered genetic testing for SDH complex mutations. This helps in defining the risk of functional tumour to the patient and in developing genetic screening programmes for other members of the kindred. SDH gene mutations may be found in some 30% of patients presenting with apparent sporadic head and neck paraganglioma.[58,61]

Neurofibromatosis type 1 (NF1)

NF1 is an autosomal dominant multisystem disorder with predominant neurological, cutaneous, ophthalmic and skeletal manifestations. Prevalence is estimated at 1 in 3500. Fifty percent of cases are sporadic, and the disease is usually 100% penetrant by 5 years of age. NF1 can be segmental, due to a postzygotic somatic mutation. Expression is variable.

Two or more of the following criteria are required for a diagnosis of NF1:

- six or more café-au-lait macules >5 mm prepubertal or >15 mm postpubertal;
- axillary or inguinal freckling;
- two or more neurofibromas or a single plexiform neurofibroma;
- two or more Lisch nodules;
- optic pathway glioma;
- sphenoid wing dysplasia, thinning of long cortical bones or pseudoarthrosis;
- a first-degree relative with NF1.

Phaeochromocytoma occurs in approximately 1% of patients with NF1. It is rare in adolescence and extremely rare in children with NF1. Tumours can be bilateral. An increased risk of carcinoid tumour and gastrointestinal stromal timour is also reported. Neurofibromatosis type 2 is not associated with phaeochromocytoma.

Genetics

The NF1 gene is located on the long arm of chromosome 17 (17q11.2). It is a large gene with no mutation hotspots. Sequence analysis is not guaranteed to be clinically useful given the difficulties of identifying a mutation. Mutations in NF1 result in loss of function of the protein product (neurofibromin), in keeping with NF1 being a tumour suppressor gene. There is some evidence of a more severe phenotype for those with an intragenic deletion, and in this group it may be useful to identify the mutation as it could influence management. Neurofibromin functions as a GTPase-activating protein (GAP) downregulating RAS activity. Loss of neurofibromin function leads to unopposed RAS activity and dysregulated cell proliferation.

Presentation

Phaeochromocytoma in NF1 can present in the same manner as sporadic disease, or be detected on routine endocrine surveillance. Patients with NF1 are also at risk of renal artery stenosis. Hypertension is therefore neither sensitive nor specific as a sign of phaeochromocytoma in NF1.

Management

Management should follow the same principles as that of sporadic disease (see Chapter 3). Patients with NF1 should have annual biochemical screening for phaeochromocytoma with analysis of timed overnight urine catecholamine production.

Familial adrenocortical disease

Familial predisposition to adrenocortical carcinoma

Adrenocortical carcinoma (ACC) is very unusual in children and young adults. When it does occur in childhood, a tumour predisposition syndrome is likely. ACC in this context is often a manifestation of the Li–Fraumeni syndrome: an autosomal dominant familial cancer syndrome caused by heterozygosity for germ-line loss of function mutations in the *TP53* tumour supressor gene. In a series of 14 such cases, nine were shown to be due to *TP53* and two were likely to have *TP53* mutations that could not be identified. The one case not due to a *TP53* mutation occurred in a child with Beckwith–Wiedemann syndrome: a familial cancer predisposition syndrome resulting in over-expression of the paracrine growth factor insulin-like growth factor 2 (IGF-2).

Carney syndrome

Carney syndrome is a multiple neoplasia syndrome with cardiac, cutaneous, endocrine and nervous system manifestations.[62] It is inherited in an autosomal dominant manner. Fifty percent of affected kindreds harbour an inactivating mutation in the tumour suppressor gene *PRKAR1A*, which codes for the type 1a regulatory subunit of protein kinase A.[63]

Presentation

Carney syndrome can present with single or multiple, synchronous or metachronous clinical and pathological features, each of which are unusual in isolation:

- Spotty pigmentation – hypermelanosis; lentigines; blue naevi; combined naevi.
- Myxomas – cardiac (any chamber and possibly multiple); cutaneous; breast; oral cavity.
- Endocrinopathy – Cushing's syndrome due to primary pigmented nodular adrenal disease; GH-secreting pituitary tumour; large-cell Sertoli cell tumour of testis; Leydig cell tumour; thyroid tumours; ovarian cysts.
- Psammomatous melanotic schwannoma – sympathetic chain; gastrointestinal tract.
- Ductal adenoma of breast.

Adrenocorticotropin (ACTH)-independent Cushing's syndrome is the most common endocrinopathy in Carney syndrome, and is present in up to 30% of cases. Presentation is generally in childhood and young adulthood. The underlying pathology, primary pigmented nodular adrenal hyperplasia (PPNAD), rarely occurs outside the disease. The adrenal glands are not enlarged and contain multiple pigmented nodules scattered throughout a characteristically atrophic cortex. These nodules may be visible on preoperative imaging. Acromegaly develops in 10% of cases and has been mainly due to pituitary macroadenoma. Prospective screening may alter this pattern. Testicular tumours occur in 30% of affected males and may lead to precocious puberty. Thyroid and ovarian tumours also develop with increased frequency.

Management

Individual features of the syndrome should be managed as in sporadic disease. Presentation of cortisol excess may be atypical and indolent. Diagnosis of Carney syndrome should trigger periodic clinical, biochemical and radiological screening for additional features with the aim of reducing associated morbidity. Genetic testing is not widely available, placing the emphasis on careful clinical review of affected kindreds.

Familial ACTH-independent adrenal hyperplasia

The hypothalamo-pituitary regulation of gluco-corticoid production is mediated though ACTH binding to its cognate G-protein-coupled receptor on the plasma membrane of steroidogenic cells of the zona fasciculata and reticularis of the adrenal cortex. Introduction of other, non-ACTH G-protein-coupled receptors to the regulatory pathway controlling steroidogenesis within the adrenal cortex would uncouple the process from the negative feedback loops that maintain normal glucocorticoid production. ACTH-independent macronodular adrenal hyperplasia (AIMAH) leading to cortisol excess can result from the inherited ectopic expression of G-protein-coupled receptors on adrenocortical cells that activate steroidogenesis but are not under the influence of negative feedback.[64] Although unusual, elucidation of the molecular mechanisms underpinning regulation of adrenocortical function are set to highlight further examples of complex gene–environment interactions that impact on familial predisposition to adrenocortical disease.[65]

Familial hyperaldosteronism

Familial hyperaldosteronism type 1 (FHA1) and type 2 (FHA2) are rare autosomal dominant disorders of aldosterone excess.

Presentation

FHA1 constitutes 1–3% of all cases of primary hyperaldosteronism.[66] Unlike other forms of hyper-aldosteronism, it is present from birth and has no gender bias. It is characterised by moderate to severe hypertension and elevated aldosterone/renin ratios (though this is not specific). Many patients are normokalaemic. The diagnosis should be considered in any patient presenting with hypertension under the age of 25 years. A strong family history of hypertension is not always apparent. There may be a prominent family history of haemorrhagic stroke. Many patients do not respond to conventional antihypertensive agents, or develop hypokalaemia on potassium-wasting diuretics. Diagnosis is supported by suppression of aldosterone to undetectable levels during a low-dose dexamethasone suppression test (0.5 mg dexamethasone 6-hourly for 48 hours), giving rise to the alternative terms for this condition of glucocorticoid-remediable aldosteronism and steroid-suppressible hyperaldosteronism.

FHA2 is not suppressible by dexamethasone and is mechanistically distinct from FHA1, although its precise molecular basis remains unclear. It is clinically, biochemically and pathologically indistinguishable from non-familial primary hyperaldosteronism.[67]

Management

Traditional therapy for FHA1 has been with glucocorticoids to suppress adrenocorticotropin drive to the chimaeric 11-β-hydroxylase-aldosterone synthase gene. Long-standing hypertension may not respond fully to this approach. Moreover, excessive suppression with glucocorticoids may result in comorbidity, especially in young children. Mineralocorticoid antagonists and dihydropyridine calcium-channel blockers are alternative approaches.

Management of FHA2 should follow the same principles as that of primary hyperaldosteronism, balancing surgical and medical approaches dependent upon localisation studies against the response to antihypertensive therapy with amiloride, mineralocorticoid antagonists and/or dihydropyridine calcium-channel blockers (see Chapter 3).

Key points

- Inherited endocrine syndromes are rare.
- Multiple endocrine glands are often involved, either synchronously or metachronously.
- A multidisciplinary approach to these conditions involving endocrinologist, clinical geneticist and endocrine surgeon is essential.
- Risk-reducing surgery in at-risk individuals on the basis of genetic predisposition testing is an acceptable way to manage these patients.

References

1. Hannan FM, Nesbit MA, Christie PT et al. Familial isolated primary hyperparathyroidism caused by mutations of the *MEN1* gene. Nature Clin Pract Endocrinol Metab 2008; 4:53–8.

2. Chandrasekharappa SC, Guru SC, Mannickam P et al. Positional cloning of the gene for multiple endocrine neoplasia type 1. Science 1997; 276: 404–6.

3. Bertolino P, Tong W-M, Galendo D et al. Heterozygous *Men1* mutant mice develop a range of endocrine tumours mimicking multiple endocrine neoplasia type 1. Molec Endocrinol 2003; 17: 1880–92.

4. Kaji H, Canaff L, Lebrun JJ et al. Inactivation of menin, a Smad3-interacting protein, blocks transforming growth factor type beta signalling. Proc Natl Acad Sci USA 2001; 98:3837–42.

5. Scacheri et al. Genome-wide analysis of menin binding provides insights into MENI tumorigenesis. PLoS Genet 2006; 2:e51.

6. Macens A, Schaaf L, Karges W et al. Age-related penetrance of endocrine tumours in multiple endocrine neoplasia type 1 (MEN1): a multicente study of 258 gene carriers. Clin Endocrinol 2007; 67:613–22.

7. Guo SS, Wu AY, Sawicki MP. Deletion of chromosome 1, but not mutation of MEN-1, predicts prognosis in sporadic pancreatic endocrine tumours. World J Surg 2002; 26:843–7.

8. Eng C, Clayton D, Schuffenecker I et al. The relationship between specific RET proto-oncogene mutations and disease phenotype in multiple endocrine neoplasia type 2. JAMA 1996; 276(19): 1575–9.

9. Verges B, Boureille F, Goudet P et al. Pituitary disease in MEN type 1 (MEN1): data from the France–Belgium MEN1 multicenter study. J Clin Endocrinol Metab 2002; 87:457–65.

10. Stratakis CA, Schussheim DH, Freedman SM et al. Pituitary macroadenoma in a 5-year-old: an early expression of multiple endocrine neoplasia type 1. J Clin Endocrinol Metab 2000; 85:4776–80.

11. Richards ML, Gauger P, Thompson NW et al. Regression of type II gastric carcinoids in multiple endocrine neoplasia type 1 patients with Zollinger–Ellison syndrome after surgical excision of all gastrinomas. World J Surg 2004; 28:652–8.

12. Gibril F, Chen Y-J, Schrump D et al. Prospective study of thymic carcinoids in patients with multiple endocrine neoplasia type 1. J Clin Endocrinol Metab 2003; 88:1066–81.

13. Langer P, Cupisti K, Bartsch DK et al. Adrenal involvement in MEN type 1. World J Surg 2002; 26:891–6.

14. Burgess JR, Harle RA, Tucker P et al. Adrenal lesions in a large kindred with multiple endocrine neoplasia type 1. Arch Surg 1996; 131:699–702.

15. Brandi LB, Gagel RF, Angeli A et al. Guidelines for the diagnosis and therapy of MEN type 1 and type 2. J Clin Endocrinol Metab 2001; 86:5658–71.

16. Hai N, Aoki N, Shimatsu A et al. Clinical features of multiple endocrine neoplasia type 1 (MEN1) phenocopy without germline MEN1 gene mutations: analysis of 20 Japanese sporadic cases without MEN1. Clin Endocrinol 2000; 52:509–18.

17. Dean PG, van Heerden JA, Farley DR et al. Are patients with multiple endocrine neoplasia type 1 prone to premature death? World J Surg 2000; 24:1437–41.

18. Skogseid B. Multiple endocrine neoplasia type 1. Br J Surg 2003; 90:383–5.

19. Arnalsteen LC, Alesina PF, Quiereux JL et al. Long term results of less than total parathyroidectomy for hyperparathyroidism in multiple endocrine neoplasia type 1. Surgery 2002; 132:1119–24.

20. Norton JA, Fraker DL, Alexander HR et al. Surgery to cure the Zollinger–Ellison syndrome. N Engl J Med 1999, 341:644–53.

21. Norton JA, Alexander HR, Fraker DL et al. Comparison of surgical results in patients with advanced and limited disease with multiple endocrine neoplasia type 1 and Zollinger–Ellison syndrome. Ann Surg 2001; 234:495–505.

22. Norton JA, Fraker DL, Alexander HR et al. Surgery increases survival in patients with gastrinoma. Ann Surg 2006; 244:410–19.

23. Gibril F, Venzon DJ, Ojeaburu JV et al. Prospective study of the natural history of gastrinoma in patients with MEN1: definition of an aggressive and a nonaggressive form. J Clin Endocrinol Metab 2001; 86:5282–93.

24. Gauger PG, Scheiman JM, Wamsteker E-J et al. Endoscopic ultrasound helps to identify and resect MEN-1 endocrine pancreatic tumours at an early stage. Br J Surg 2003; 90:748–54.

25. Akerstrom G, Hessman O, Hellman P et al. Pancreatic tumours as part of the MEN-1 syndrome. Best Pract Res Clin Gastroenterol 2005; 19:819–30.

26. Ullrich A, Schlessinger J. Signal transduction by receptors with tyrosine kinase activity. Cell 1990; 61:203–12.

27. Santoro M, Carlomango F, Romano A et al. Activation of RET as a dominant transforming gene by germ-line mutations of MEN2A and MEN2B. Science 1995; 267:381–3.

28. Weber F, Eng C. Editorial: germline variants within RET – clinical utility or scientific playtoy? J Clin Endocrinol Metab 2005; 88:5438–43.

29. Tamanaha R, Cleber P, Camacho CP et al. Y791F RET mutation and early onset medullary thyroid carcinoma in a Brazilian kindred: evaluation of phenotype-modifying effect of germline variants. Clin Endocrinol 2007; 67:806–8.

30. Machens A, Nicolli-Sire P, Hoegel J et al. Early malignant progression of hereditary medullary thyroid cancer. N Engl J Med 2003; 349:1517–25.

This paper outlines the evidence base for the timing of thyroidectomy in patients with MEN 2 based on the age of expression of extrathyroidal MTC. Such data are key to the basis of clinical approaches to management of the condition based on early molecular diagnostics and tailored intervention.

31. Kahraman T, de Groot JWB, Rou WEC et al. Acceptable age for prophylactic surgery in children with multiple endocrine neoplasia type 2a. Eur J Surg Oncol 2003; 29:331–5.

32. Sherman SI. Thyroid carcinoma. Lancet 2003; 361:501–11.

33. Vestergard P, Vestergard EM, Brockstedt H et al. Codon Y791F mutation in a large kindred: is prophylactic thyroidectomy always indicated? World J Surg 2007; 31:996–1001.

34. Costante G, Meringolo D, Durante C et al. Predictive value of serum calcitonin levels for preoperative diagnosis of medullary thyroid carcinoma in a cohort of 5817 consecutive patients with thyroid nodules. J Clin Endocrinol Metab 2007; 92:450–5.

35. Gourgiotis L, Sarlis NJ, Reynolds JC et al. Localization of medullary thyroid carcinoma metastasis in a multiple endocrine neoplasia type 2A patient by 6-[^{18}F]-fluorodopamine positron emission tomography. J Clin Endocrinol Metab 2003; 88:637–41.

36. Sclumberger M, Carlomagno F, Baudin E et al. Novel therapeutic approaches to treat medullary thyroid carcinoma. Nature Clin Pract Endocrinol Metab 2008; 4:22–32.

37. Grossman A, Pacak K, Sawka A et al. Biochemical diagnosis and localization of phaeochromocytoma. Can we reach a consensus? Ann NY Acad Sci 2006; 1073:332–347.

This paper outlines a consensus approach established as an outcome of the first International Phaeochromocytoma Workshop, presenting the relative merits of a number of alternative testing strategies.

38. Neumann HPH, Bausch B, McWhinney SR et al. Germ-line mutations in non-syndromic phaeochromocytoma. N Engl J Med 2002; 346:1459–66.

39. Marx SJ, Spiegel AM, Brown EM et al. Family studies in patients with primary parathyroid hyperplasia. Am J Med 1997; 62:698–706.

40. Perrier ND, Villablanca A, Larsson C et al. Genetic screening for MEN-1 mutations in families presenting with familial primary hyperparathyroidism. World J Surg 2002; 26:907–13.

41. Chen JD, Morrison C, Zhang C et al. Hyperparathyroidism–jaw tumour syndrome. J Intern Med 2003; 253:634–42.

42. Cetani F, Pardi E, Giovannetti A et al. Genetic analysis of the MEN1 and HPRT2 locus in two Italian kindreds with familial isolated hyperparathyroidism. Clin Endocrinol 2002; 56: 457–64.

43. Shattuck TM, Valimaki S, Obara T et al. Somatic and germ-line mutations of the HRPT2 gene in sporadic parathyroid carcinoma. N Engl J Med 2003; 349:1722–9.

44. Hanssen AMN, Fryns JP. Syndrome of the month: Cowden syndrome. J Med Genet 1995; 32: 117–19.

45. Gujrati M, Thomas C, Zelby A et al. Bannayan Zonana syndrome: a rare autosomal dominant syndrome with multiple lipomas and haemangiomas: a case report and review of the literature. Surg Neurol 1998; 50:164–8.

46. Celebi JT, Tsou HC, Chen FF et al. Phenotypic findings of Cowden syndrome and Bannayan–Zonaz syndrome in a family associated with a single germline mutation in PTEN. J Med Genet 1999; (36):360–4.

47. Li D-M, Sun H. PTEN/MMAC1/TEP1 suppresses the tumorigenicity and induces G1 cell cycle arrest in human glioblastoma cells. Proc Natl Acad Sci USA 1998; 95:15406–11.

48. Bulow C, Bulow S, Group LCP. Is screening for thyroid carcinoma indicated in familial adenomatous polyposis. Int J Colorectal Dis 1997; 12:240–2.

49. Lonser RR, Glen GM, Walther M et al. Von Hippel–Lindau disease. Lancet 2003; 361:2059–67.

50. Friedrich CA. Genotype–phenotype correlation in von Hippel Lindau syndrome. Hum Molec Genet 2001; 10(7):763–7.

51. Hes FJ, Hoppener JWM, Lips CJM. Phaeochromocytoma in von Hippel–Lindau disease. J Clin Endocrinol Metab 2003; 88:969–74.

52. Koch CA, Mauro D, Walhter MM et al. Phaeochromocytoma in von Hippel–Lindau disease: distinct histopathologic phenotype compared to phaeochromocytoma in multiple endocrine neoplasia type 2. Endocr Pathol 2002; 13:17–27.

53. Eisenhofer G, Walther MM, Huynh T-T et al. Phaeochromocytomas in von Hippel–Lindau syndrome and multiple endocrine neoplasia type 2 display distinct biochemical and clinical phenotypes. J Clin Endocrinol Metab 2001; 86: 1999–2008.

54. Maher ER, Eng C. The pressure rises: update on the genetics of phaeochromocytoma. Hum Molec Genet 2002; 11(20):2347–54.

55. Nderveen FH, Korpershoek E, Lenders JWM et al. Somatic SDHB mutation in an extraadrenal phaeochromocytoma. N Engl J Med 2007; 357: 306–8.

56. McWhinney SR, Pasini B, Stratakis CA. Familial gastrointestinal stromal tumours and germ-line mutations. N Engl J Med 2007; 357:1054–6.

57. Astuti D, Latif F, Dallol A et al. Gene mutations in the succinate dehydrogenase subunit SDHB cause

susceptibility to familial phaeochromocytoma and to familial paraganglioma. Am J Hum Genet 2002; 69:49–54.

58. Peczkowska M, Cascon A, Prejbbisz A et al. Extra-adrenal and adrenal pheochromocytomas associated with a germline *SDHC* mutation. Nature Clin Pract Endocrinol Metab 2008; 4:1111–15.

59. Astuti D, Douglas F, Lennard TWJ et al. Germline SDHD mutation in familial phaeochromocytoma. Lancet 2001; 357:1181–2.

60. Kaltsas GA, Mukherjee JJ, Foley R et al. Treatment of metastatic phaeochromocytoma with ^{131}I-metaiodobenzylguanidine (MIBG). Endocrinologist 2003; 13:321–33.

61. Baysal BE, Willet-Brozick JE, Lawrence EC et al. Prevalence of SDHB, SDHC and SDHD germline mutations in clinic patients with head and neck paragangliomas. J Med Genet 2002; 39:178–183.

62. Carney JA. Discovery of the Carney complex, a familial lentiginosis–multiple endocrine neoplasia syndrome: a medical odyssey. Endocrinologist 2003; 13:23–30.

63. Stratakis CA, Kirschner LS, Carney JA. Clinical and molecular features of the Carney complex: diagnostic criteria and recommendations for patient evaluation. J Clin Endocrinol Metab 2001; 86:4041–6.

64. Vezzosi D et al. Familial adrenocorticotropin-independent macronodular adrenal hyperplasia with aberrant serotonin and vasopressin adrenal receptors. Eur J Endocrinol 2007; 156:21–31.

65. Stratakis CA, Boikos SA. Genetics of adrenal tumours associated with Cushing's syndrome: a new classification for bilateral adrenocortical hyperplasias. Nature Clin Pract Endocrinol Metab 2007; 3:748–57.

66. Jackson RV, Lafferty A, Torpy DJ et al. New genetic insights in familial hyperaldosteronism. Ann NY Acad Sci 2002; 970:77–88.

67. Stowasser M, Gunasekera TG, Gordon R. Familial varieties of primary aldosteronism. Clin Exp Pharmacol Physiol 2001; 28:1087–90.

5

Endocrine tumours of the pancreas

Robin M. Cisco
Jeffrey A. Norton

Introduction

Pancreatic endocrine tumours may be broadly classified into two groups: functional tumours, which cause clinical syndromes due to ectopic hormone secretion; and non-functional tumours, which cause symptoms only through mass effect and not through hormone production. All of these tumours arise from neuroendocrine cells, display characteristic ultrastructural features, and biochemically consist of amine precursor uptake and decarboxylation (APUD) cells. Functional pancreatic endocrine tumours are predominantly gastrinomas and insulinomas, but a variety of other rarer tumours also occur (Table 5.1). Identification of clinical syndromes and detection of hormones produced allow the classification of functional pancreatic endocrine tumours into specific types. Potentially life-threatening situations caused by hormone overproduction are a major reason to identify and resect these neoplasms. Additionally, except for insulinomas, pancreatic endocrine neoplasms are predominantly malignant. However, they are low-grade tumours such that aggressive surgical extirpation is beneficial in most instances.

Insulinoma

Endogenous hyperinsulinism was first described in 1927, and was the first syndrome of excessive pancreatic hormone production to be recognised.[1]

Hyperinsulinaemia and consequent hypoglycaemia is the major cause of morbidity and potential mortality associated with insulinoma, a neoplasm arising from the pancreatic insulin-producing β cells. Insulinoma occurs in approximately one person per million population per year (Table 5.1).[1] Hyperinsulinaemic hypoglycaemia associated with insulinoma is not well controlled by medical therapy, and surgery has remained the cornerstone of treatment over the past 80 years. Insulinomas are unique among pancreatic endocrine tumours because 90% of insulinomas are benign, solitary growths that occur uniformly throughout and almost exclusively within the pancreas, without evidence of local invasion or loco-regional lymph node metastases. Tumours may be as small as 6 mm in diameter and are usually less than 2 cm in size, making localisation difficult in many cases.[2]

Presentation

Excessive and physiologically uncontrolled secretion of insulin by the tumour causes episodes of acute symptomatic hypoglycaemia and leads patients to present for medical evaluation. Acute neuroglycopenia induces anxiety, dizziness, obtundation, confusion, unconsciousness, personality changes and seizures.[2] Symptoms commonly occur during early morning hours, when glucose reserves are low after a period of overnight

Table 5.1 • Features of endocrine tumours of the pancreas

Tumour	Incidence (people per million per year)	Hormone secreted	Signs or symptoms	Diagnosis	Location (%) Duodenum	Location (%) Pancreas	Malignant (%)	MEN 1 (%)
Gastrinoma	0.1–3	Gastrin	Ulcer pain diarrhoea, oesophagitis	Fasting serum gastrin >100 pg/mL Basal acid output >15 mEq/h	38	62	60–90	20
Insulinoma	1	Insulin	Hypoglycaemia	Standard fasting test	0	>99	5	5–10
VIPoma		Vasoactive intestinal peptide (VIP)	Watery diarrhoea, hypokalaemia, hypochlorhydria	Fasting plasma VIP >250 pg/h	15	85	60	<5
Glucagonoma		Glucagon	Rash, weight loss, malnutrition, diabetes	Fasting plasma glucagon >500 pg/h	0	>99	70	<5
Somatostatinoma		Somatostatin	Diabetes, cholelithlasis, steatorrhoea	Increased fasting plasma somatostatin concentration	50	50	70	<5
GRFoma	0.2	Growth hormone-releasing factor (GRF)	Acromegaly	Increased fasting plasma GRF concentration	0	100	30	30
ACTHoma		Adrenocorticotropic hormone (ACTH)	Cushing's syndrome	24-hour urinary free cortisol >100 μg, plasma ACTH >50 pg/h no dexamethasone suppression, **no CRH suppression**	0	100	100	<5

Tumour		Hormone	Symptoms	Diagnosis				
PTH-like-oma		Parathyroid hormone (PTH)-like factor	Hypercalcaemia, bone pain	Serum calcium >11 mg/dL, serum PTH undetectable, increased serum PTH-like factor	0	100	100	<5
Neurotensinoma		Neurotensin	Tachycardia, hypotension, hypokalaemia	Increased fasting plasma neurotensin concentration	0	100	>80	<5
Calcitonin-secreting PET		Calcitonin	Diarrhoea		Rare			
Non-functioning (PPoma)	1–2	Pancreatic polypeptide (PP), chromogranin A, neurone-specific enolase	Pain, bleeding mass	Increased plasma concentration of PP, chromogranin A or neuron-specific enolase	0	>99	>60	80–100

fasting during which endogenous insulin over-production has continued. Most patients (80%) experience major weight gain and may first present with symptoms of hypoglycaemia when food intake is decreased in an attempt to lose weight. A majority (60–75%) of patients are women, and many have undergone extensive psychiatric evaluation. Many patients will have been misdiagnosed with neurological conditions such as seizure disorders, cerebrovascular accidents or transient ischaemic attacks. Potentially life-threatening symptoms may be present for several years before the correct diagnosis is considered.[2] In a review of 59 patients with insulinoma, the interval from onset of symptoms to time of diagnosis ranged from 1 month to 30 years, with the median time to diagnosis being 2 years.[3] Because insulinoma is rare and neuroglycopenic symptoms are relatively non-specific, a high index of suspicion for insulinoma is necessary when other explanations for these symptoms are not evident. The identification of symptomatic patients and the liberal use of simple and precise biochemical tests results in accurate diagnosis of insulinoma prior to life-threatening sequelae.

Screening for multiple endocrine neoplasia type 1 (MEN 1)

Approximately 5–10% of patients with insulinoma also have MEN 1 (Table 5.1; see Chapter 4). These patients must be recognised because they frequently have multiple pancreatic tumours, and this greatly influences operative management.[4] MEN 1 is inherited as an autosomal dominant disease, and tumours develop in several endocrine organs. Sporadic primary hyperparathyroidism (PHP) due to multiglandular disease in patients younger than age 40 years may be the first organ manifestation, and these patients should be screened for MEN 1. Virtually all (96%) MEN 1 patients have four-gland parathyroid hyperplasia, up to 75% develop pancreatic islet cell tumours, and pituitary tumours (usually prolactinomas) occur in less than 50% of patients. The most common pancreatic endocrine tumour in MEN 1 is the non-functional tumour. Gastrinomas are the most common functional pancreatic endocrine tumour, with insulinoma second in incidence.[1] Islet cell tumours of different types may occur simultaneously in a patient with MEN 1. Patients also have an increased incidence of carcinoid tumours, thyroid adenomas, adrenocortical tumours and lipomas.

Diagnosis

> The diagnosis of insulinoma is established through a 72-hour supervised fast. The most definitive biochemical result for insulinoma is a plasma insulin concentration above 5 μU/mL in the presence of symptomatic hypoglycaemia.[2,5] Factitious hypoglycaemia must be excluded.[6]

The classic diagnostic triad, proposed by Whipple in 1935 based on his observations in 32 patients, consists of symptoms of hypoglycaemia during a fast, a concomitant blood glucose concentration less than 3 mmol/L and relief of the hypoglycaemic symptoms after glucose administration.[1]

Factitious hypoglycaemia due to clandestine administration of exogenous insulin or oral hypoglycaemic drugs may present with exactly the same symptoms as an insulinoma and may lead to an inappropriate diagnosis.[6] Factitious hypoglycaemia classically occurs in patients associated with the medical profession (such as nurses) or patients who have relatives with diabetes. The diagnosis of insulinoma must be reached in each patient by performing a 72-hour supervised fast with appropriate biochemical measurements. Urinary sulphonylurea concentrations (to exclude oral hypoglycaemic drugs) should be measured by gas chromatography–mass spectroscopy; they are undetectable in patients with insulinoma.

Supervised standard fasting test

The standard fasting test is carried out in a hospital setting and begins with a baseline examination in which memory, calculations and coordination are documented (**Fig. 5.1**). An intravenous catheter with a heparin lock is then placed, and the patient is allowed to drink only non-caloric beverages. Close observation is necessary. Blood is collected every 6 hours for measurement of serum glucose and immunoreactive insulin concentrations. As the blood glucose level falls below 3 mmol/L, blood samples are collected more frequently (every hour or less), and the patient is observed more closely. When neuroglycopenic symptoms appear, blood is collected immediately for determination of serum insulin, glucose, C-peptide and proinsulin concentrations (Fig. 5.1). Glucose is then administered, and the fast is terminated. If a patient remains symptom-free for the entire 72 hours, the test is terminated and the above blood concentrations are measured.

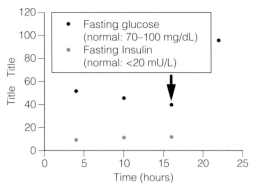

Figure 5.1 • Results of supervised fast in a patient with insulinoma. The patient, a 48-year-old woman, experienced acute onset of confusion and blurred vision 16 hours into a supervised fast in the ICU (arrow). Plasma glucose was 40 mg/dL at this time and plasma insulin was 12 μU/mL. Proinsulin measured simultaneously was 87 pmol/L (normal: 3–20 pmol/L). Symptoms rapidly resolved following intravenous administration of dextrose. The most diagnostic biochemical result in a patient with insulinoma is an inappropriately increased plasma insulin concentration above 5 μU/mL at the time of documented hypoglycaemia and symptoms.

Neuroglycopenic symptoms manifest in approximately 60% of patients with insulinomas within 24 hours after fasting begins.[5] Approximately 16% of patients with insulinoma develop symptoms when the blood glucose concentration is greater than 2.5 mmol/L.[2] The blood glucose concentration eventually decreases below 2.5 mmol/L in approximately 85% of patients with insulinomas during the 72-hour fast (Table 5.2). The most definitive diagnostic biochemical test for insulinoma is an inappropriately increased plasma immunoreactive insulin concentration above 5 μU/mL at the time of documented hypoglycaemia and symptoms.[5] The plasma insulin concentration is usually greater than 10 μU/mL.[2] Although prolonged

maximal stimulation of insulin secretion in normal subjects does not cause the release of the insulin precursor molecule proinsulin, some insulinomas secrete large amounts of uncleaved proinsulin. Patients with high proinsulin-producing tumours may remain euglycaemic and asymptomatic for longer periods during the fast because proinsulin is not biologically active. The proinsulin-like component (PLC) is measured at the time of symptomatic hypoglycaemia and termination of the fast. A value greater than 25% or an increased PLC:total immunoreactive insulin ratio is abnormal and consistent with the diagnosis of insulinoma.[2,5] Hypersecretion of endogenous insulin also results in increases of the circulating concentration of C-peptide, a biologically inactive by-product of enzymatic insulin cleavage from the precursor proinsulin molecule. Most patients with insulinomas have C-peptide concentrations greater than 1.7 ng/mL.[2]

Increased serum concentrations of proinsulin or C-peptide during hypoglycaemia effectively exclude the diagnosis of factitious hypoglycaemia because exogenously administered insulin does not contain these proteins and actually suppresses their production. However, approximately 13–22% of patients with insulinoma do not have increased serum proinsulin or C-peptide concentrations, and a supervised fast prohibiting exogenous insulin administration remains the best test to diagnose insulinoma and conclusively exclude factitious hypoglycaemia. The biochemical parameters measured during the standard fasting test cannot discriminate between patients with MEN 1 and ones with sporadic insulinoma.[5]

Nesidioblastosis

Because of differences in their surgical management, insulinoma must be distinguished from nesidioblastosis,

Table 5.2 • Standard fasting test results and the differentiation of insulinoma from factitious hypoglycaemia

Blood measurement	Fasting normal range	Result with insulinoma	Result with factitious hypoglycaemia	Test sensitivity (%)
Glucose	90–150 mg/dL	<40 mg/dL	<40 mg/dL	99
Immunoreactive insulin (IRI)	<5 μU/mL	Increased	Increased (usually >10 μU/mL)	100
C-peptide	<1.7 ng/mL	Increased	Normal range	78
Direct proinsulin-like component (PLC)	<0.2 ng/mL	Increased	Normal range	85
PLC/total IRI	<25%	Increased	Normal range	87

a condition of islet cell dysmaturation or malregulation that occurs primarily in infants and causes hyperinsulinaemic hypoglycaemia. Age at the time of presentation is the most important distinguishing factor, as nesidioblastosis occurs most commonly in children under the age of 18 months. Approximately half of infants with nesidioblastosis require a spleen-preserving near-total pancreatectomy, in which 95% of the pancreas is removed, because this disorder affects the entire pancreas diffusely.[7,8]

Adult nesidioblastosis has been reported and was recently described in a series of adult patients following gastric bypass surgery for morbid obesity.[9] However, nesidioblastosis in adults is exceedingly rare. In a review of over 300 cases of hyperinsulinaemic hypoglycaemia at the Mayo Clinic since 1927, only five adult patients had a reasonably confirmed diagnosis of nesidioblastosis.[10] Furthermore, biochemical tests (blood glucose, insulin and C-peptide) do not reliably distinguish hyperinsulinaemic hypoglycaemia caused by an insulinoma from that attributed to nesidioblastosis, and an insulinoma may be present in a patient who has islet cell hyperplasia. Therefore the diagnosis of nesidioblastosis in the adult must be critically suspect and should not preclude attempts to localise an insulinoma.

Management

Medical management of hypoglycaemia

Medical management aims to prevent hypoglycaemia caused by hyperinsulinism so that symptoms and life-threatening sequelae are avoided. In patients with acute hypoglycaemia, blood glucose concentrations are normalised initially with an intravenous dextrose infusion. To prevent hypoglycaemic episodes during diagnosis, tumour localisation and the preoperative period, euglycaemia is maintained by giving frequent feeds of a high-carbohydrate diet, including a night meal. Cornstarch may be added to food for prolonged slow absorption. For patients who continue to become hypoglycaemic between feedings, diazoxide may be added to the treatment regimen at a dose of 400–600 mg orally each day. Diazoxide inhibits insulin release in approximately 50% of patients with insulinoma; however, side-effects of oedema, weight gain and hirsutism occur in 50% of patients, and nausea occurs in over 10%.[10] Diazoxide should be discontinued 1 week prior to surgery to avoid intraoperative hypotension.

Calcium-channel blockers or phenytoin may also suppress insulin production in some patients. Long-term control of hypoglycaemic symptoms with medical management has generally been ineffective for patients with insulinoma. Knowledge of the patient's response to medical management is important for the surgeon so that the urgency and potential benefits of surgery can be determined.

Octreotide is a synthetic, long-acting (half-life >100 min) analogue of the naturally occurring hormone somatostatin. Octreotide binds to and activates somatostatin receptors on cells expressing them, inhibiting the secretion of many gastrointestinal peptides. Octreotide may be useful for treating symptoms caused by VIPomas and carcinoid tumours but is not generally recommended for insulinomas because its efficacy in inhibiting insulin release is unpredictable.[11] The usefulness of radiolabelled octreotide in imaging insulinomas has been equally disappointing. Therefore, long-term medical management of hypoglycaemia in patients with insulinomas generally is reserved for the few patients (<5%) with unlocalised, unresected tumours after thorough preoperative testing and exploratory laparotomy and for patients with metastatic, unresectable malignant insulinoma. Patients with malignant insulinomas and refractory hypoglycaemia may even require the placement of implantable glucose pumps for continuous glucose infusion.[10]

Preoperative tumour localisation

Virtually all insulinomas may be localised by the experienced surgeon through the combination of preoperative modalities and intraoperative ultrasound.[12] Blind pancreatic resection is not indicated.

After definitive diagnosis the tumour must be localised and the presence of unresectable metastatic disease excluded. Accurate tumour localisation is the most difficult aspect of management because the tumours are usually small and solitary.

Non-invasive imaging studies

An initial attempt should be made to localise the tumour and identify metastatic disease by using non-invasive tests. Computed tomography (CT) and magnetic resonance imaging (MRI) are both able to identify pancreatic tumours as small as 1 cm in diameter (Table 5.3). If CT is elected, a pancreatic protocol study with biphasic contrast injection

Table 5.3 • Sensitivities of localisation studies for insulinomas and gastrinomas

| | | % of tumours localised | | | |
| | | | Gastrinoma | | |
Study	Insulinoma	Overall	Pancreas	Duodenum	Liver metastases
PREOPERATIVE					
Non-invasive					
Abdominal CT	40–80	50	80	35	50
Abdominal MRI	11–43	25			83
Octreoscan	0–50	88			
Invasive					
Endoscopic ultrasonography	70–90	85	88–100	<5	<5
Selective arteriography	40–70	68		34	86
+ calcium stimulation	88–94	–	–	–	–
+ secretin injection	–	90–100			
Unlocalised primary tumour	10–20	15			
INTRAOPERATIVE					
Palpation	65	65	91	60	
Intraoperative ultrasonography	75–100	83	95	58	
Duodenotomy	–	–	–	100	
Unlocalised primary tumour	1	5			

and fine cuts through the pancreas should be used. Tumours will appear hypervascular on arterial phase images (**Fig. 5.2**a). The sensitivity of CT for insulinoma is 40–80% in recent series.[13,14] MRI may image an islet cell tumour based on increased signal intensity (brightness) on T2-weighted images (Fig. 5.2b). The sensitivity of MRI is equivalent to that of CT and, as expected, the accuracy of both CT and MRI increases with larger tumour size, achieving a sensitivity of 100% as tumour size increases to 6 cm.[15]

Malignant insulinomas are almost always very large (>4 cm) and are easily imaged by CT or MRI. The extent of bulky metastatic tumour deposits and hepatic metastases are also usually readily identifiable by CT or MRI. Metastases should be identified preoperatively so that the operative approach can be planned or, in the case of unresectability, unnecessary surgery avoided.

Somatostatin receptor scintigraphy (SRS), or octreoscan, utilises octreotide labelled with a radioactive tracer and is given intravenously (Table 5.3). The radiolabelled octreotide binds to tumours with somatostatin receptors, causing the tumour to appear as a 'hotspot' on whole-body gamma camera scintigraphy. Thus, SRS depends on the ability of a particular islet cell tumour to express somatostatin receptors. Some islet cell tumours, such as gastrinomas, express somatostatin receptors and are nearly always imaged by labelled octreotide. However, less than 50% of insulinomas are imaged by SRS because they do not consistently express high levels of somatostatin receptors. Thus SRS is not recommended for localising insulinomas.

Invasive localising procedures

Approximately 50% of patients have small (<2 cm) insulinomas that are not detected by non-invasive imaging, and a variety of more sensitive invasive tests are used to localise these tumours preoperatively. Endoscopic ultrasound (EUS) is safe and highly effective in experienced hands and is the modality of choice for patients whose insulinoma is not localised by CT.[16] It has been demonstrated to detect tumours as small as 2–3 mm, well below the limits of detection of CT or MRI,[17,18] and it is the most sensitive modality for detection of intrapancreatic tumours.

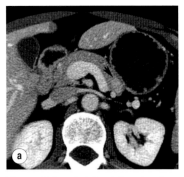 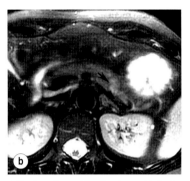 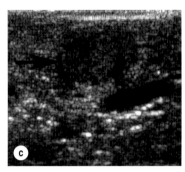

Figure 5.2 • A 1.3 × 1.3 cm insulinoma at the junction of the body and tail of pancreas as visualised on preoperative and intraoperative imaging (tumour is identified by arrows). **(a)** Pancreatic protocol CT demonstrates the hypervascular tumour following administration of intravenous contrast. **(b)** On T2-weighted MRI images the tumour has increased signal intensity (brightness). **(c)** Intraoperative ultrasound demonstrates the insulinoma, which is sonolucent compared with the more echodense pancreas.

To perform EUS of the pancreas the endoscope is passed into the duodenum and a saline-filled balloon is inflated against the intestinal wall. A 5- to 10-MHz transducer is used to generate an image of the pancreas through the intestinal and stomach walls. Tumours as small as 2–3 mm in diameter can be identified at the pancreatic head by moving the transducer through the duodenum at the junction with the pancreas. The endoscope must be passed well into the third portion of the duodenum to adequately visualise the uncinate process. Insulinomas in the pancreatic body and tail are imaged by positioning the transducer in the stomach and scanning through its posterior wall. Insulinomas will appear homogeneously hypoechoic, well circumscribed and round, and are typically easily distinguishable from the surrounding pancreatic parenchyma. Sensitivity of EUS for insulinoma ranges from 70% to 94%.[19,20] Rates of detection are highest in the head of the pancreas (83–100%) because the head can be viewed from three angles (from the third portion of the duodenum, through the bulb of the duodenum and through the stomach). They are lower (37–60%) in the body and tail, which can only be viewed through the stomach.[21]

Despite the tremendous potential and proven benefit of EUS for insulinoma, there are some limitations. First, there may be false positives, which include accessory spleens and intrapancreatic lymph nodes. Further, EUS is limited in assessment of malignancy, identification of pedunculated tumours, and differentiation of large tumours from the pancreatic parenchyma.[22]

In patients with negative results after non-invasive imaging studies and EUS, calcium arteriography may be helpful (**Fig. 5.3**). This study relies on the functional activity of the insulinoma (i.e. excessive insulin production) and not on the ability to image the tumour (i.e. tumour size). Arteries that perfuse the pancreatic head (gastroduodenal artery and superior mesenteric artery) and the body/tail (splenic artery) are selectively catheterised sequentially, and a small amount of calcium gluconate (0.025 mEq Ca^{2+}/kg body weight) is injected into each artery during different runs. A catheter positioned in the right hepatic vein is used to collect blood for measurement of insulin concentrations 30–60 seconds after the calcium injection. Calcium stimulates a marked increase in insulin secretion from the insulinoma. A greater than twofold increase in the hepatic vein insulin concentration indicates localisation of the tumour to the area of the pancreas being perfused by the injected artery (Fig. 5.3). In this way, calcium provocation may identify the region of the pancreas containing the tumour (head, body or tail). Additionally, injection of contrast may reveal a tumour blush, confirming the location of the insulinoma by imaging the tumour. These combined features are particularly useful in identifying the insulinoma in patients with MEN 1 who may have multiple imaged pancreatic endocrine tumours. The reported sensitivity of calcium stimulation is between 88% and 94% and few false-positive results occur (Table 5.3).[23]

A small proportion of insulinomas will remain unlocalised even after all preoperative studies are

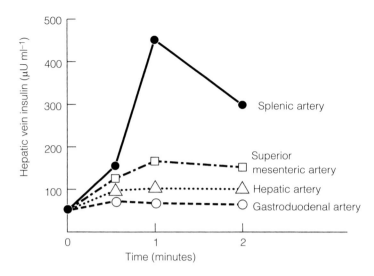

Figure 5.3 • Calcium angiogram in a patient with an insulinoma localised to the pancreatic tail. Intra-arterial calcium was selectively injected into splenic, superior mesenteric, hepatic and gastroduodenal arteries in four different runs. Blood samples were taken serially from hepatic vein and insulin concentrations measured at 0, 1 and 2 minutes before and after calcium injection. After injection into the splenic artery there was a rapid marked increase in hepatic vein insulin concentrations at 1 and 2 minutes. This finding localised the insulinoma to the pancreatic tail.

obtained, and such tumours are therefore considered occult. When the diagnosis is certain on the basis of the results of the supervised fast, surgical exploration with careful inspection, palpation and intraoperative ultrasonography (IOUS) of the pancreas is still indicated. Most of these patients (>90%) will still have an insulinoma identified and removed by experienced surgeons.[1,24] Retrospective reviews have shown that the combination of careful surgical exploration with IOUS will identify almost all insulinomas.[21,25]

Operative management

Surgery is the only curative therapy for insulinoma. Blind pancreatic resection is no longer indicated, and IOUS should be used to clearly identify the tumour and preserve as much normal pancreatic tissue as possible. Accurate preoperative localisation correlates with a high probability of cure. However, even with successful preoperative localisation, a careful pancreatic exploration should be performed at the time of surgery, including palpation and IOUS. The possibility of multiple insulinomas or a false-positive result from a preoperative localisation test may result in surgical failure. IOUS also helps to define the relationship of the tumour to the common bile duct, pancreatic duct, portal vein and adjacent blood vessels. As previously stated, adequate mobilisation of the pancreas with use of IOUS results in successful identification and resection of the insulinoma in nearly all cases, even in the absence of preoperative localisation.

Operative approach

If distal pancreatectomy with splenectomy is planned, then pneumococcal, meningococcal and *Haemophilus* influenza vaccines should be administered preoperatively. A standard midline laparotomy or bilateral subcostal incision is recommended to give adequate exposure. The entire abdomen, including regional lymph nodes, is initially inspected for potential metastases, which occur in 10% of sporadic cases. Metastatic insulinoma deposits on the surface of the liver typically appear as firm nodules. IOUS with a 5-MHz transducer may be helpful in identifying deep hepatic metastases.

Suspicious hepatic lesions that are small and peripheral should be excised by wedge resection, and larger or deeper lesions should be biopsied. Samples are sent for immediate frozen-section analysis to exclude tumour. In general, resection of localised tumour metastases is indicated to decrease symptoms associated with hyperinsulinaemia, which may be poorly controlled by medical means. To expose the pancreas adequately, the hepatic and splenic flexures of the colon are mobilised out of the upper abdomen, and the gastrocolic ligament is divided to open the lesser sac.

Pancreatic mobilisation

In contradistinction to gastrinomas, virtually all insulinomas are located within the pancreas and are uniformly distributed throughout the entire gland.[2] Therefore, the head, body and tail of the pancreas must be sufficiently mobilised to permit evaluation of the entire organ. This requires an extended Kocher manoeuvre, to lift adequately the head of the pancreas out of the retroperitoneum, and division of attachments at the inferior and posterior border of the pancreas, to permit evaluation of the posterior body and tail (**Fig. 5.4**). Because the head of the pancreas is thick, small tumours that are centrally located may not be easily palpated. The entire pancreatic head must be sufficiently mobilised so that the posterior surface can be adequately examined visually and palpated between the thumb and forefinger. The splenic ligaments may be divided to completely mobilise the spleen

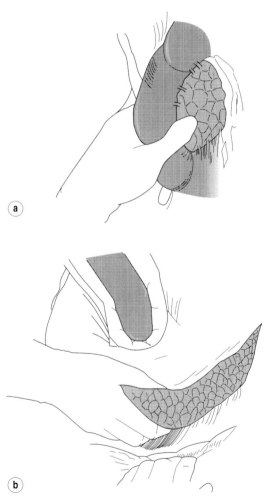

(a)

(b)

Figure 5.4 • Intraoperative manoeuvres to identify insulinoma. **(a)** Kocher manoeuvre with careful palpation of head of pancreas. **(b)** Opening gastrocolic ligament, superior retraction of stomach, inferior retraction of transverse colon, and careful palpation of body and tail of pancreas after incision along inferior border.

out of the retroperitoneum for full examination and palpation of the pancreatic tail.

Intraoperative manoeuvres to find insulinoma

Direct inspection of the entire pancreatic surface is carried out first because an insulinoma may appear as a brownish-red purple mass, like a cherry. Most insulinomas are encompassed by pancreatic parenchyma and may not be directly visible, but careful palpation of the pancreas between the thumb and forefinger may identify some of these. The tumour feels like a firm, nodular and discrete mass. Tumours are more difficult to identify when the pancreas is scarred from previous surgery or alcoholism and when tumours arise centrally within the thick pancreatic head.

IOUS is the best intraoperative method to find and remove insulinoma. It is performed by placing the transducer on the surface of the pancreas, which is covered in a pool of saline to maximise image quality. A 10- or 7.5-MHz real-time probe is used, which has a short focal length and high resolution. An insulinoma appears as a sonolucent mass with margins distinct from the uniform, more echodense pancreatic parenchyma (Fig. 5.2c).

IOUS can localise an occult insulinoma that has not been identified preoperatively and can identify tumours that are not visible or palpable.[26] It is particularly helpful in evaluation of the pancreatic head.[2,24] In conjunction with simultaneous palpation, ultrasonography further clarifies lesions. The sensitivity for detecting insulinomas using IOUS is greater than 75%[13,25] and approaches 100%[2,27] (Table 5.3). A study of 37 consecutive patients showed that intraoperative ultrasound correctly identified 35 (95%), and the two tumours that were missed were in the pancreatic tail.[12]

Insulinoma resection

Enucleation means excision only of the adenoma with minimal normal pancreatic tissue. It is the operation of choice for benign insulinomas. Tumour size, location and surrounding anatomy determine whether enucleation or pancreatic resection is performed. It is important to consider the relationship of the tumour to the pancreatic duct by imaging both structures with IOUS prior to tumour excision. Small tumours that are separated from the pancreatic duct and major vessels by normal pancreas can be safely enucleated. IOUS allows a precise, safe tumour enucleation and helps plan the shortest, most direct route to the tumour while avoiding the pancreatic duct. If a clear margin of normal pancreatic tissue does not exist between the insulinoma and other structures, then a spleen-preserving distal or subtotal pancreatectomy is advised.[12,26] Ductal injury in an attempt to resect a tumour in close proximity to the pancreatic duct results in significant postoperative morbidity. Evidence of malignancy, such as involvement of peripancreatic lymph nodes or tumour invasion, mandates pancreatic resection and not enucleation. Large tumour size may also be an indication for pancreatic resection. Rarely, pancreatico-duodenectomy is indicated if enucleation cannot be performed safely. Frozen-section confirmation of neuroendocrine tumour is traditionally used as the end-point of surgery.

Insulinoma and MEN 1

Approximately 10% of insulinomas occur in the setting of MEN 1, and 20% of patients with MEN 1 develop insulinomas. Insulinomas in MEN 1 may be multiple and may occur simultaneously and diffusely throughout the pancreas. The goal of treatment is to ameliorate the hypoglycaemia by eliminating the source of insulin hypersecretion. Difficulty arises in identifying which tumour or tumours produce the excessive insulin, but there is usually a dominant large tumour (>3 cm) that is readily identified on abdominal CT. Calcium angiogram is useful to determine if the dominant imaged tumour is responsible for the excessive secretion of insulin. Other small islet cell tumours may also be identified, but these are most likely clinically insignificant. If the insulinoma(s) arises within the body or tail of the pancreas, then a subtotal or distal pancreatectomy is indicated because multiple other islet cell tumours are virtually always present. A tumour that arises in the head of the pancreas is enucleated, if possible, or alternatively resected by pancreatico-duodenectomy. Medical management for this condition is reserved for those occasional patients who have failed surgical therapy, those who are poor surgical risks or those in whom a single source of hyperinsulinism cannot be found.[28]

Laparoscopic surgery

Laparoscopic surgery offers many advantages to patients, including shorter hospital stay, reduced pain, smaller incisions and faster recovery. Because insulinomas are usually small, benign and almost always located within the pancreas, laparoscopic surgery with laparoscopic IOUS is a logical

approach to treat these patients. Both enucleation and distal pancreatectomy are performed.[29,30] Good candidates for a minimally invasive approach have benign-appearing tumours that are well localised on preoperative studies. Some recommend that candidates have tumour confined to the body and tail of the pancreas; however, it is also possible to laparoscopically enucleate an insulinoma in the pancreatic head. Even after successful preoperative localisation, tumour location should be confirmed intraoperatively through the use of laparoscopic IOUS. Several published series indicate that laparoscopic pancreatic resection is safe in experienced hands, although operation times are typically longer than for an open procedure.[31,32] Complications include pancreatic fistula, and some procedures will require conversion to open surgery.

Outcome

Most patients with insulinoma are cured of hypoglycaemia and return to a fully functional lifestyle with normal long-term survival (Table 5.4). Appropriate localisation of sporadic insulinoma and complete surgical resection results in a cure rate of greater than 95%.[2,12] Symptoms resolve

Table 5.4 • Results of recent series for insulinoma and localised gastrinoma

Series	n	Tumour found (%)	Initial remission (%)
Insulinoma			
Brown et al.	36	100	100
Huai et al.	28	100	100
Hashimoto and Walsh	21	95	94
Lo et al.	27	100	96
Doherty et al.[2]	25	96	96
Grant et al.[13]	36	100	97
Hiramoto et al.[12]	37	37	100
Gastrinoma			
Norton et al.[62]	123	86/100*	51†
Mignon et al.	125	81	26
Howard et al.	11	91	82
Thompson et al.[57]	5	100	100

* Gastrinomas were found in 86% of initial explorations and 100% of subsequent explorations.
† Five-year-disease-free survival was maintained at 49%.

postoperatively and the fasting serum concentration of glucose normalises. Although successful resection of the tumour(s) responsible for hyperinsulinism renders most MEN 1 patients asymptomatic postoperatively,[33] persistent or recurrent hypoglycaemia due to a missed insulinoma or metastatic disease from the original tumour may develop.

Gastrinoma

Each year, approximately 0.1–3 people per million population develop gastrinoma, the second most common functional pancreatic endocrine tumour (Table 5.1).[34] The clinical features of this tumour were first described by Zollinger and Ellison in 1955.[35] Because of an increased awareness of Zollinger–Ellison syndrome (ZES) and the widespread availability of accurate immunoassays to measure serum concentrations of gastrin, gastrinoma is increasingly diagnosed and treated at an early stage of disease. However, the mean time from symptoms to diagnosis is 8 years in many studies, so improvements in detection are needed.

Patient presentation

Gastrinomas secrete excessive amounts of the hormone gastrin, causing acid hypersecretion which results in epigastric pain, diarrhoea and oesophagitis. The most common presenting symptoms are those of peptic ulcer disease. Diarrhoea, caused by gastrin-induced hypersecretion and increased bowel motility, is the second most common symptom and may be the only manifestation of ZES in 20% of patients. Oesophagitis with or without stricture occurs with more severe forms of the syndrome. Approximately 20% of patients with ZES will have it as part of MEN 1,[1] and this syndrome must always be excluded. A significant family history of ulcers, peptic ulceration occurring at a young age, and peptic ulcers in association with hyperparathyroidism or nephrolithiasis may all suggest MEN 1.

Patients with ZES usually present with a solitary ulcer in the proximal duodenum, similar to patients with peptic ulcer disease unrelated to gastrinoma, and 'typical' ulceration does not exclude ZES. All patients with peptic ulcer disease severe enough to require surgery should be screened pre-operatively for gastrinoma by obtaining a fasting serum gastrin concentration. Recurrent ulceration after appropriate medical treatment, or peptic ulceration in multiple locations or unusual locations such as distal duodenum or jejunum, should raise suspicion of ZES. In addition patients with peptic ulcer disease in the presence of persistent diarrhoea or the absence of *H. pylori* should be investigated.[36] However, not all patients with ZES have peptic ulcer disease: 20% of patients with ZES have no evidence of peptic ulceration at the time of presentation.[37]

Diagnosis

The evaluation of a patient in whom ZES is suspected begins by obtaining a fasting serum concentration of gastrin (**Fig. 5.5**). Hypergastrinaemia occurs in almost all patients with ZES and is defined as a serum gastrin concentration >100 pg/mL.[38] Therefore, a normal fasting serum gastrin concentration effectively excludes ZES. Antacid medications like proton-pump inhibitors (PPIs) or H_2-receptor antagonists may cause a false-positive increase in serum gastrin concentration and should be withheld for at least 1 week before measurement of the serum gastrin concentration.

Achlorhydria is a common cause of hypergastrinaemia, and gastric acid secretion is measured to exclude this condition (Fig. 5.5). A basal acid output (BAO) greater than 15 mEq/h (>5 mEq/h in patients who have undergone previous acid-reducing operations) is abnormal and occurs in 98% of patients with ZES. Measurement of gastric pH is a simpler but less accurate indicator of gastric acid hypersecretion. A gastric pH > 3 essentially excludes ZES, whereas a pH ≤ 2 is consistent with ZES.

A markedly increased fasting serum gastrin concentration (>1000 pg/mL) in the presence of an elevated BAO (>15 mEq/L) is diagnostic of ZES. However, many patients with ZES have gastric acid hypersecretion and moderately increased fasting serum gastrin concentrations (100–1000 pg/mL). For these patients, the secretin stimulation test is the provocative test of choice.[1] The secretin test is carried out after an overnight fast; secretin, 2 U/kg i.v. injection, is administered, and blood samples are collected immediately before and at 2, 5, 10 and 15 minutes after giving the secretin. A 200 pg/mL increase of gastrin concentration above baseline is diagnostic of

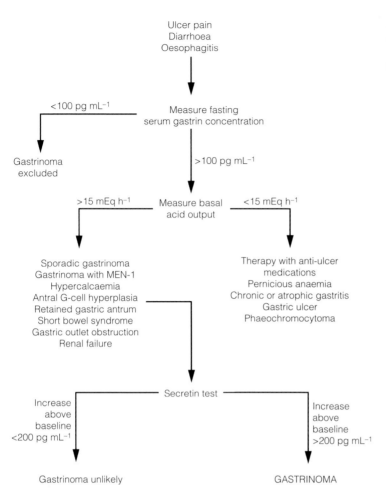

Figure 5.5 • Flow diagram for diagnosis and evaluation of patients with suspected Zollinger–Ellison syndrome.

ZES. The test sensitivity is not 100%, and approximately 15% of patients with gastrinoma may have a negative secretin test.

Management

Medical control of gastric acid hypersecretion

The management of patients with gastrinoma consists of two phases: control of the symptoms associated with acid hypersecretion and removal of the tumour, which is potentially malignant and life-threatening. The development of H_2-receptor antagonists and PPIs has made medical control of gastric acid hypersecretion possible in all patients. Patients with ZES typically require 2–5 times the usual dose of anti-ulcer medications to keep the BAO <15 mEq/h. Omeprazole at 20–40 mg p.o.

twice a day will usually control acid hypersecretion. Patients who have reflux oesophagitis or who have had prior operations to reduce acid secretion, such as subtotal gastrectomy, should have the acid output maintained at <5 mEq/h. The intravenous PPI pantoprazole should be administered at the same dose throughout the perioperative period. Once acid hypersecretion is controlled, epigastric discomfort resolves and ulcers heal in virtually all patients.[39,40] Because of the effective medical treatment of peptic ulcer disease, total gastrectomy is no longer indicated in patients with gastrinoma.

Adequate medical control of gastric acid hypersecretion with resolution of symptoms and decreased ulcerogenic complications has resulted in increased concern about the potential malignancy of the primary tumour. The most important determinant of long-term survival in patients with ZES is the growth of the primary tumour and its metastatic spread.

Tumour progression accounts for most deaths when patients are followed long term. Development of liver metastases is associated with subsequent death from tumour, and surgical resection of the primary can reduce the incidence of liver metastases. Hepatic metastases developed in only 3% of patients with gastrinoma treated by surgical excision of the primary compared with 23% managed without surgery.[41] Therefore, the current goal of surgery for ZES has shifted away from controlling gastric acid hypersecretion to aggressive resection of the primary tumour as well as localised metastatic disease. Surgical intervention can also normalise gastrin levels and lessen the requirement for long-term medical therapy. This is an important benefit since long-term hypergastrinaemia is associated with the development of gastric carcinoid tumours.[42]

The natural history of long-standing ZES in patients in whom the excessive acid secretion is controlled is largely unclear, primarily because effective medical therapy is relatively new. A longitudinal study of 212 patients with ZES and well-controlled acid secretion showed that none of these patients died of acid-related complications.[43] This study evaluated the long-term clinical course of patients with gastrinoma. Pancreatic location of tumour and a tumour diameter >3 cm were found to be associated with an increased risk of death from gastrinoma, and higher serum gastrin concentrations correlated with more malignant disease and a shortened survival time. Extensive liver metastases also had a negative impact on survival, as did the development of bone metastases or ectopic Cushing's syndrome. These results lend further support to early surgical intervention (as surgery decreases the rate of development of liver metastases), as well as aggressive surgical therapy of limited hepatic metastases.

Preoperative tumour localisation

Somatostatin receptor scintigraphy is the preoperative study of choice for localisation of gastrinoma.[44,45]

In contradistinction to insulinoma, gastrinoma is malignant in 60–90% of patients.[46] Duodenal gastrinomas as small as 2 mm in diameter may have associated regional lymph node metastases.[47] At the time of diagnosis, approximately 25–40% of patients have liver metastases.[48] Imaging studies must carefully assess the liver, and all patients

with ZES should undergo preoperative testing to localise the tumour and to define the extent of disease so that appropriate surgical treatment can be undertaken.

Non-invasive tumour-localising studies

Initial tumour localisation studies should be non-invasive and should adequately assess the liver for metastases. Primary gastrinomas that arise within the pancreas are identified much more reliably than those in extrapancreatic, extrahepatic locations (80% vs. 35%). Abdominal CT detects approximately 50% of gastrinomas overall (**Fig. 5.6**), but sensitivity depends greatly on tumour size, tumour location and the presence of metastases.[49] Gastrinomas >3 cm in diameter are reliably detected by CT, whereas tumours <1 cm in diameter are rarely detected. Abdominal MRI has a low sensitivity (25%) in localising primary gastrinomas but is excellent for detection of hepatic metastases (Table 5.3). Gastrinoma metastases in the liver appear bright on dynamic T2-weighted MRI images and show a distinct ring with gadolinium enhancement. MRI is especially useful to differentiate gastrinoma metastases within the liver from haemangiomas.

The use of somatostatin receptor scintigraphy (SRS) has significantly improved the preoperative localisation of gastrinomas.[50] SRS images gastrinomas on the basis of the density of somatostatin type 2 receptors (Fig. 5.6). Because a high proportion of gastrinomas have type 2 receptors, approximately 80% of primary tumours can be identified, and the true extent of metastatic disease is delineated more accurately than by CT or MRI.[50] SRS is now the non-invasive imaging modality of choice for gastrinomas.

Several prospective studies have evaluated the utility of SRS compared with conventional imaging. In a prospective study of 35 patients, SRS had a greater sensitivity than all other modalities combined (angiography, MRI, CT, ultrasonography).[44] The rate of detection correlated closely with tumour size: 30% of gastrinomas <1.1 cm in diameter and 96% of those >2 cm were detected. A positive SRS study strongly predicts the presence of tumour, but the inconsistent negative predictive value (33–100%) cautions against excluding a tumour on the basis of a negative study.[51] Another prospective study of 146 patients with gastrinoma found a sensitivity of 71%, specificity of 86%, positive predictive value of 85% and a negative predictive

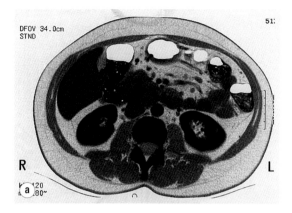

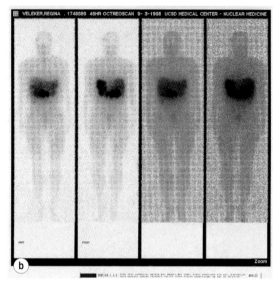

Figure 5.6 • CT scan **(a)** and somatostatin receptor scintigraphy **(b)** preoperatively identified large gastrinomas in this patient.

value of 52%. These 146 patients underwent 480 SRS studies, with a false-positive localisation rate of 12%. Extra-abdominal false-positive localisation studies were more common than intra-abdominal false-positive scans and were attributed to thyroid, breast or granulomatous lung disease.[52] The most common causes of false-positive intra-abdominal SRS scans were accessory spleens, localisation to prior operative sites and renal parapelvic cysts. Only 2.7% of these false-positive studies actually altered management, suggesting the importance of a high awareness of other potential causes for a positive SRS scan in the clinical setting.

Invasive tumour-localising modalities

Although non-invasive imaging studies are important to exclude unresectable metastatic disease,

these studies may fail to image the primary gastrinoma. Invasive modalities may be useful to localise the primary tumour prior to surgery. As discussed previously, EUS is highly sensitive for detecting intrapancreatic endocrine tumours. It has a reported sensitivity of 75–94% for identification of gastrinomas located within the pancreas.[20] It has also been reported to precisely identify the location of small lymph node metastases in patients with gastrinoma. Sensitivity for duodenal wall gastrinoma has been disappointing, however (11–50%).[53] This represents a significant limitation of EUS, as the majority of gastrinomas are located within the duodenum.

Previously, selective angiography was commonly used to localise gastrinomas. Selective arterial secretin injection (SASI) was performed, with collection of blood for measurement of gastrin from both a hepatic vein and a peripheral site. This allowed identification of the arterial distribution containing the gastrinoma. However, SASI currently has limited utility in patients with ZES because it is now recognised that occult gastrinomas are nearly always located within the duodenum.

Surgery for tumour eradication

If preoperative imaging studies reveal no evidence of unresectable metastatic disease, then patients with sporadic gastrinoma and acceptable risk should undergo abdominal exploration for tumour resection and possible cure.

Operative approach

The surgeon should be prepared for hepatic resection if unsuspected liver metastases are identified intraoperatively. An upper abdominal incision that provides adequate exposure for exploration of the entire pancreas, regional lymph nodes and liver is necessary. The abdomen is initially inspected for metastases, with particular attention to possible ectopic sites of tumour such as the ovaries, jejunum and omentum. The entire surface of the liver is then palpated for metastatic lesions. Metastases typically appear tan in colour and feel firm. Deep hepatic metastases may be identified by using IOUS with a 5-MHz transducer. All suspicious hepatic lesions must be either excised or biopsied to exclude malignant gastrinoma. In general, liver metastases that are not identified preoperatively by abdominal MRI or SRS are small and potentially resectable at the time of operation. Similarly, hilar, coeliac and peripancreatic regional lymph nodes are carefully sampled for metastatic disease.

Intraoperative manoeuvres to find
the primary gastrinoma

 Duodenotomy has been demonstrated to improve
cure rates in surgery for gastrinoma[54] and
should be performed during every exploration
for Zollinger–Ellison syndrome.

Successful intraoperative localisation and resection of tumours may be extremely challenging because gastrinomas only 2 mm in diameter may reside in the wall of the duodenum. There is also a high rate of associated lymph node metastases and even the posibility of primary gastrinomas arising within lymph nodes.[55,56] The initial finding of a single involved lymph node may therefore represent a primary tumour or metastatic disease from a very small, unlocalised primary tumour. Preoperative studies, such as SRS, accurately localise the primary gastrinoma and metastases and greatly facilitate the operative management, allowing a surgical approach directed to the area containing the tumour. Intraoperative localisation is still necessary because 20–40% of patients in whom the tumour is not apparent with preoperative studies will still have tumour identified at surgery.

Successful intraoperative tumour identification requires knowledge of where primary gastrinomas arise. The so-called 'gastrinoma triangle', bounded by the neck and body of the pancreas medially, the junction of the cystic and common bile ducts superiorly, and the second and third portions of the duodenum inferiorly, contains more than 80% of primary gastrinomas.[57] Most gastrinomas arise within the duodenum. The head of the pancreas and duodenum are first exposed by mobilising the hepatic flexure of the colon out of the upper abdomen and dividing the gastrocolic ligament to open the lesser sac. A Kocher manoeuvre is performed to lift the head of the pancreas out of the retroperitoneum. The entire pancreatic surface is carefully examined visually and palpated between the thumb and forefinger. IOUS is very useful for localising intrapancreatic gastrinomas (Table 5.3). The body and tail of the pancreas may be mobilised and similarly examined after dividing the inferior and posterior pancreatic attachments to find the few gastrinomas that may arise in the distal pancreas.

Primary gastrinomas have increasingly been recognised as occurring in extrapancreatic locations, most significantly the duodenum.[57–60] IOUS

is poor at detecting duodenal gastrinomas (Table 5.3), and the surgeon must rely on inspection, palpation and duodenotomy to find these tumours. These gastrinomas are usually very small – <6 mm – and are difficult to palpate. They are concentrated more proximally in the duodenum, decreasing in density as one moves distally (**Fig. 5.7**). Duodenotomy is necessary to allow direct inspection of the duodenal mucosa. A review of 143 patients with sporadic ZES who underwent surgical exploration revealed a significantly higher cure rate following duodenotomy, both immediately and in the long term. Duodenotomy was particularly important in the detection of small duodenal tumours, allowing localisation of 90% of tumours <1 cm versus only 50% discovered on preoperative imaging. Duodenotomy is the intraoperative procedure of choice for detection of gastrinoma and should be performed in all surgical explorations for gastrinoma. Gastrinomas will ultimately be found by an experienced surgeon in >95% of patients.[54,57,61,62] Further, duodenotomy is associated with a higher rate of finding gastrinoma and a higher rate of cure.[54]

Approximately 5–24% of gastrinomas are found in extrapancreatic, extraintestinal lymph nodes only, with no identifiable primary pancreatic or duodenal tumour.[55,63–67] Whether these represent lymph node primary tumours or metastases from occult pancreatic or intestinal primary tumours is controversial. In one series of patients who underwent exploration for gastrinoma, 10% of patients (13/138) with sporadic ZES met the criteria for lymph node primary gastrinoma in that they achieved long-term

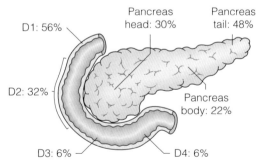

Figure 5.7 • Distribution of gastrinomas throughout the duodenum and pancreas. Duodenal gastrinomas are concentrated in the proximal duodenum and become progressively less frequent in the distal duodenum. Pancreatic gastrinomas are most commonly found in the tail of the pancreas.

cure after resection of a lymph node only. These patients were followed for a mean of 10 years, suggesting that these tumours represent true lymph node primary gastrinoma.[55] The discovery that neuroendocrine cells may be found within abdominal lymph nodes offers a possible explanation for the origin of these tumours.[56]

A prospective study found eight patients to have extrapancreatic, extraduodenal, extralymphatic primary gastrinomas. These tumours were located in the liver (three patients), common bile duct (one), jejunum (one), omentum (one), pylorus (one) and ovary (one).[68] A gastrinoma has been reported in the interventricular septum of the heart.[69] It is reasonable to conclude the surgical exploration for gastrinoma if careful exploration with duodenotomy does not reveal a primary tumour, all involved lymph nodes have been resected, and other ectopic sites have been carefully examined.

Tumour resection

As described for insulinoma, tumour enucleation remains the preferred approach for sporadic gastrinomas. Tumours that arise within the pancreas and that are not near the pancreatic duct or major vessels are safely enucleated. Large pancreatic tumours with vital structures in close proximity must be removed by pancreatic resection. Duodenal gastrinomas may be precisely resected following duodenotomy to localise the tumour. Some normal duodenal wall around the tumour is removed, but as much of the duodenal wall as possible is preserved to allow a non-constricting closure. Special attention is paid to avoid the ampulla of Vater. Regional lymph nodes should be systematically sampled, as lymph node metastases may be inapparent at exploration and will be found in 55% of patients with duodenal tumours. Although most gastrinomas are malignant, performing a more radical pancreatic resection (e.g. pancreatico-duodenectomy) is currently not indicated. Small tumours can be easily enucleated and because of the slow progression of disease, symptomatic relief with medical treatment is easily achieved. However, pancreatico-duodenectomy (Whipple procedure) can be performed with acceptable morbidity and mortality and may be indicated for patients with larger, locally aggressive tumours. Further, the morbidity and mortality of a Whipple procedure are decreasing, making this a potentially acceptable operative procedure for locally advanced gastrinomas and other islet cell tumours.[70]

The presence of lymph node metastases at the time of operation should not discourage an aggressive surgical approach to remove all gross tumour. Gastrinoma is associated with lymph node involvement in 50–80% of patients and, unlike many other types of cancer, lymph node involvement alone without hepatic or distant metastases does not appear to decrease survival.[71,72] Resection of all apparent tumour to eradicate disease increases disease-free survival and may extend overall survival. The development of hepatic and distant metastatic disease occurs in 25–90% of patients and is the most common cause of morbidity and mortality associated with tumour.[71,73] Patients should be carefully followed by screening for recurrent disease because if a patient develops an increased serum gastrin concentration in conjunction with a tumour that has been imaged, re-operation should be considered. Approximately one-third of patients with a recurrence can be rendered free of disease.[74]

Gastrinoma and MEN 1

Parathyroidectomy should be performed first in patients with MEN 1 who have hyperparathyroidism and ZES, because normalisation of the serum calcium concentration usually results in a marked decrease in serum gastrin, allowing better medical control of the symptoms of ZES.[75] Whether patients should undergo abdominal exploration is controversial. Earlier surgical series suggest that resecting gastrinoma does not cure these patients of ZES. Some studies suggest that aggressive surgical approaches may result in normalisation of serum gastrin concentrations in MEN 1 patients. However, prospective studies with strict criteria for cure indicate that few, if any, patients with ZES and MEN 1 are cured. Preoperative abdominal CT is necessary to identify hepatic metastases and plan surgical resection. SRS is also useful in determining the true extent of disease. In patients with MEN 1, 70% of gastrinomas are found within the duodenum, and approximately 50% of patients may have multiple duodenal tumours.[76] We advocate performing routine duodenotomy and peripancreatic lymph node sampling during exploration for gastrinoma in a patient with MEN 1, as well as enucleation of palpable tumours in the pancreas.

The appropriate extent of surgical resection in patients with ZES and MEN 1 is controversial, with only a few studies having enough patients to allow for analysis of surgical outcome. Thompson argues for an aggressive surgical approach.[77] In a series of 34 patients with ZES and MEN 1 who had undergone surgery, 68% remained eugastrinaemic, with a 15-year survival rate of 94%. He recommends performing a distal pancreatectomy (because of the concomitant neuroendocrine tumours in the neck, body and tail of the pancreas in these patients), enucleation of any tumours in the pancreatic head or uncinate process, duodenotomy and exision of any tumours from the first to fourth portions of the duodenum, and a peripancreatic lymph node dissection.[77,78] We, however, found that patients with MEN 1 and ZES rarely became free of disease despite extensive duodenal exploration, with only 16% of patients free of disease immediately after surgery and only 6% at 5 years. This is in contrast to a surgical cure of approximately 40% of patients with sporadic gastrinomas.[62] We therefore recommend surgical exploration only for those patients with ZES/MEN 1 and an imageable tumour >2 cm. The indication in this case is to prevent metastatic spread of tumour to the liver, not to cure ZES.

Outcome

Surgical exploration for cure is recommended for all patients with sporadic ZES. In addition, surgery has been demonstrated to improve long-term survival in patients with sporadic ZES and patients with MEN 1/ZES and tumour >2.5 cm.

In patients with sporadic ZES, an immediate postoperative cure rate of 60% can be obtained if all identifiable tumour is resected, and approximately 40% of these patients remain free of disease at 5-year follow-up.[62] With regard to tumour-related mortality, surgery to remove gastrinoma has been shown to improve survival in patients with sporadic ZES and patients with MEN 1/ZES who have tumour >2.5 cm. Specifically, surgery for gastrinoma has been demonstrated to result in a lower rate of liver metastasis (5% vs. 29%, $P = 0.0002$) and lower rate of disease-related death (1% vs. 23%, $P < 0.00001$), translating into a statistically significant 15-year survival difference of 93% vs. 73% ($P = 0.0002$).[79] These data were collected prospectively from groups with equivalent patient and tumour characteristics,

who differed only in whether or not they underwent surgery. Patients who have liver metastases at time of presentation have an overall survival of only 20–38%.[71] Therefore surgical exploration can be recommended for all patients with sporadic ZES, and all patients with MEN 1/ZES who have a tumour larger than 2.5 cm.

Non-functional pancreatic endocrine tumours

Pancreatic endocrine tumours that do not cause a syndrome of hormone excess occur with an incidence of 1–2 cases per million population per year.[80] These are the most common pancreatic endocrine tumour in individuals with MEN 1, occurring in up to 80–100% of cases in pathological studies.[4] Although commonly classified as non-functional pancreatic endocrine tumours (NFPETs), these tumours may in fact produce multiple hormones and peptides, including neurotensin, pancreatic polypeptide, chromogranin A and neuron-specific enolase.[80] On immunohistochemistry they may also stain for insulin, gastrin or somatostatin, although serum levels of the hormones are not elevated and associated clinical syndromes are absent. Plasma levels of chromogranin A are elevated in 60–100% of patients with NFPETs and may be useful to follow disease progression, relapse and response to therapy.[81,82]

Because they do not cause a clinical syndrome of hormone excess, NFPETs are typically larger at presentation than functional pancreatic endocrine tumours. Patients present with symptoms of mass effect, including abdominal pain, jaundice and obstruction. Greater than 60% will have liver metastases at the time of diagnosis. Because aggressive surgical management including resection of localised liver metastases is indicated for NFPET, it is important to distinguish this tumour from pancreatic adenocarcinoma. SRS and biopsy are useful in this regard.[83] With the increasing frequency of cross-sectional imaging, NFPETs are also sometimes diagnosed as an incidental small pancreatic mass and should be resected because of their potential for malignancy. As with functional pancreatic endocrine tumours, development of liver metastases is the most important determinant of survival, and preventing metastasis is the primary goal of surgical resection.

Other rare endocrine tumours of the pancreas

Other pancreatic endocrine tumours include vaso-active intestinal peptide (VIP)-oma, glucagonoma, somatostatinoma, growth hormone-releasing factor (GRF)-oma, adrenocorticotropic hormone (ACTH)-oma, parathyroid hormone (PTH)-like-oma and neurotensinoma (Table 5.1). These neoplasms occur in less than 0.2 persons per million per year. In general, these tumours resemble gastrinoma in that all are associated with a high incidence of malignancy. Each can also arise in association with MEN 1. The hormones, symptoms and signs, diagnostic tests, sites of occurrence, proportions malignant and frequency of associated MEN 1 for each tumour are given in Table 5.1.

Glucagonomas produce a characteristic rash called necrolytic migratory erythema (NME). These patients commonly have type 2 diabetes mellitus, weight loss, anaemia, stomatitis, glossitis, thromboembolism, and other gastrointestinal and neuropsychiatric symptoms. The rash is secondary to severe hypoaminoacidaemia and zinc deficiency. These tumours are commonly malignant and are not often resectable for cure. However, in some instances all tumour can be removed surgically, which leads to complete amelioration of symptoms.

For all of these tumours, preoperative abdominal CT is necessary to localise the primary tumour and exclude liver metastases. The goals of surgical treatment are to control symptoms caused by excessive hormone production and to potentially cure or decrease disease bulk. The only potentially curative treatment for malignant endocrine tumours is surgical resection. Patients with extensive bilobar hepatic metastases are typically not candidates for surgery, and symptoms may respond to chemotherapy, interferon α or octreotide.

Occult pancreatic endocrine tumours

An 'occult' islet cell tumour is an unlocalised tumour that occurs in a patient with a definitively diagnosed clinical hormonal syndrome, such as hyperinsulinaemic hypoglycaemia or ZES. The tumour is biochemically proven, but its anatomical site remains unclear. Approximately 10–20% of insulinomas and 15% of gastrinomas are occult.

Patients with insulinoma should undergo a calcium angiogram preoperatively in an attempt to localise the tumour to a specific anatomical area. Patients with occult gastrinomas need not undergo a regional localisation study as these tumours are nearly always in the duodenum within the gastrinoma triangle. Exploratory laparotomy is then the last resort to identify the location of the tumour and to resect it. Surgery should not be performed in patients with insulinoma unless IOUS is available, given its advantages in finding small tumours within the pancreas. Surgery in patients with occult gastrinoma should focus on the duodenum and should include duodenotomy.

Abdominal exploration by an experienced pancreatic endocrine surgeon, knowledge of the sites of occurrence of specific tumours and the use of IOUS results in identification and removal of the tumour in all but a few patients. In the rare instance that a tumour remains unlocalised and unresected after thorough exploration, the decision whether to perform a pancreatectomy depends on the particular patient's response to medical management and the results of the preoperative regional localisation study. Pancreatic resection is not indicated if the patient's hormonal syndrome can be well controlled by medical management. When medical management is unsatisfactory, the only alternative is to perform a pancreatectomy on the basis of the regional localisation data. Blind pancreatectomy is never indicated.

Malignant pancreatic endocrine tumours

With improved medical management of endocrine hypersecretion, metastatic spread has become the primary source of morbidity and mortality from pancreatic endocrine tumours. Except for insulinomas, which are malignant in only 5–10% of cases, more than 60% of pancreatic endocrine tumours overall are malignant. Data concerning the management of these patients are mainly derived from experience with malignant gastrinomas, which occur more commonly than other more obscure pancreatic neuroendocrine tumours.

No diagnostic histological criteria from examination of tumour biopsy samples or resected primary tumours exist to define malignancy for pancreatic endocrine tumours. Malignancy is definitively established with surgical exploration and histological evidence of tumour remote from the primary lesion, usually in peripancreatic lymph nodes or the liver. Recurrence of tumour at a location distant from a resected primary tumour site also definitively indicates malignancy. Gross invasion of blood vessels, surrounding tissues or adjacent organs usually suggests a malignant tumour. IOUS showing a pancreatic tumour with indistinct margins may imply local invasion and malignancy. Very large tumours (>5 cm) have an increased risk of being malignant.[46] Tumour DNA ploidy and tumoral growth fraction determined by flow cytometry may provide an indication of biological behaviour of some of these tumours. Because islet cell tumours generally grow slowly, metastases may not become evident until years after the initial primary tumour resection.

Evaluation of metastatic disease

Evaluation of a patient with a malignant neuroendocrine tumour begins by assessing the extent of disease using radiological imaging studies. SRS seems to be the single best imaging study to select patients for aggressive surgery to remove metastatic disease.[1] If the tumour binds this isotope, then disease anywhere in the body can be identified. Miliary or extensive bilobar hepatic disease and distant metastases are considered inoperable and, if identified preoperatively, can prevent unnecessary surgery. CT or MRI may identify disease in the chest and abdomen. Specific complaints of bone pain are elicited and, if present, evaluated with bone scan and radiography.

Malignant primary insulinomas are relatively large (≈6 cm) and can usually be readily detected by non-invasive imaging studies.[24] Gastrinomas may metastasise to regional lymph nodes when only millimetres in size. In one study, duodenal primary gastrinomas have been found to have a higher incidence of lymph node metastases (55%) than pancreatic gastrinomas (22%).[1] Some suggest that rare gastrinomas to the left of the superior mesenteric artery in the pancreatic tail are always malignant and more commonly produce liver metastases. Metastatic tumour must be distinguished from multiple tumours, which occur simultaneously. If multiple insulinomas or gastrinomas are found in a patient, then MEN 1 should be suspected.

Surgical management

Pancreatic neuroendocrine carcinomas have a better prognosis than adenocarcinoma of the exocrine pancreas and are often managed with aggressive surgical resection.[73] Surgery is undertaken to decrease tumour bulk so that hormonal syndromes are more effectively controlled by medical management, to relieve symptoms of mass effect, and/or to eliminate cancerous tissue and improve disease-free or overall survival. Preoperative staging studies are important to exclude patients from surgery who would not benefit from resection.

Limited metastases as well as the primary tumour should be resected to adequately debulk tumour and to eliminate the hormonal syndrome. Some patients with MEN 1 and ZES have had more aggressive tumours, as evidenced by larger size, liver metastases and higher serum levels of gastrin. Resection of advanced disease, including vascular reconstruction, has been performed safely and is suggested to improve survival.[84] Incomplete tumour resection may improve the ability to control the hormonal syndrome medically. For medically fit patients with metastatic insulinoma in whom hypoglycaemia is poorly controlled by medical management, tumour debulking may control symptoms for prolonged time periods, even in the setting of distant metastases. Approximately 50% of patients with metastatic insulinoma undergoing resection have complete biochemical remission.[85] Surgical resection of the primary tumour and aggressive resection of liver metastases are both associated with prolonged survival.

Although treatment is generally palliative and not curative for patients with locally advanced tumours and limited metastatic disease, surgery may be the only therapy that effectively ameliorates life-threatening symptoms. It may also increase survival because these tumours are generally indolent, slow-growing neoplasms. Limited regional metastatic disease can often be successfully resected and may be curative if no liver metastases are present. Complete resection of localised or regional nodal metastases with negative margins at the initial surgery provides the highest probability of cure.[1] Although disease-free survival is prolonged in most patients, most eventually develop recurrent tumour.

Approximately 30% of patients with metastatic insulinoma can undergo complete resection of tumour.[86] Median survival is increased from 11 months in patients with metastatic insulinoma who cannot undergo resection to 4 years in those in whom tumour debulking is possible. Palliative re-resection of recurrent tumour extends median survival from 11–19 months to 4 years.[87] Surgery may also be the most effective treatment for patients with metastatic gastrinoma if most or all of the tumour can be resected.[1] Aggressive resection of liver metastases of gastrinoma, considered resectable by preoperative radiological imaging studies, improves 5-year survival from 28% in patients with inoperable metastases to 79–85%.[88,89] Surgical resection of other liver metastatic neuroendocrine tumours besides gastrinoma is also associated with a 5-year survival of 73%.[90]

Non-surgical management

Symptoms from extensive metastases may respond to chemotherapy or octreotide, but these treatments are not curative.[1] Treatment with octreotide results in unpredictable responses, causing decreased tumour growth in some patients and having no effect in others.[91] The addition of interferon α to octreotide therapy may benefit a subgroup of patients with advanced metastatic disease that is unresponsive to octreotide monotherapy.[92] Octreotide may ameliorate symptoms, especially in patients with malignant VIPoma (**Fig. 5.8**), and when symptoms are adequately controlled, patients can live comfortably and productively for many years despite metastatic disease.

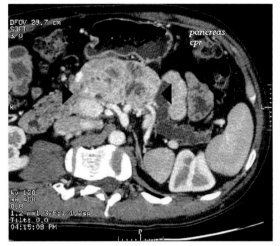

Figure 5.8 • Pancreatic protocol CT scan of a glucagonoma within the body of the pancreas (arrows). The tumour was abutting the superior mesenteric vein and causing obstruction of the pancreatic duct with atrophy of the tail of the pancreas.

Key points

- With the exception of insulinomas, most pancreatic endocrine tumours are malignant.
- The diagnosis of insulinoma is established through a supervised 72-hour fast.
- Virtually all insulinomas may be localised by the experienced surgeon with the aid of preoperative and intraoperative modalities. Blind distal pancreatectomy is never indicated.
- Medical control of acid hypersecretion in ZES should be achieved with a PPI to maintain BAO <15 mEq/h.
- Somatostatin receptor scintigraphy is the first-line preoperative localisation study for gastrinoma.
- Duodenotomy has been shown to improve cure rates in ZES and should be performed during every exploration for gastrinoma.
- Surgical exploration for cure is recommended for all patients with sporadic ZES. In addition, surgery has been demonstrated to improve long-term survival in patients with sporadic ZES and patients with MEN 1/ZES and tumour >2.5 cm.
- Patients with pancreatic endocrine tumours that are locally advanced or have limited metastatic spread appear to benefit from aggressive surgical resection.

References

1. Norton JA. Neuroendocrine tumors of the pancreas and duodenum. Curr Probl Surg 1994; 31(2):77–156.

2. Doherty GM, Doppman JL, Shawker TH et al. Results of a prospective strategy to diagnose, localize, and resect insulinomas. Surgery 1991; 110(6):989–996; discussion 996–7.

   Excellent paper describing the results of diagnostic testing in 25 patients with insulinoma.

3. Dizon AM, Kowalyk S, Hoogwerf BJ. Neuroglycopenic and other symptoms in patients with insulinomas. Am J Med 1999; 106(3):307–10.

4. Thompson NW, Lloyd RV, Nishiyama RH et al. MEN I pancreas: a histological and immunohistochemical study. World J Surg 1984; 8(4): 561–74.

5. Gorden P, Skarulis MC, Roach P et al. Plasma proinsulin-like component in insulinoma: a 25-year experience. J Clin Endocrinol Metab 1995; 80(10): 2884–7.

6. Grunberger G, Weiner JL, Silverman R et al. Factitious hypoglycemia due to surreptitious administration of insulin. Diagnosis, treatment, and long-term follow-up. Ann Intern Med 1988; 108(2):252–7.

7. Glaser B, Hirsch HJ, Landau H. Persistent hyperinsulinemic hypoglycemia of infancy: long-term octreotide treatment without pancreatectomy. J Pediatr 1993; 123(4):644–50.

8. Thornton PS, Alter CA, Katz LE et al. Short- and long-term use of octreotide in the treatment of congenital hyperinsulinism. J Pediatr 1993; 123(4):637–643.

9. Service GJ, Thompson GB, Service FJ et al. Hyperinsulinemic hypoglycemia with nesidioblastosis after gastric-bypass surgery. N Engl J Med 2005; 353(3):249–54.

10. Grant CS. Insulinoma. Surg Oncol Clin North Am 1998; 7(4):819–44.

11. Arnold R, Frank M, Kajdan U. Management of gastroenteropancreatic endocrine tumors: the place of somatostatin analogues. Digestion 1994; 55(Suppl 3):107–13.

12. Hiramoto JS, Feldstein VA, LaBerge JM et al. Intraoperative ultrasound and preoperative localization detects all occult insulinomas. Arch Surg 2001; 136(9):1020–1025; discussion 1025–6.

13. Grant CS, van Heerden J, Charboneau JW et al. Insulinoma. The value of intraoperative ultrasonography. Arch Surg 1988; 123(7):843–48.

14. Rodallec M, Vilgrain V, Zins M et al. Helical CT of pancreatic endocrine tumors. J Comput Assist Tomogr 2002; 26(5):728–33.

15. Boukhman MP, Karam JM, Shaver J et al. Localization of insulinomas. Arch Surg 1999; 134(8):818–822; discussion 822–3.

16. Owens LV, Huth JF, Cance WG. Insulinoma: pitfalls in preoperative localization. Eur J Surg Oncol 1995; 21(3):326–8.

17. Gauger PG, Scheiman JM, Wamsteker EJ et al. Role of endoscopic ultrasonography in screening and treatment of pancreatic endocrine tumours in asymptomatic patients with multiple endocrine neoplasia type 1. Br J Surg 2003; 90(6):748–54.

18. Kann PH, Rothmund M, Zielke A. Endoscopic ultrasound imaging of insulinomas: limitations and clinical relevance. Exp Clin Endocrinol Diabetes 2005; 113(8):471–4.

19. Glover JR, Shorvon PJ, Lees WR. Endoscopic ultrasound for localisation of islet cell tumours. Gut 1992; 33(1):108–10.

20. Rosch T, Lightdale CJ, Botet JF et al. Localization of pancreatic endocrine tumors by endoscopic ultrasonography. N Engl J Med 1992; 326(26): 1721–6.

21. McLean AM, Fairclough PD. Endoscopic ultrasound in the localisation of pancreatic islet cell tumours. Best Pract Res Clin Endocrinol Metab 2005; 19(2):177–93.

22. Richards ML, Gauger PG, Thompson NW et al. Pitfalls in the surgical treatment of insulinoma. Surgery 2002; 132(6):1040–49; discussion 1049.

23. Cohen MS, Picus D, Lairmore TC et al. Prospective study of provocative angiograms to localize functional islet cell tumors of the pancreas. Surgery 1997; 122(6):1091–100.

24. Norton JA, Cromack DT, Shawker TH et al. Intraoperative ultrasonographic localization of islet cell tumors. A prospective comparison to palpation. Ann Surg 1988; 207(2):160–8.

25. Gianello P, Gigot JF, Berthet F et al. Pre- and intraoperative localization of insulinomas: report of 22 observations. World J Surg 1988; 12(3): 389–97.

26. Norton JA, Sigel B, Baker AR et al. Localization of an occult insulinoma by intraoperative ultrasonography. Surgery 1985; 97(3):381–4.

27. Doppman JL, Chang R, Fraker DL et al. Localization of insulinomas to regions of the pancreas by intra-arterial stimulation with calcium. Ann Intern Med 1995; 123(4):269–73.

28. Veldhuis JD, Norton JA, Wells SA Jr et al. Surgical versus medical management of multiple endocrine neoplasia (MEN) type I. J Clin Endocrinol Metab 1997; 82(2):357–64.

29. Dexter SP, Martin IG, Leindler L et al. Laparoscopic enucleation of a solitary pancreatic insulinoma. Surg Endosc 1999; 13(4):406–8.

30. Gagner M, Pomp A, Herrera MF. Early experience with laparoscopic resections of islet cell tumors. Surgery 1996; 120(6):1051–4.

31. Pierce RA, Spitler JA, Hawkins WG et al. Outcomes analysis of laparoscopic resection of pancreatic neoplasms. Surg Endosc 2007; 21(4):579–86.

32. Toniato A, Meduri F, Foletto M et al. Laparoscopic treatment of benign insulinomas localized in the body and tail of the pancreas: a single-center experience. World J Surg 2006; 30(10):1916–19; discussion 1920–1.

33. Sheppard BC, Norton JA, Doppman JL et al. Management of islet cell tumors in patients with multiple endocrine neoplasia: a prospective study. Surgery 1989; 106(6):1108–17; discussion 1117–18.

34. Eriksson B, Oberg K, Skogseid B. Neuroendocrine pancreatic tumors. Clinical findings in a prospective study of 84 patients. Acta Oncol 1989; 28(3): 373–77.

35. Zollinger RM, Ellison EH. Primary peptic ulcerations of the jejunum associated with islet cell tumors of the pancreas. Ann Surg 1955; 142(4): 709–23; discussion 724–8.

36. Cisco RM, Norton JA. Surgery for gastrinoma. Adv Surg 2007; 41:165–76.

37. Norton JA, Doppman JL, Jensen RT. Curative resection in Zollinger–Ellison syndrome. Results of a 10-year prospective study. Ann Surg 1992; 215(1): 8–18.

38. Wolfe MM, Jensen RT. Zollinger–Ellison syndrome. Current concepts in diagnosis and management. N Engl J Med 1987; 317(19):1200–9.

39. Fox PS, Hofmann JW, Decosse JJ et al. The influence of total gastrectomy on survival in malignant Zollinger–Ellison tumors. Ann Surg 1974; 180(4): 558–66.

40. Zollinger RM, Ellison EC, O'Dorisio TM et al. Thirty years' experience with gastrinoma. World J Surg 1984; 8(4):427–35.

41. Fraker DL, Norton JA, Alexander HR et al. Surgery in Zollinger–Ellison syndrome alters the natural history of gastrinoma. Ann Surg 1994; 220(3): 320–328; discussion 328–30.

42. Norton JA, Melcher ML, Gibril F et al. Gastric carcinoid tumors in multiple endocrine neoplasia-1 patients with Zollinger–Ellison syndrome can be symptomatic, demonstrate aggressive growth, and require surgical treatment. Surgery 2004; 136(6):1267–74.

43. Yu F, Venzon DJ, Serrano J et al. Prospective study of the clinical course, prognostic factors, causes of death, and survival in patients with long-standing Zollinger–Ellison syndrome. J Clin Oncol 1999; 17(2):615–30.

44. Alexander HR, Fraker DL, Norton JA et al. Prospective study of somatostatin receptor scintigraphy and its effect on operative outcome in patients with Zollinger–Ellison syndrome. Ann Surg 1998; 228(2):228–38.

45. Lamberts SW, Bakker WH, Reubi JC et al. Somatostatin-receptor imaging in the localization of endocrine tumors. N Engl J Med 1990; 323(18): 1246–49.

Original description of somatostatin receptor scintigraphy.

46. Peplinski GR, Norton JA. Gastrointestinal endocrine cancers and nodal metastasis: biologic significance and therapeutic implications. Surg Oncol Clin North Am 1996; 5(1):159–71.

47. Thompson NW, Pasieka J, Fukuuchi A. Duodenal gastrinomas, duodenotomy, and duodenal exploration in the surgical management of Zollinger–Ellison syndrome. World J Surg 1993; 17(4):455–62.

48. Sutliff VE, Doppman JL, Gibril F et al. Growth of newly diagnosed, untreated metastatic gastrinomas and predictors of growth patterns. J Clin Oncol 1997; 15(6):2420–31.

49. Wank SA, Doppman JL, Miller DL et al. Prospective study of the ability of computed axial tomography to localize gastrinomas in patients with Zollinger–Ellison syndrome. Gastroenterology 1987; 92(4): 905–12.

50. Gibril F, Reynolds JC, Doppman JL et al. Somatostatin receptor scintigraphy: its sensitivity compared with that of other imaging methods in detecting primary and metastatic gastrinomas. A prospective study. Ann Intern Med 1996; 125(1): 26–34.

51. Meko JB, Doherty GM, Siegel BA et al. Evaluation of somatostatin-receptor scintigraphy for detecting neuroendocrine tumors. Surgery 1996; 120(6): 975–983; discussion 983–4.

52. Gibril F, Reynolds JC, Chen CC et al. Specificity of somatostatin receptor scintigraphy: a prospective study and effects of false-positive localizations on management in patients with gastrinomas. J Nucl Med 1999; 40(4):539–53.

53. McLean AM, Fairclough PD. Endoscopic ultrasound in the localisation of pancreatic islet cell tumours. Best Pract Res Clin Endocrinol Metab 2005; 19(2):177–93.

54. Norton JA, Alexander HR, Fraker DL et al. Does the use of routine duodenotomy (DUODX) affect rate of cure, development of liver metastases, or survival in patients with Zollinger–Ellison syndrome? Ann Surg 2004; 239(5):617–25; discussion 626.

Demonstrates that duodenotomy not only localises more gastrinomas, but also improves cure rates.

55. Norton JA, Alexander HR, Fraker DL et al. Possible primary lymph node gastrinoma: occurrence, natural history, and predictive factors: a prospective study. Ann Surg 2003; 237(5):650–657; discussion 657–9.

56. Perrier ND, Batts KP, Thompson GB et al. An immunohistochemical survey for neuroendocrine cells in regional pancreatic lymph nodes: a plausible explanation for primary nodal gastrinomas? Mayo

Clinic Pancreatic Surgery Group. Surgery 1995; 118(6):957–965; discussion 965–6.

57. Thompson NW, Vinik AI, Eckhauser FE. Microgastrinomas of the duodenum. A cause of failed operations for the Zollinger–Ellison syndrome. Ann Surg 1989; 209(4):396–404.

58. Pipeleers-Marichal M, Donow C, Heitz PU et al. Pathologic aspects of gastrinomas in patients with Zollinger–Ellison syndrome with and without multiple endocrine neoplasia type I. World J Surg 1993; 17(4):481–8.

59. Stabile BE, Morrow DJ, Passaro E Jr. The gastrinoma triangle: operative implications. Am J Surg 1984; 147(1):25–31.

60. Pipeleers-Marichal M, Somers G, Willems G et al. Gastrinomas in the duodenums of patients with multiple endocrine neoplasia type 1 and the Zollinger–Ellison syndrome. N Engl J Med 1990; 322(11):723–7.

61. Frucht H, Norton JA, London JF et al. Detection of duodenal gastrinomas by operative endoscopic transillumination. A prospective study. Gastroenterology 1990; 99(6):1622–7.

62. Norton JA, Fraker DL, Alexander HR et al. Surgery to cure the Zollinger–Ellison syndrome. N Engl J Med 1999; 341(9):635–44.

    Results of a prospective surgical trial to cure ZES.

63. Bornman PC, Marks IN, Mee AS et al. Favourable response to conservative surgery for extra-pancreatic gastrinoma with lymph node metastases. Br J Surg 1987; 74(3):198–201.

64. Norton JA, Doppman JL, Collen MJ et al. Prospective study of gastrinoma localization and resection in patients with Zollinger–Ellison syndrome. Ann Surg 1986; 204(4):468–79.

65. Wolfe MM, Alexander RW, McGuigan JE. Extrapancreatic, extraintestinal gastrinoma: effective treatment by surgery. N Engl J Med 1982; 306(25):1533–6.

66. Arnold WS, Fraker DL, Alexander HR et al. Apparent lymph node primary gastrinoma. Surgery 1994; 116(6):1123–1129; discussion 1129–30.

67. Herrmann ME, Ciesla MC, Chejfec G et al. Primary nodal gastrinomas. Arch Pathol Lab Med 2000; 124(6):832–35.

68. Wu PC, Alexander HR, Bartlett DL et al. A prospective analysis of the frequency, location, and curability of ectopic (nonpancreaticoduodenal, nonnodal) gastrinoma. Surgery 1997; 122(6):1176–82.

69. Noda S, Norton JA, Jensen RT et al. Surgical resection of intracardiac gastrinoma. Ann Thorac Surg 1999; 67(2):532–3.

70. Ahn YJ, Kim SW, Park YC et al. Duodenal-preserving resection of the head of the pancreas and pancreatic head resection with second-portion duodenectomy for benign lesions, low-grade malignancies, and early carcinoma involving the periampullary region. Arch Surg 2003; 138(2):162–8; discussion 168.

71. Ellison EC. Forty-year appraisal of gastrinoma. Back to the future. Ann Surg 1995; 222(4):511–21; discussion 521–4.

72. Kisker O, Bastian D, Bartsch D et al. Localization, malignant potential, and surgical management of gastrinomas. World J Surg 1998; 22(7):651–57; discussion 657–8.

73. Norton JA, Sugarbaker PH, Doppman JL et al. Aggressive resection of metastatic disease in selected patients with malignant gastrinoma. Ann Surg 1986; 203(4):352–9.

74. Jaskowiak NT, Fraker DL, Alexander HR et al. Is reoperation for gastrinoma excision indicated in Zollinger–Ellison syndrome? Surgery 1996; 120(6):1055–62; discussion 1062–3.

75. Norton JA, Cornelius MJ, Doppman JL et al. Effect of parathyroidectomy in patients with hyperparathyroidism, Zollinger–Ellison syndrome, and multiple endocrine neoplasia type I: a prospective study. Surgery 1987; 102(6):958–66.

76. MacFarlane MP, Fraker DL, Alexander HR et al. Prospective study of surgical resection of duodenal and pancreatic gastrinomas in multiple endocrine neoplasia type 1. Surgery 1995; 118(6):973–79; discussion 979–80.

77. Thompson NW. Current concepts in the surgical management of multiple endocrine neoplasia type 1 pancreatic-duodenal disease. Results in the treatment of 40 patients with Zollinger–Ellison syndrome, hypoglycaemia or both. J Intern Med 1998; 243(6):495–500.

78. Thompson NW. Management of pancreatic endocrine tumors in patients with multiple endocrine neoplasia type 1. Surg Oncol Clin North Am 1998; 7(4):881–91.

79. Norton JA, Fraker DL, Alexander HR et al. Surgery increases survival in patients with gastrinoma. Ann Surg 2006; 244(3):410–19.

    Study demonstrating improved survival in patients who undergo surgical resection for gastrinoma.

80. Jensen RT. Pancreatic endocrine tumors: recent advances. Ann Oncol 1999; 10(Suppl 4):170–6.

81. Baudin E, Gigliotti A, Ducreux M et al. Neuron-specific enolase and chromogranin A as markers of neuroendocrine tumours. Br J Cancer 1998; 78(8):1102–7.

82. Nobels FR, Kwekkeboom DJ, Bouillon R et al. Chromogranin A: its clinical value as marker of neuroendocrine tumours. Eur J Clin Invest 1998; 28(6):431–40.

83. van Eijck CH, Lamberts SW, Lemaire LC et al. The use of somatostatin receptor scintigraphy in the differential diagnosis of pancreatic duct cancers and islet cell tumors. Ann Surg 1996; 224(2):119–24.

84. Gibril F, Venzon DJ, Ojeaburu JV et al. Prospective study of the natural history of gastrinoma in patients with MEN1: definition of an aggressive

and a nonaggressive form. J Clin Endocrinol Metab 2001; 86(11):5282–93.

85. Rothmund M, Stinner B, Arnold R. Endocrine pancreatic carcinoma. Eur J Surg Oncol 1991; 17(2):191–9.

86. Modlin IM, Lewis JJ, Ahlman H et al. Management of unresectable malignant endocrine tumors of the pancreas. Surg Gynecol Obstet 1993; 176(5):507–18.

87. Zogakis TG, Norton JA. Palliative operations for patients with unresectable endocrine neoplasia. Surg Clin North Am 1995; 75(3):525–38.

88. Danforth DN Jr, Gorden P, Brennan MF. Metastatic insulin-secreting carcinoma of the pancreas: clinical course and the role of surgery. Surgery 1984; 96(6):1027–37.

89. Norton JA, Doherty GM, Fraker DL et al. Surgical treatment of localized gastrinoma within the liver: a prospective study. Surgery 1998; 124(6): 1145–52.

90. Norton JA, Warren RS, Kelly MG et al. Aggressive surgery for metastatic liver neuroendocrine tumors. Surgery 2003; 134(6):1057–63; discussion 1063–5.

91. Mozell E, Woltering EA, O'Dorisio TM et al. Effect of somatostatin analog on peptide release and tumor growth in the Zollinger–Ellison syndrome. Surg Gynecol Obstet 1990; 170(6):476–84.

92. Frank M, Klose KJ, Wied M et al. Combination therapy with octreotide and alpha-interferon: effect on tumor growth in metastatic endocrine gastroenteropancreatic tumors. Am J Gastroenterol 1999; 94(5):1381–7.

6

Gastrointestinal carcinoids

Göran Åkerström
Per Hellman
Ola Hessman

Introduction

In 1907 Oberndorfer first used the name carcinoid to describe rare ileal tumours with less malignant behaviour than common large-bowel carcinomas. Subsequently it has become a common name for tumours derived from a widely distributed neuro-endocrine cell system, with a typical positive silver staining reaction histologically, termed argyrophilia. The carcinoids have been classified according to embryological origin into **foregut carcinoids** (lungs, thymus, stomach, duodenum, pancreas), **midgut carcinoids** (small bowel to proximal colon) and **hindgut carcinoids** (distal colon and rectum), and each of these tumour groups have displayed variable microscopic staining characteristics and clinical features. The midgut carcinoids, originating from intestinal enterochromaffin (EC) cells, have been named classical carcinoids because of their positive argentaffin silver staining reaction (positive Masson stain), due to serotonin production in the tumour cells.

Carcinoids are relatively rare neuroendocrine tumours with an incidence of 1.2–2.1 per 100 000 population per year.[1] Nearly 70% of carcinoids occur in the gastrointestinal tract (Table 6.1).[1] Many carcinoids are clinically silent and subclinical carcinoids have been detected at autopsy with an incidence of 8.4%. Appendiceal carcinoids have been common in autopsy studies and previous clinical series, and recent reports indicate an increase in pulmonary, small-intestinal and gastric carcinoids, due to increased awareness and improved detection.[1]

Under a new classification the term 'carcinoid tumour' is reserved for classical midgut carcinoid tumours secreting serotonin, often demonstrated histologically by specific immunoreactivity. Other types of carcinoids are more properly named neuroendocrine tumours of the respective organ of origin. They are further classified into the categories well-differentiated neuroendocrine tumours, well-differentiated endocrine carcinoma, poorly differentiated endocrine carcinomas, and mixed exocrine–endocrine tumours (Box 6.1).[2,3] The classification is based on histological appearance, mitotic index (number of mitoses per $2\,mm^2$ or 10 high-power fields), and proliferation index established by Ki67/Mib-1 antibody staining (of the proliferation antigen).[4] The well-differentiated tumours have a low rate of mitosis and low proliferation index (generally <2%). Most poorly differentiated tumours have an increased rate of mitosis and higher proliferation index of around 20–40%, but a subgroup has intermediate proliferation with an index of 5–15%, indicating variable rate of tumour progression. The Ki67 proliferation index has become of increased importance in clinical planning.[1,4,5] Extensive surgery is more likely to be beneficial for

Table 6.1 • Distribution of carcinoid tumours by site[1]

Site	Occurrence (%)
Extragastrointestinal (lung, thymic, ovary, uterus)	33
Oesophagus	<1
Stomach	4–8
Duodenum/pancreas	<2
Small intestine	30
Appendix	8
Colon	10
Rectum	11

Box 6.1 • Alternative classification of endocrine tumours, including the carcinoids[3]

Well-differentiated neuroendocrine tumour (carcinoid)

Benign behaviour: confined to mucosa–submucosa, non-angioinvasive, ≤1 cm in size and non-functioning.
Uncertain behaviour: confined to mucosa–submucosa, >1 cm in size or angioinvasive.

Well-differentiated endocrine carcinoma (malignant carcinoid)

Low-grade malignant, deeply invasive (muscularis propria or beyond) or with metastases.
Non-functioning or **functioning**

Poorly differentiated endocrine carcinoma – small-cell carcinoma

High-grade malignant, usually non-functioning (occasionally with ectopic Cushing's syndrome).

Mixed exocrine–endocrine tumours

differentiated tumours with low proliferation, in contrast to chemotherapy, which generally has little effect in low proliferating carcinoids. Chromogranin A and synaptophysin immunostains, which identify proteins of neurosecretory granules, are now commonly used instead of silver stains to identify neuroendocrine tumours. Antibodies against cytosolic markers – neurone-specific enolase (NSE) and PGP9.5 – have also been used to assist in the identification of these tumours, but have generally not been as specific.[5] In poorly differentiated lesions chromogranin staining is variable and involves only subsets of cells. Synaptophysin reactivity alone in the absence of chromogranin staining may indicate an exocrine tumour with endocrine differentiation, the so-called mixed exocrine–endocrine carcinoma. Dominant secretion (e.g. serotonin, histamine, gastrin, somatostatin) may also be detected in neuroendocrine tumours, and occasionally ectopic hormone production, such as adrenocorticotropic hormone (ACTH) and corticotropin-releasing factor (CRF), is seen. The latter two sometimes cause an ectopic Cushing's syndrome in association with foregut carcinoids (Table 6.2).[5]

This chapter will for clarity utilise the traditional classification, and the term midgut carcinoids will mainly refer to the majority of jejuno-ileal tumours. Patients with any of the carcinoid tumours may be at increased risk for a second malignancy, mainly colorectal cancers, but also breast and prostate carcinoma, and although this has been disputed it should be considered during long-term patient follow-up.

Table 6.2 • Classification of carcinoid tumours, hormone production and syndromes[5]

Category	Localisation	Hormone production*	Syndrome
Foregut carcinoids	Thymus	ACTH, CRF	Ectopic Cushing's syndrome, acromegaly, atypical carcinoid syndrome
	Lung	ACTH, CRF, ADH, GRH, gastrin, PP, hCG-α/β, serotonin	A typical carcinoid syndrome
	Stomach	Gastrin, histamine (serotonin)	Zollinger–Ellison syndrome
	Duodenum	Gastrin, somatostatin (Serotonin)	(Carcinoid syndrome)
	Pancreas		
Midgut carcinoids	Jejunum–ileum	Serotonin, NKA	Classical carcinoid syndrome (Carcinoid syndrome)
	Prox. colon	Substance P, bradykinin, prostaglandins	
	Appendix	No hormone production (serotonin)	
Hindgut carcinoids	Colon	PYY	
	Rectum	CG-α/β	

*ACTH, adrenocorticotropic hormone; ADH, antidiuretic hormone (vasopressin); CRF, corticotropin-releasing factor; GRH, growth hormone; hCG, human choriogonadotropin (α/β subunits); NKA, neurokinin A; PP, pancreatic polypeptide; PYY, peptide YY.

Oesophageal carcinoids

Oesophageal carcinoids are exceedingly rare, and occur with male predominance at an age of around 60 years.[1] Most tumours are found in the lower third of the oesophagus or in the gastro-oesophageal junction. Symptoms are non-specific and similar to adenocarcinoma or squamous carcinoma, and patients rarely exhibit a carcinoid syndrome. Lymph node metastases have been present at diagnosis in 50% of patients; survival rates correlate with stage of the disease, and overall is poor.

Gastric carcinoids

Gastric carcinoids are rare tumours, constituting less than 1% of gastric neoplasms and approximately 8% of all carcinoids (Table 6.1).[1,6,7] Most of these tumours are derived from argyrophilic enterochromaffin-like (ECL) cells of the gastric fundus and corpus. The majority of gastric carcinoids occur secondary to hypergastrinaemia in patients with chronic atrophic gastritis (CAG). These carcinoids are typically multicentric and develop concomitant with ECL cell hyperplasia in the fundus and corpus, or occasionally in the transitional zone to the antrum[6,7] (**type 1 gastric carcinoids**). Similar non-antral and multicentric argyrophilic carcinoids and ECL cell hyperplasia are occasionally seen in patients with hypergastrinaemia and multiple endocrine neoplasia type 1 (MEN 1)-related Zollinger–Ellison syndrome (ZES) (**type 2 gastric carcinoids**). Less common are gastric carcinoids that develop as sporadic, generally solitary tumours, without concomitant argyrophilic cell hyperplasia (**type 3 gastric carcinoids**). These sporadic carcinoids are often large when detected, and more frequently associated with metastases. Like the other gastric carcinoids, the sporadic tumours most often develop from ECL cells, but may also originate in argentaffin (serotonin-producing) cells, or contain a mixture with other endocrine cell types. The ECL cells have the ability to secrete histamine, and disseminated lesions of the solitary type may occasionally be associated with an atypical carcinoid syndrome. Exceptionally, prepyloric or antral sporadic tumours may produce gastrin and should therefore more appropriately be named gastrinomas. Another group of gastric neuroendocrine tumours consists of undifferentiated tumours, composed of intermediate-sized or small cells (**poorly differentiated neuroendocrine carcinoma**).

The incidence of gastric carcinoids has increased, due to more frequent gastroscopic examinations, for example during population screening for gastric cancer, or when screening studies have been performed in patients with atrophic gastritis or pernicious anaemia.

Histology

Different histological patterns have been defined in ECL hyperplasia, and used to depict the stepwise progression through dysplasia to the formation of carcinoid tumours.[3,6,7] **Simple or diffuse hyperplasia** is defined as increased density of often hypertrophic, argyrophilic ECL cells; **linear hyperplasia** consists of ECL cell trabeculae along the basement membrane or gastric glands; **micronodular hyperplasia** depicts clusters or nodules of such cells and, together with linear hyperplasia, is common in CAG patients with advanced hypergastrinaemia; **adenomatoid hyperplasia** consists of collections of several micronodules often found in cases with CAG or MEN 1/ZES.

Dysplastic or precarcinoid ECL cell lesions also appear with different histological patterns, but generally consist of larger collections of slightly atypical endocrine cells with enlarged nuclei and reduced reactivity for secretory granule markers. These lesions are non-invasive and do not infiltrate beyond the muscularis mucosae, but constitute markers for neoplastic alterations, since they coexist with carcinoids in CAG and MEN 1/ZES.[6]

When nodules are larger than 0.5 mm the lesions are classified as **carcinoid tumours**. Gastric carcinoids are generally composed of regular-shaped tumour cells with round nuclei and mainly characterised by microlobules and trabeculae. In histological grading, grades 1 and 2 correspond to 'typical' and 'atypical' carcinoids, and grade 3 to the poorly differentiated neuroendocrine carcinomas.[2] Mitoses are absent or rare in **grade 1** lesions, occur with cellular atypia in **grade 2**, and are abundant with poor differentiation, severe atypia and cell necrosis in **grade 3**.[2]

ECL cell tumours are strongly agyrophilic and immunoreactive to chromogranin A and histamine, and are reported to be identified with the marker vesicular monoamine transporter isoform

2 (VMAT2),[8] which also may be positive in midgut carcinoids. Immunoreactivity to hormonal products such as serotonin, gastrin, somatostatin, pancreatic polypeptide (PP) or α-subunit of human choriogonadotropin (hCG-α) is absent or focal.[3] Grade 1 lesions with a proliferation index <1–2%, size less than 1 cm, and no invasion beyond the mucosa are mostly benign, whereas tumours with histological grade 2 and 3, size 3 cm, and with higher mitotic and proliferation index (Ki67 >5%) are more commonly malignant.[2]

Type 1: gastric carcinoids associated with chronic atrophic gastritis

These tumours account for 70–80% of gastric carcinoids (Table 6.3). They occur occasionally in young individuals, but most commonly in older patients, with a mean age around 65 years, and there is a 3:1 female to male predominance.[7]

The carcinoids develop in patients with autoimmune CAG type A,[7] where atrophy of the fundic mucosa is accompanied by pentagastrin-resistant achlorhydria and vitamin B_{12} malabsorption. More than half of the patients also have pernicious anaemia (Table 6.3). Reduction of gastric acid and increase in pH stimulates gastrin secretion from gastrin (G) cells in the antrum, and the resulting hypergastrinaemia induces hyperplasia of the fundic ECL cells. Diffuse argyrophilic hyperplasia of the non-antral mucosa occurs in 65% of patients with

CAG, and micronodular/adenomatoid hyperplasia in 30%, whereas the precarcinoid and dysplastic, enlarged micronodules develop mainly in patients with gross carcinoids. The tumour development progresses from the specified stages of hyperplasia, through dysplastic stages, to neoplastic intramucosal or invasive carcinoids.[6,7]

It is important to emphasise that, although CAG is common in elderly individuals, only few affected patients (1%) ultimately develop gastric carcinoids. The tumours occur mainly in patients with a long duration of a markedly raised serum gastrin, and who have more prevalent hyperplastic changes. The CAG-associated carcinoids contain predominantly ECL cells, intermingled with other specific or poorly defined endocrine cells.

The argyrophilic gastric carcinoids are predominantly located within the body or the fundus of the stomach, or in the transitional zone to the antrum.[7,9] They are frequently multicentric, consisting of multiple, small gastric polyps and invariably associated with ECL cell hyperplasia and microscopic tumours. The number of gross lesions can, however, be limited and some tumours may thus appear as solitary. Individual tumours can present as broad-based, round polypoid lesions, reddish to yellowish, depending on the thickness of the covering mucosa. Some carcinoids can be flat and broad, or appear as discoloured spots or simply as slight mucosal protrusions. Only a few are ulcerated or bleeding. The number and size vary from innumerable pinpoint-size tumours to a few or solitary prominent lesions ranging from a few millimetres up to 1–1.5 cm,

Table 6.3 • Gastric carcinoid tumours

	Type 1 (70–80%)	Type 2 (6–8%)	Type 3 (15–20%)
Description	Chronic atrophic gastritis (type A), pernicious anaemia	MEN 1-associated Zollinger–Ellison syndrome	Sporadic
Tumour site in stomach	Fundus and body	Fundus and body	Fundus, body and antrum
Characteristics	Usually multiple polyps (often <1 cm, occasionally 1–2 cm)	Usually multiple polyps (<1–2 cm), occasionally larger	Single, solitary (2–5 cm)
Histopathology*/gastric fundal biopsy	ECL cell lesion; progression: hyperplasia–dysplasia–neoplasia	ECL cell lesion; progression: hyperplasia–dysplasia–neoplasia	ECL, EC or other cells; normal adjacent mucosa
Biological behaviour	Slow growth, rarely metastasise	Usually slow growth, lymph node metastases 30%, liver metastases 10–20%	Aggressive, frequent metastases to regional nodes (71%) and liver (69%)
Plasma gastrin	Elevated	Elevated	Normal
Acid output	Low or absent	High	Normal or low

* EC, enterochromaffin; ECL, enterochromaffin-like.

and only occasionally larger tumours (>2 cm). The tumours are generally benign, without signs of invasion beyond the submucosa. Infiltration of the muscularis propria is found in a minority (<10%). The polypoid carcinoids may be difficult to distinguish from hyperplastic polyps, which are also more frequent in patients with CAG.

CAG-associated carcinoids have a lower incidence of metastases and more favourable outcome than other types of gastric carcinoids. Metastases to regional lymph nodes occur in <5% and distant metastases in around 2%.[7] However, earlier reports with a greater proportion of large lesions described more frequent metastases.[10] Disease-related deaths are exceptional.

Occasional CAG patients have harboured larger, considerably more invasive tumours, representing poorly differentiated neuroendocrine carcinomas or composite endocrine tumours/adenocarcinoma (see below). All these have an unfavourable prognosis.

Type 2: carcinoids associated with ZES in MEN 1 patients

These gastric carcinoids constitute 6–8%[8] of all gastric carcinoids, and are thus much less common than those associated with atrophic gastritis (Table 6.3). They occur in patients with MEN 1 and gastrin-producing tumours as a cause of ZES, with equal female:male distribution, at a mean age of 45–50 years.[7]

ECL cell hyperplasia is found in almost 80% of MEN 1 patients with ZES, and fundic gastric carcinoids develop in 5–30% of these patients.[11] In addition to the hyperplasia and dysplasia of ECL cells in the fundic mucosa, the oxyntic mucosal thickness is invariably increased, in contrast to the atrophy of type 1 lesions. These carcinoids also develop in a hyperplasia–dysplasia–neoplasia sequence, but have mainly been associated with diffuse hyperplasia and precarcinoid lesions, and less evident micronodular changes. However, gastric carcinoids in sporadic ZES have been rare, and only ZES in association with MEN 1 seems to promote growth of gastric carcinoids.[12] The MEN 1 syndrome is caused by an inherited mutation of the *MEN1* tumour suppressor gene located on chromosome 11q13 (see Chapter 4). As in other MEN 1 lesions, the gastric carcinoids in MEN 1 lose their single remaining functional copy of the *MEN1* gene by chromosomal deletions.[13]

In MEN 1 patients without ZES, gastric carcinoids are extremely rare.[14] Thus, hypergastrinaemia seems to be required for development of gastric carcinoids from ECL hyperplasia. However, additional factors are obviously needed for tumour formation, since only 1% of patients with hypergastrinaemia due to atrophic gastritis and <1% of patients with sporadic ZES develop gastric carcinoids.[11,14,15]

The type 2 gastric carcinoids are located in the gastric body and fundus, and occasionally in the antrum, and have been composed mainly of ECL cells with sparse other cell types. They are most often multiple and small (73% are smaller than 1.5 cm), although often larger than type 1 tumours, with a size varying from 0.5 to 2 cm. Occasionally there are markedly larger tumours. The malignant potential is intermediate between that of CAG-associated gastric carcinoids and sporadic carcinoids, and 90% will not have infiltrated beyond the submucosa. However, lymph node metastases are present in up to 30% of the patients and distant metastases, assumed to originate from gastric carcinoids, occur in 10–20%. MEN 1 patients develop distant metastases from other MEN 1-associated tumours as well, and the gastric carcinoids are not the most likely origin. The overall prognosis will depend more on the other MEN 1 lesions, and the prognosis is usually rather favourable for the type 2 carcinoids.[12] However, rare cases of highly malignant neuroendocrine gastric carcinomas with poor prognosis have also occurred in some MEN 1/ZES patients.[14]

Type 3: sporadic carcinoid tumours

Tumours with no association to hypergastrinaemia account for 15–20% of the gastric carcinoids and have features that markedly differ from type 1 and type 2 lesions (Table 6.3).[7] They occur sporadically, are usually solitary, and grow much more aggressively. Many are already disseminated at diagnosis.[7] These carcinoids have a male predominance, with a male:female ratio of 3:1; mean age of presentation is around 50 years of age. The sporadic gastric carcinoids occur in non-atrophic gastric mucosa, without endocrine cell proliferation. Determination of serum calcium and examination of the family history may help exclude the MEN 1 syndrome, which should be suspected in all patients with foregut carcinoids unrelated to atrophic gastritis.

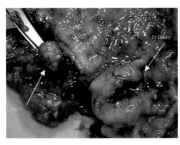

Figure 6.1 • Sporadic, solitary gastric carcinoid with lymph gland metastasis removed by gastric resection.

The sporadic tumours are often large; one-third exceed 2 cm (**Fig. 6.1**). Two-thirds of the lesions will have infiltrated the muscularis propria and 50% invaded all layers of the gastric wall. Some tumours occur in the antral, prepyloric regions, although the majority are located in the body and fundus of the stomach. Most tumours originate in argyrophilic ECL cells, but a mixture of other cell types and EC cells may be present, and are associated with a less favourable prognosis. Regional lymph node metastases have been described in 71% of these patients and liver metastases ultimately develop in 69% of the patients. Half of patients are alive after follow-up of 5 years, but patients with distant metastases have a 10% 5-year survival.[1,16]

The sporadic carcinoids may have typical or atypical histology. Atypical implies marked nuclear pleomorphism with irregular hyperchromatic nuclei, increased number of mitoses and frequent areas of necrosis. The atypical tumours are larger, more frequently invasive and commonly associated with metastases at diagnosis.[2] A series of sporadic gastric carcinoids with atypical morphology reported a mean size of 5 cm and unfavourable survival.[17]

An **atypical carcinoid syndrome** occurs in 5–10% of the patients with sporadic gastric carcinoids, and is associated with tumour release of histamine. The syndrome is characterised by bright-red cutaneous flushing, often with a patchy 'geographic' distribution, cutaneous oedema, intense itching, bronchospasm, salivary gland swelling and lacrimation.[7] The atypical carcinoid syndrome is related to histamine secretion, and urinary estimates of the histamine metabolite methylmidazoleacetic acid (MelmAA) may serve as tumour marker. Most gastric carcinoid tumours are deficient in the enzyme L-amino acid decarboxylase, and only a few patients have elevated levels of serotonin. Urinary excre-

tion of the serotonin metabolite 5-hydroxyindole-acetic acid (5-HIAA) is therefore less appropriate as a tumour marker.[9] However, the precursor 5-hydroxytryptophan (5-HTP) may be excreted and partly decarboxylated in the kidney, and the patients with disseminated sporadic gastric carcinoids may exhibit some elevated urinary 5-HIAA values.

Gastrinoma

Tumours with sparse staining for gastrin may occur in association with chronic atrophic gastritis. Tumours with intense positive staining for gastrin are rare in the stomach, and are more commonly located in the prepyloric mucosa close to the duodenum. Few gastric carcinoids cause hypergastrinaemia and peptic ulcer disease, but they still represent an exceptional but possible origin of gastrin excess and ZES.[9] Rare tumours may present with ectopic Cushing's syndrome due to ACTH secretion.

Poorly differentiated neuroendocrine carcinomas

The poorly differentiated neuroendocrine carcinomas are highly malignant neoplasms, with generally extensive local invasion and metastases already at diagnosis. They are not associated with the carcinoid syndrome and occur at a mean age of 60–70 years, with male predominance.[18] Atrophic gastritis is present in half of the patients, but is not believed to cause the tumour, since only a minority of patients have hypergastrinaemia. The majority of tumours are located in the gastric corpus or fundus, but 10–20% may occur in the antrum.[18] The tumours are generally large, with median size of around 4–5 cm, invariably deeply invading the gastric wall and associated with metastases. The majority of lesions appear as ulcerated tumours and a quarter are fungating.[18] They all tend to be of histological grade 3, and often have solid structures with necrosis, a high degree of atypia, frequent mitoses and high proliferation index in Ki67 staining (generally around 20–40%). Almost all tumours show vascular and perineural invasion. In contrast to the well-differentiated gastric carcinoids, the poorly differentiated neuroendocrine carcinomas may have sparse immunoreactivity to chromogranin A, at least in the majority of tumour cells.[2] Immunoreactivity to synaptophysin (and possibly NSE or PGP9.5) may verify the neuroendocrine differentiation and separate these tumours from exocrine carcinomas. The prognosis is poor with a median survival of 8 months, albeit some individuals are reported to be still alive after follow-up of 10–15 years.[2,18]

The possibility of progression from well-differentiated gastric carcinoids, especially type 3 lesions, to neuroendocrine carcinomas has been suggested by a few cases with coexisting well- and poorly differentiated gastric neuroendocrine tumours.[2,3,14]

Aberration of the *p53* tumour suppressor gene and chromosomal deletion of the long arm of chromosome 18 are common in poorly differentiated neuroendocrine carcinomas, and occasionally found also in type 3 sporadic gastric carcinoids.[2] These genetic defects occur in gastrointestinal exocrine carcinomas and may promote aggressive tumour growth. Genetic studies of rare mixed neuroendocrine–exocrine gastric carcinomas suggest that the endocrine tumour component may originate in adenocarcinoma cells.

Clinical evaluation

Symptoms and patient history

The majority of gastric carcinoids found in elderly patients with atrophic gastritis are detected incidentally by gastroscopy evaluation for anaemia or uncharacteristic abdominal symptoms, or by routine endoscopic screening. Bleeding and anaemia may occur, generally with the larger, mainly sporadic carcinoids. The poorly differentiated tumours especially may mimic gastric carcinoma, with gastric outlet obstruction. Some become apparent because of metastases, and a few disseminated sporadic carcinoids present with the atypical carcinoid syndrome.

Patient history should explore the presence of CAG or pernicious anaemia or MEN 1-related endocrinopathies (hyperparathyroidism, endocrine pancreatic or pituitary tumours) both in the patient and family members.

Diagnosis

Diagnosis of CAG carcinoids is based on demonstration of high levels of serum gastrin, lack of gastric acid secretion and demonstration of atrophy of the oxyntic mucosa, with concomitant ECL cell hyperplasia in mucosal biopsies from the fundus (Table 6.3). The serum levels of gastrin are also high

in patients with MEN 1 gastrinomas, although these patients have contrasting high gastric acidity.

Thorough gastroscopic examination should be performed to evaluate multiplicity and size of the carcinoid tumours. Tumour biopsies should be stained with specific endocrine tumour markers and proliferation markers (chromogranin A, Ki67 staining), and should carefully investigate infiltrative depth and possible vascular invasion. In addition, multiple biopsies from the fundus region, away from the tumour(s), are crucial to reveal concomitant ECL cell hyperplasia or dysplasia, the presence of atrophic gastritis, or the contrasting increased oxyntic mucosa thickness of rare MEN 1/ZES (Table 6.3). Multiple carcinoid polyps in the gastric fundus in an elderly individual are most likely to represent CAG-associated carcinoids, since MEN 1-associated carcinoids are rare. A larger, solitary tumour is more likely to be sporadic (Fig. 6.1), and the largest ulcerating and most prominent lesions poorly differentiated. Endoscopic ultrasound added to the gastroscopic examination may give information about infiltrative depth, reveal associated lesions in the pancreas or duodenum in MEN 1 patients, and also show metastases to regional lymph nodes or the liver.[19]

Biochemical screening for other MEN 1 endocrinopathies should include analysis of serum calcium and parathyroid hormone, pituitary-related hormones such as growth hormone, prolactin and insulin-like growth factor 1 (IGF-1), and pancreatic hormones (Box 6.2). For cases with the atypical carcinoid syndrome, screening should include urinary analysis of the histamine metabolite MelmAA. Serum values of chromogranin A are generally raised in patients with CAG and ECL hyperplasia. These values are also the most important tumour markers, and since they tend to reflect the tumour load,

---

Box 6.2 • Biochemical screening for the MEN 1 syndrome (serum estimates)

- Serum calcium
- Parathyroid hormone
- Chromogranin A
- Pancreatic polypeptide (PP)
- Gastrin
- Insulin, proinsulin/glucose
- Glucagon
- Prolactin
- Somatomedin C (IGF-1)

they are often used to monitor patients undergoing treatment for advanced gastric carcinoids.[20]

Computed tomography (CT) with contrast enhancement is routinely performed for tumour delineation and to detect regional lymph node or liver metastases. Scintigraphy using [^{111}In]octreotide scintigraphy (OctreoScan) can often efficiently reveal metastatic spread from differentiated carcinoids.[21]

Treatment

CAG-associated type 1 gastric carcinoids

These may disappear spontaneously, and few show more marked progression.[7,9,15] Small, multicentric lesions may be followed with annual repeated endoscopy.

For larger type 1 carcinoids close to and above 1 cm endoscopic mucosal resection is recommended for up to six polyps not involving the muscularis propria layer. Endoscopic ultrasound (EUS) is necessary for evaluation of invasiveness.[22–25] Local surgical tumour excision is performed for larger tumours or those with muscularis layer invasion. In case of malignant development or recurrence despite local surgical resection, partial or total gastrectomy with lymph node dissection is recommended.[25]

Antrectomy has been recommended for treatment of CAG-associated gastric carcinoids, with the aim of inhibiting antral overproduction of gastrin.[26] The antrectomy is claimed to cause regression of ECL dysplasia and small carcinoids; however, large, invasive or metastatic lesions may remain unaffected.[26,27] Resection of the antrum may therefore be considered for multicentric or recurrent tumour, and is often combined with surgical excision of larger type 1 carcinoids, but results and morbidity of this versus repeated endoscopic excision remain unclear.[16,27]

MEN 1-related type 2 gastric carcinoids

These are more malignant than CAG-associated carcinoids. Surgical treatment should focus both on removal of the source of hypergastrinaemia and on excision of the gastric carcinoids. Concomitant

exposure of both pancreas and duodenum, via duodenotomy, is done to locate both gastrinomas and possible MEN 1 pancreatic lesions, and 80% distal pancreatic resection is most often performed.[14,28] In type 2 ECLomas >1 cm local excision is recommended. Gastric resection with regional lymph node clearance is advocated for larger tumours.[7,25]

Gastrectomy may occasionally be required for very large tumours, although gastrin excess in MEN 1 gastrinoma is generally efficiently treated by proton-pump inhibitors.

Sporadic type 3 gastric carcinoids

These are clearly malignant, with high risk of metastases also for rare small tumours. Most tumours are large and require operative excision, often performed as gastric resection, combined with regional lymph node clearance. Tumours >2 cm or those with atypical histology, gastric wall invasion or local metastases are most appropriately dealt with by gastrectomy.[9,16,25]

In cases with metastases, tumour debulking of lymph gland and liver metastases may alleviate symptoms of an associated carcinoid syndrome and apparently improve survival.[7] Hepatic metastases may be treated with liver resection, hepatic artery embolisation or chemoembolisation, and radiofrequency (RF) ablation (see below). The somatostatin analogue octreotide may palliate symptoms in patients with the carcinoid syndrome. Chemotherapy is likely to be valuable when the proliferation index exceeds 5%, and has response rates of 20–40%. Chemotherapy can be combined with other treatment modalities.[29]

Poorly differentiated neuroendocrine tumours

These generally have a dismal prognosis, with a median survival of only 8 months.[2,24,25] The tumours are rarely suitable for radical surgery and recurrence should be checked for after gastric resection. However, aggressive surgery together with chemotherapy may be an option to consider, especially in patients with mixtures of well- and poorly differentiated tumours.[2]

Duodenal carcinoids

Carcinoids of the duodenum are rare, and comprise less than 2% of all gastrointestinal neuroendocrine tumours.[9,30] Duodenal adenomas or adenocarcinomas are much more frequent. However, the endocrine tumours are important to recognise because of a possible association with hormonal or hereditary syndromes and the consequential requirements of treatment. Duodenal carcinoids are so rare that it is difficult to identify prognostic factors and decide optimal treatment on an evidence base.

Gastrinomas

Gastrin-cell (G-cell) tumours – gastrinomas – are the most prevalent and constitute 60% of the duodenal neuroendocrine tumours; 15–30% of G-cell tumours cause clinical ZES, the remainder are clinically silent.[9,30] Most gastrinomas are located in the first and second parts of the duodenum. They are frequently small (often around 0.5 cm or smaller), with early metastases to regional lymph nodes reported in 30–70% of patients.[31,32] The regional lymph node metastases may be considerably larger than the primary tumours, which sometimes may be difficult to detect even at operation. There is generally considerable delay before liver metastases develop, and this is claimed to provide a favourable interval for surgical treatment. It has been recognised that 40–60% of gastrinomas responsible for ZES are located within the duodenal submucosa.[31,32] In nearly 90% of cases, MEN 1/ZES patients have multifocal duodenal gastrinomas.[33,34] The duodenal gastrinomas in ZES are slow-growing, indolent malignancies despite their tendency to spread with local lymph node metastases. Duodenal gastrinomas in ZES are rarely identified by endoscopy because of their small size, and they are also often difficult to visualise during surgery. Endoscopic transillumination has been advocated, but it is more efficient to perform a long duodenotomy, allowing discovery of gastrinomas after inversion and palpation of the duodenal mucosa.[32,33]

Duodenal tumours smaller than 5 mm can be enucleated with the overlying mucosa; larger tumours are excised with full thickness of the duodenal wall. Careful exploration is undertaken for the removal of lymph gland metastases around the pancreatic head. The duodenal gastrinoma has been considered as a potentially curable cause of ZES, especially for non-MEN 1/ZES. The prognosis is favourable after resection of duodenal gastrinomas in both sporadic and MEN 1/ZES patients, with survival reaching 60–85% after 10 years.[31–34]

Somatostatin-rich carcinoids

Carcinoids with somatostatin reactivity comprise 15–20% of duodenal neuroendocrine tumours. These tumours are most often clinically hormonally non-functioning.[30,35,36] They occur almost exclusively in the ampulla of Vater, causing obstructive jaundice, pancreatitis or bleeding. The tumours appear as 1- to 2-cm homogeneous ampulla nodules, which only occasionally are polypoid, larger or ulcerated. Regional lymph node or liver metastases are present in nearly 50% of patients. Unlike conventional carcinoids, these tumours have a glandular growth pattern and characteristically contain special laminated psammoma bodies. They are neither argyrophilic nor argentaffin but can be identified with special silver staining or chromogranin stain. One-third of these lesions are associated with von Recklinghausen's neurofibromatosis (neurofibromatosis type 1, NF1) and occasionally with phaeochromocytoma.[35] Depending on the size of the tumours and the age of the patient, the somatostatin-rich carcinoids may be locally excised or removed by pancreatico-duodenectomy.

Gangliocytic paragangliomas

Gangliocytic paragangliomas are rare tumours, occurring almost exclusively in the second portion of the duodenum, and are sometimes associated with neurofibromatosis (NF1). The tumours consist of a mixture of paraganglioma, ganglioneuroma and carcinoid tissue with reactivity for somatostatin and pancreatic polypeptide (PP). The tumours are generally benign, recognised only incidentally or because of bleeding, and have an excellent prognosis following surgical excision.

Other carcinoids

More unusual well-differentiated duodenal carcinoids may display reactivity for other hormones, such as calcitonin, PP and serotonin. Most of these tumours are found in the proximal part of the duodenum as small polyps (<2 cm). Multiple tumours should raise suspicion of an associated MEN 1 syndrome. The majority of these tumours are low-grade malignant and often suitable for local surgical excision. Only rarely do large tumours require pancreatico-duodenectomy.

A distinct group of duodenal carcinoids without release or staining for hormones is also recognised. These tumours have a somewhat different biology and metastasise less often than the gastrinomas and somatostatinomas.[37] Some of them are asymptomatic and incidentally found at endoscopic examination. Others present with non-specific abdominal symptoms, gastrointestinal bleeding and sometimes with vomiting or weight loss.[37] Most tumours are located in the first portion of the duodenum, occasionally in the second part and rarely in the third portion (horizontal duodenum). The majority stain for chromogranin A, and some for synaptophysin and/or NSE.[37] Up to one-third of the patients have had other primary malignancies as well, including adenocarcinomas of the gastrointestinal tract, prostate or other organs.[37]

More than half of the tumours are smaller than 2 cm, and generally have a good prognosis after resection. Size >2 cm, invasion beyond the submucosa or presence of mitotic figures are independent risk factors for metastases.[30] Tumours with these risk factors are likely to recur after apparently curative surgery, even if no lymph node metastases have been detected, whereas lesions smaller than 2 cm rarely metastasise.[37]

Lesions smaller than 1 cm can be endoscopically excised, but re-examination with follow-up endoscopy is required to ensure complete removal.[37] Tumours smaller than 2 cm, without signs of invasion of the muscularis, can be safely treated by open local excision. The treatment suggested for larger tumours is segmental resection or pancreatico-duodenectomy in order to decrease the risk of recurrence.[37] Periampullary tumours behave in a malignant fashion and need more radical surgery. Patients with metastasising duodenal carcinoids may survive for decades, substantiating that these neuroendocrine tumours are less aggressive than adenocarcinomas.

Neuroendocrine carcinomas

Poorly differentiated neuroendocrine carcinomas in the duodenum are exceptionally rare. Most occur in the ampulla of Vater, and the patients present with obstructive jaundice and invariably with a rapidly fatal course.[9]

Pancreatic carcinoids

Pancreatic islet cell tumours are generally classified according to their dominant hormone secretion, or depicted as clinically non-functioning if not associated with any clinical syndrome of hormone excess. These tumours should not be included among carcinoids in the presence of minimal serotonin immunoreactivity. Exceptionally, endocrine tumours of the pancreas stain intensely for serotonin (and may also contain other biogenic amines).[9] They appear histologically as classical carcinoids, but few have been associated with the carcinoid syndrome. The tumours are managed surgically according to guidelines similar to those for other malignant endocrine pancreatic tumours. Hepatic metastases and a carcinoid syndrome may be treated with somatostatin analogues and interferon, or chemotherapy in the presence of a higher proliferation rate.

Jejuno-ileal/midgut carcinoids

The midgut carcinoids originate from intestinal enterochromaffin (EC) cells in intestinal crypts. They have been named classical carcinoids, and typically display both an argyrophilic and argentaffin silver staining reaction (positive Masson stain) due to serotonin production in the tumour cells.[38] The small-intestinal carcinoids have increased in frequency and constitute 25–30% of carcinoids.[1] This syndrome requires somewhat complicated and often combined specialist medical and surgical treatment.[38] The small-intestinal carcinoids account for 25% of small-bowel neoplasms, and have been diagnosed at an average age of 65 years, with slight male predominance.

Morphological features

The primary small-intestinal carcinoid is most commonly located in the terminal parts of the ileum, often appearing as a small, flat and fibrotic submucosal tumour, measuring around 1 cm or less (**Fig. 6.2**),[38] occasionally with some central navelling. Sometimes the tumour is so tiny that it is difficult to detect at

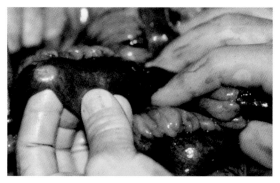

Figure 6.2 • Small-intestinal carcinoid, unusual entity with liver metastases but no mesenteric tumour. Reproduced from Åkerström G, Hellman P, Öhrvall U. Midgut and hindgut carcinoid tumors. In: Doherty GM, Skogseid B (eds) Surgical endocrinology, 1st edn. Philadelphia: Lippincott Williams & Wilkins, 2001; pp. 448–52. With permission from Lippincott Williams & Wilkins.

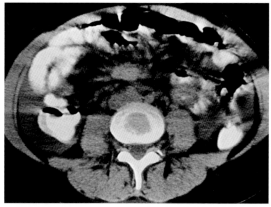

Figure 6.3 • Computed tomography image of mesenteric metastasis from a midgut carcinoid tumour, typically surrounded by fibrosis (appearing like 'hurricane centre'). Reproduced from Åkerström G, Hellman P, Öhrvall U. Midgut and hindgut carcinoid tumors. In: Doherty GM, Skogseid B (eds) Surgical endocrinology, 1st edn. Philadelphia: Lippincott Williams & Wilkins, 2001; pp. 448–52. With permission from Lippincott Williams & Wilkins.

surgery, appearing only as a limited area of fibrosis or circumscribed thickening of the intestinal wall. In up to one-third of patients, multiple smaller carcinoid polyps occur in the nearby intestine, most likely caused by lymphatic dissemination. In a few cases additional larger carcinoid polyps have been found in proximal parts of the intestine, and these represent additional primary tumours. Among patients subjected to surgery, mesenteric metastases have been found at a high frequency. When growing close to the intestinal wall such metastases have sometimes been mistaken for primary tumours. In contrast to carcinoids located elsewhere in the gastrointestinal tract, microscopic or gross metastases have also occurred in association with the smallest primary tumours.[38] Unusual large primary tumours sometimes extend directly into a conglomerate of mesenteric lymph gland metastases. The mesenteric metastases typically grow conspicuously larger than the primary tumour, and characteristically evoke a marked desmoplastic reaction with pronounced mesenteric fibrosis (**Fig. 6.3**). The fibrosis might result from local effects of serotonin, growth factors and other substances secreted from the carcinoid metastases.[38,39]

With more extensive fibrosis the distal ileal mesentery often becomes contracted and tethers the mesenteric root to the retroperitoneum, with fibrous bands attaching to the serosa of the horizontal duodenum. Occasionally fibrosis and tumour extend over parts of the transverse or the sigmoid colon.[38]

The mesenteric tumour and fibrosis can often cause partial or complete small-intestinal obstruc-

tion by kinking and fibrotic entrapment of the intestine, whereas the primary tumour only occasionally is large enough to obstruct the intestinal lumen.[38] Obstruction of the duodenum tends to occur at advanced stages. The mesenteric vessels are often encased or occluded by the growing mesenteric tumour, with resulting local venous stasis and ischaemia in the small intestine, and occasionally frank impairment of the intestinal circulation. Variable segments of the small intestine thus appear dark blue to reddish due to incipient venous gangrene (**Fig. 6.4**), or occasionally pale and cyanotic due to deficient arterial circulation.[38] A specific angiopathy, called vascular elastosis, occurs with advanced midgut carcinoids and causes marked thickening of mesenteric vessel walls due to elastic tissue proliferation in the adventitia; this contributes to the intestinal vascular impairment.[40] However, compression by tumour and fibrosis has in our experience been the obvious cause in patients where intestinal ischaemia was revealed at operation.[38]

Fibrotic attachments between intestines invariably become more pronounced after surgery and frequently create a conglomerate of distal small-intestinal loops and caecum, which becomes fixed to the posterior and anterior abdominal wall.

Distant metastases from small-intestinal carcinoids occur most commonly in the liver and the patients then often present with variable features of

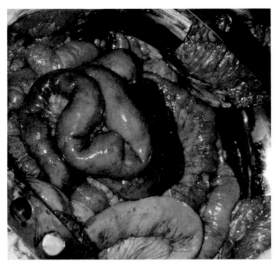

Figure 6.4 • Intestinal venous ischaemia due to midgut carcinoid. Reproduced from Åkerström G, Hellman P, Öhrvall U. Midgut and hindgut carcinoid tumors. In: Doherty GM, Skogseid B (eds) Surgical endocrinology, 1st edn. Philadelphia: Lippincott Williams & Wilkins, 2001; pp. 448–52. With permission from Lippincott Williams & Wilkins.

the carcinoid syndrome. Liver metastases are often bilateral and diffusely spread; approximately 10% of the patients have fewer or dominant lesions, sometimes with conspicuous growth of individual lesions. Around 10% of patients present with liver metastases, without mesenteric lesions. Spread to extra-abdominal sites can involve the skeleton (spine and orbital framing are predilection sites), the lungs, CNS, mediastinal and peripheral lymph nodes, ovaries, breast and the skin.[38] A neck lymph gland metastasis can sometimes be the primary clinical sign of a disseminated tumour.

Clinical symptoms

The carcinoid tumours grow slowly and many patients have experienced long periods of prodromal symptoms before the disease has been clinically recognised.[38] Some patients have had symptoms of borborygmia or episodic abdominal pain, others have had unrecognised features of the carcinoid syndrome, with diarrhoea, discrete flush, palpitations or intolerance for specific food or alcohol. Intestinal bleeding is generally rare with small-intestinal carcinoids due to the moderate size and submucosal location of the primary tumour. Bleeding has been

mainly encountered at later stages, with larger, ulcerating primary tumours, or if mesenteric metastases have grown in the intestinal wall.[38] Such metastases have a special tendency to grow into the horizontal duodenum and have sometimes caused bleeding. In other cases bleeding has occurred as a result of intestinal venous stasis.

Intermittent attacks of abdominal pain may initially occur, and increase in frequency until the patient develops obvious subacute or acute intestinal obstruction requiring surgery. In 30–45% of patients the small-intestinal carcinoids are thus revealed at operation for intestinal obstruction, where the patients often have been submitted to surgery without awareness of the diagnosis.[38] In another 50% of patients the diagnosis becomes evident after detection of liver metastases, and some of the patients have features of the carcinoid syndrome.

Carcinoid syndrome

The carcinoid syndrome occurs in approximately 20% of patients with jejuno-ileal carcinoids.[1] Monoamine oxidase activity in the liver can generally detoxify substances released from the intestinal and mesenteric tumours, and symptoms associated with the carcinoid syndrome generally imply that the patient has liver metastases. Occasionally the syndrome may be encountered in patients with large retroperitoneal or ovarian lesions, where secretory products exceed the capacity of detoxification or can bypass the liver and drain directly into the systemic circulation. The syndrome includes flushing, diarrhoea, right-sided valvular heart disease and bronchoconstriction. The aetiology of the carcinoid syndrome is related to release of serotonin, bradykinin, tachykinins (substance P, neuropeptide K), prostaglandins and growth factors such as platelet-derived growth factor (PDGF) and transforming growth factor β (TGF-β), as well as noradrenaline (norepinephrine).

Secretory diarrhoea is the most common feature of the syndrome, but it may sometimes be mild and non-specific initially. Diarrhoea is often most prevalent in the morning, and often meal related. The diarrhoea may, however, have many causes in carcinoid patients, especially when they have been previously operated upon or have reached advanced disease stages.[38] Resection of the distal small intestine may cause moderate diarrhoea due to reduced bile salt absorption; other causes are a short bowel or partial intestinal obstruction. In patients with large mesenteric tumours intestinal venous stasis or ischaemia may often contribute significantly to stool frequency. Severe watery diarrhoea and malnutrition can occasionally occur due to occlusion of main mesenteric veins, which has caused severely oedematous, fluid-leaking intestinal segments of variable length.[38,41]

Cutaneous flushing generally affects the face, neck and upper chest, and is the most typical feature of the carcinoid syndrome. Flushing may, however, be overlooked especially in females at menopause. The flush may be provoked by stress, alcohol, certain food, aged cheese or coffee. It is often of short duration, lasting for 1–5 minutes, but may occasionally be prolonged for several hours or even days. Flushing may be severe, and when the flush has been long-standing there may be frequent telangiectases and persistent blue-cyanotic discoloration of the skin of the nose and chin.

Heart valve fibrosis, affecting tricuspid and pulmonary valves with plaque-like fibrotic endocardial thickening, is a serious and late consequence of a severe and long-standing carcinoid syndrome.[5,42] Serotonin and tachykinins may influence the heart and cause fibrosis and valvular thickening with retraction and fixation of the heart valves and subsequently regurgitation and stenosis. As many as 65% of patients with the carcinoid syndrome have tricuspid valve abnormalities, and 19% had pulmonary valve regurgitation in one series. In less than 10%, the pulmonary degradation by monoamine oxidase activity is exceeded, and the fibrosis may also involve the left-sided heart valves and possibly contribute to bronchoconstriction.

The carcinoid heart disease may cause progressive cardiac insufficiency with typically right-sided heart failure and severe lethargy, and used to be an important cause of death in patients with the carcinoid syndrome.[5,42] However, nowadays, after introduction of somatostatin analogues, patients more often die of progressive tumour.[5] Affected patients may require heart surgery and replacement of fibrotic heart valves with prostheses.[5,42] This operation may lead to substantial improvement, but can be associated with complications, especially in older persons. The heart disease can be diagnosed by echocardiography, which should always be performed prior to major abdominal surgery.

Bronchial constriction as part of the carcinoid syndrome caused by midgut carcinoids is rare.

Diagnosis

Biochemistry

The biochemical diagnosis of small-intestinal carcinoids is often based on the demonstration of raised concentrations of the serotonin metabolite **5-HIAA** excreted in 24-hour urine samples. The raised 5-HIAA values are specific for carcinoids, but occur only at advanced disease stages and generally imply the presence of liver metastases.[5,38]

Determination of **plasma chromogranin A** is a more sensitive measure, which may be used for the early diagnosis of persistent or recurrent carcinoid disease. Circulating chromogranin A levels reflect the tumour load, and serial measurements have become the most important parameter for monitoring disease spread and to follow results of treatment.[5,38] The chromogranin values may also predict prognosis. However, it is a non-specific marker for any neuroendocrine tumour and false-positive values occur with liver or kidney failure, inflammatory bowel disease, atrophic gastritis or chronic use of proton-pump inhibitors.

Human choriogonadotropin (hCG-α/β) α and β subunits may be predictors of poor prognosis.[5] Exceptionally, carcinoids secrete enteroglucagon and pancreatic polypeptide (PP), but PP is a non-specific marker, which may be raised in any patients with diarrhoea.[5]

Pentagastrin provocation test

Pentagastrin injection has occasionally been used to verify the presence of occult carcinoid disease by inducing flushing and a rise in plasma peptides.[5]

Radiology

The primary midgut carcinoids are generally too small to be diagnosed with conventional **bowel contrast studies**.[5,38] At more advanced disease stages typical arcading of entrapped intestines with segments of partial obstruction may be visualised, and occasionally signs of chronic obstruction with thickened bowel wall. In patients with large-bowel symptoms entrapment of the sigmoid or transverse colon may be important to identify prior to surgery. Concomitant colorectal adenocarcinoma has been reported in 10–15%, and it may sometimes be necessary to exclude coexisting rectosigmoid adenocarcinoma by endoscopy prior to surgery, or during follow-up of a small-intestinal carcinoid.

Computed tomography

CT can very infrequently visualise a primary midgut carcinoid tumour, but often efficiently demonstrates mesenteric lymph node metastases, retroperitoneal extension of such masses, and liver metastases. The presence of a circumscribed mesenteric mass with radiating densities is very suspicious of a midgut carcinoid mesenteric metastasis[38] (Fig. 6.3).

Dynamic CT with contrast enhancement is of particular value for planning surgery, when the relation between the mesenteric metastases and the main mesenteric artery and vein is crucially important to visualise. In cases with advanced intestinal ischaemia, CT may reveal a characteristic image of universally dilated peripheral mesenteric vessels and sometimes oedematous loops of intestine. CT with contrast enhancement is often the primary method for visualisation of liver metastases, but may fail to identify the smallest lesions.

Magnetic resonance tomography (MRT) can sometimes be more efficient than CT for demonstration of liver metastases.

Angiography

Mesenteric angiography often shows typical features in midgut carcinoids, with calibre changes, segmental occlusions and tortuosity of mesenteric vessels, but is now seldom used due to the efficiency of dynamic CT.[38] It is important to know, however, that in patients with abdominal pain, angiography cannot discriminate between intestinal obstruction and ischaemia, because the vascular impairment generally involves peripheral vessels, and laparotomy is often required to distinguish these causes.[38]

Ultrasound

Percutaneous ultrasound is mainly utilised to visualise liver metastases or to guide fine-needle or preferably core-needle biopsy for histological diagnosis of liver metastases or the deposits in the mesentery. Ultrasound with power Doppler enhancement, and especially use of ultrasound contrast, may increase sensitivity for detection of liver metastases.

OctreoScan®

In nearly 90% of cases, small-intestinal carcinoids possess somatostatin receptors types 2 and 5, for which the somatostatin analogue octreotide has high affinity.[5] Somatostatin receptor scintigraphy (OctreoScan®) has detected carcinoid tumours with a sensitivity of 90%, and is being increasingly utilised to determine metastatic spread. OctreoScan® is especially efficient for detection of extra-abdominal metastases and can visualise bone metastases better than a routine isotope bone scan, which may miss osteolytic metastases.

Positron emission tomography (PET)

PET with the serotonin precursor 5-hydroxytryptophan, labelled with ^{11}C (5-HTP-PET), can identify the small-intestinal carcinoids with high sensitivity and has been used to monitor effects of therapy.[43] PET with [^{18}F]deoxyglucose (FDG) is rarely positive in low proliferating carcinoid tumours.

Histology

Needle biopsy specimens from metastases are often used for diagnosis. The carcinoid tumour cells stain immunocytochemically with neuroendocrine tumour markers, mainly chromogranin A and synaptophysin. Reactivity with serotonin-specific antisera implies that a primary tumour should be searched for in the midgut;[1,5,38] 85% of jejuno-ileal carcinoids show reactivity for chromogranin A and serotonin. Proliferation rate is determined with the Ki67 antibody and is invariably low in classical midgut carcinoids (<2%).[5,29]

Most jejuno-ileal carcinoids show a mixed insular and glandular growth pattern; occasional tumours have a pure insular and trabecular pattern and have been reported as having a slightly less favourable prognosis. Rarely, tumours have an undifferentiated pattern and high proliferation rate. Since they belong to the group of neurendocrine carcinomas with poor prognosis, patients with these tumours can generally not be helped by surgery.

Surgery

Many patients with midgut carcinoids will be subjected to acute laparotomy due to intestinal obstruction without suspicion of the underlying cause. It is important to appreciate then that the carcinoid is common among small-bowel neoplasms, and findings at laparotomy are often typical with a tiny ileal primary tumour, and conspicuously larger mesenteric metastases with marked mesenteric desmoplastic reaction.[38] The primary tumour and mesenteric metastases should be removed by wedge resection of the mesentery and limited intestinal resection, and lymph node metastases should be cleared as far as possible by dissection around the mesenteric artery and its branches. This procedure is generally indicated also in the presence of liver metastases. If the surgery has been inadequately performed, because the surgeon believed he or she was facing inoperable adenocarcinoma, this will result in the primary tumour and especially the bulk of mesenteric metastases not being removed. Re-operation is then strongly recommended to remove any remaining mesenteric tumour, which can otherwise be expected to cause future abdominal complications.[38]

If grossly radical removal of the primary tumour and mesenteric metastases has been accomplished, midgut carcinoid patients may often remain symptom-free for long periods. However, midgut carcinoid tumours are markedly tenacious and recurrence should be watched for, as the majority of patients (>80%) will ultimately develop liver metastases if follow-up is long enough (**Fig. 6.5**).[38,44] The midgut carcinoids are unusually slow-growing tumours, and clinically overt recurrence occurs after a median of 10 years and up to 25 years.[38,44] Earlier diagnosis of such recurrence may be more sensitively based on serum chromogranin A estimates, rather than urinary 5-HIAA measurements.

Many patients with midgut carcinoids lack acute abdominal symptoms, and instead present with liver metastases and sometimes also features of the carcinoid syndrome at the time of diagnosis. Only a few decades ago life expectancy was poor in patients with liver metastases and carcinoid syndrome, with an expected median survival of around 2 years, and abdominal surgery was not often considered.[5] Now symptoms of the carcinoid syndrome may be efficiently controlled by medical treatment with somatostatin analogues and interferon, and these and other new treatment modalities have increased life expectancy.[5,29]

Abdominal complications have become of increased concern and have appeared as a principal cause of death in patients with midgut carcinoids.[38,44] Such threatening complications have widened indications for abdominal surgery in patients undergoing medical treatment for the advanced carcinoids.

Due to continued growth and increased intestinal entrapment by mesenteric tumour or fibrosis, patients often experience abdominal pain and will require surgery for relief of partial or complete intestinal obstruction.[38,44–46] Since incipient intestinal ischaemia may cause similar symptoms of feeding-related crampy abdominal pain, laparotomy can be urgently needed to distinguish these causes. Liberal operative intervention is also indicated because incipient venous ischaemia may contribute markedly to conditions with diarrhoea and general malaise. Occasional patients present with severe abdominal pain, weight loss, and even malnutrition and cachexia due to the intestinal ischaemia (**Fig. 6.6**).[38,45–47] Abdominal pain is unlikely to occur due to the carcinoid syndrome, and weight loss and malnutrition are rarely caused merely by a large tumour burden in midgut carcinoid patients. Complications of the mesenteric tumour have been evident in a large proportion of patients with midgut carcinoids subjected to laparotomy, and are important to recognise since these patients may benefit from considerable long-term palliation following surgery.[45–47]

The natural course of the mesenterico-intestinal disease with midgut carcinoids can be variable, but surgery at an early stage is a distinct advantage, as it may provide an exceptional chance to remove the mesenteric tumour before more extensive involvement of major mesenteric vessels has occurred.[38,44–46] The authors thus advocate removal of the mesenterico-intestinal tumour as a prophylactic procedure even in asymptomatic patients considered for medical

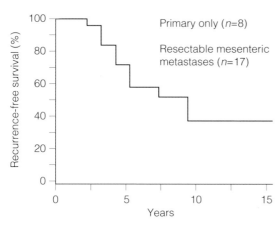

Figure 6.5 • Recurrence-free survival in midgut carcinoid patients subjected to apparently curative surgery. A majority of patients will experience recurrence during long-term follow-up. Reproduced from Åkerström G, Hellman P, Öhrvall U. Midgut and hindgut carcinoid tumors. In: Doherty GM, Skogseid B (eds) Surgical endocrinology, 1st edn. Philadelphia: Lippincott Williams & Wilkins, 2001; pp. 448–52; and Makridis C, Öberg K, Juhlin C et al. Surgical treatment of midgut carcinoid tumors. World J Surg 1990; 14:377–85. With kind permission of Springer Science and Business Media.

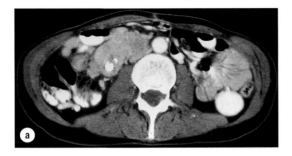

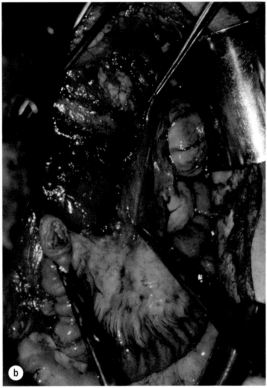

Figure 6.6 • (a) Computed tomography image of mesenteric tumour deemed inoperable at previous surgery, with resulting progressive intestinal vascular impairment, weight loss and cachexia. **(b)** Re-operation with mesenteric tumour removal and limited intestinal resection performed with alleviation of abdominal symptoms. Part (b) reproduced from Åkerström G, Hellman P, Öhrvall U. Midgut and hindgut carcinoid tumors. In: Doherty GM, Skogseid B (eds) Surgical endocrinology, 1st edn. Philadelphia: Lippincott Williams & Wilkins, 2001; pp. 448–52. With permission from Lippincott Williams & Wilkins.

therapy.[47] During periods of medical treatment patients are likely to benefit markedly from close cooperation between internists and surgeons, reflecting the multidisciplinary approach required for the optimal management of this condition.

Surgical technique

Important considerations for abdominal surgery in patients with midgut carcinoids have been outlined.[38,45] During surgical exploration advanced midgut carcinoids may seem inoperable since large mesenteric metastases with surrounding fibrosis and entrapped loops of intestine will frequently appear to encase the major intestinal vascular supply.[38,44,45] Incautious wedge resection in the fibrotic and contracted mesentery may easily compromise the main mesenteric artery and cause devascularisation of a major part of the small intestine, resulting in a short-bowel syndrome.[38,45] However, since the majority of these metastases originate from primary lesions in the most terminal parts of the ileum, they tend to be deposited mainly on the right side of the mesenteric artery, implying that they can often be removed without interfering with the main intestinal vascular supply. A procedure has been described where the right colon and the entire small-intestinal mesenteric root is mobilised from adhesions to the retroperitoneum up to the level of the horizontal duodenum and the pancreas.[38,45] A large tumour deposit in the mesenteric root and fibrosis often has to be dissected from the serosa of the horizontal duodenum. With a posterior view in the elevated mesenteric root it is possible to identify the mesenteric vessels, divide the fibrotic surroundings of the mesenteric metastases, and free-dissect and debulk a major portion, or the entire tumour, from the mesenteric root (Figs 6.6 and **6.7**). Sometimes part of the tumour may be cleaved to allow separation from the mesenteric artery and vein, since the tumour seems rarely to invade the vessel walls. The procedure can preserve the main mesenteric artery and vein, and maintain blood flow through jejunal and ileal arteries and important arcades along the intestine (Fig. 6.6). The larger of the mesenteric metastases (up to 10 cm in our experience) can occasionally be easier to dissect than the smaller and diffusely fibrotic ones, which may grow more diffusely around the mesenteric root. The procedure will generally permit a more limited small-intestinal resection, and thereby a reduced risk of creating a short bowel, which is likely to be very troublesome for the patient in combination with the carcinoid syndrome. Generally the right colon has to be removed together with the most terminal parts of the ileum, and occasionally fibrotic entrapment of the transverse or sigmoid colon has to be released. In our experience, intestinal bypasses should be avoided as far as possible, because ischaemia may

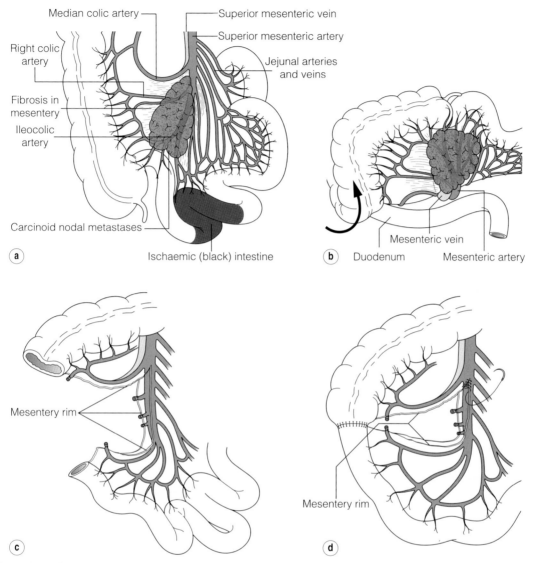

Figure 6.7 • Resection of carcinoid primary tumour and mesenteric metastasis. **(a)** Mesenteric tumour may extensively involve the mesenteric root and appear impossible to remove. **(b)** Mobilisation of caecum, terminal ileum and mesenteric root by separation of retroperitoneal attachments allows the tumour to be lifted, approached also from a posterior angle and separated from duodenum and main mesenteric vessels, with preservation of intestinal vascular supply and intestinal length. **(c,d)** Bowel anastomosed and mesenteric defect repaired. Redrawn from Åkerström G, Hellman P, Öhrvall U. Midgut and hindgut carcinoid tumors. In: Doherty GM, Skogseid B (eds) Surgical endocrinology, 1st edn. Philadelphia: Lippincott Williams & Wilkins, 2001; pp. 448–52. With permission from Lippincott Williams & Wilkins.

develop in a disengaged intestinal segment, and also because the mesenteric tumour will continue to grow and symptoms then generally progress. The bypass procedure can markedly complicate repeat surgery, which often becomes necessary in these patients.[38,45] Intestinal bypassing should be reserved for cases where extensive tumour growth, carcinoidosis or fibrosis after previous operations inhibit appropriate mesenteric dissection.

When planning dissection of mesenteric metastases it is valuable to preoperatively map the level of extension in the mesenteric root with dynamic CT investigation (**Fig. 6.8**).[38,45] For jejunal carcinoids and occasional ileal carcinoids, mesenteric metastases extend high or completely surround the mesenteric root or even extend retroperitoneally above the pancreas, and these tumours have been inoperable in our experience.

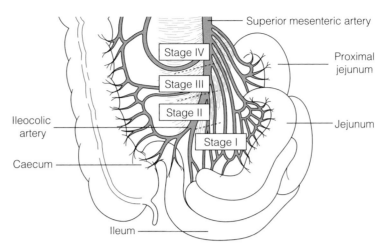

Figure 6.8 • Stages of midgut carcinoid mesenteric metastases. Stage I tumours located close to the intestine, removed by limited ileal resection. Stage II tumours involving arterial branches close to the origin in the mesenteric artery, requiring right-sided colectomy, distal ileal resection and dissection from mesenteric vessels. Stage III tumours extending along but without encircling the mesenteric trunk may be free-dissected. Stage IV tumours growing around the mesenteric trunk involving origins of proximal jejunal arteries, median colic artery or extending retroperitoneally; these tumours have proved impossible to remove. Reproduced from Öhrvall U, Eriksson B, Juhlin C et al. Method of dissection of mesenteric metastases in mid-gut carcinoid tumors. World J Surg 2000; 24: 1402-8 with permission from Springer Science and Business Media.

Repeated surgery may sometimes be required in patients with advanced midgut carcinoids, when they suffer from chronic or intermittent abdominal pain due to partial or complete intestinal obstruction, or segmental intestinal ischaemia.[38] These operations may be exceedingly difficult and time-consuming due to the presence of harsh fibrosis and carcinoidosis between loops of intestine, but nevertheless they are crucially important for the well-being of the patient. Re-operations, and indeed any surgery in patients with midgut carcinoid tumours, should be undertaken with great caution, since minor mistakes may easily cause intestinal fistulation, devascularisation of major parts of the small intestine, or creation of a short-bowel syndrome.[38,45] Duodenal fistulation can be a significant risk. Emphasising these difficulties, it is recommended that surgery for midgut carcinoids be referred to colleagues with experience in this management.

 The authors have evaluated more than 200 laparotomies in patients with advanced carcinoids, including re-operations in several patients.[44–47] Alleviation of abdominal symptoms was often efficiently achieved by surgery, with often long duration, and was especially favourable in patients with intestinal venous stasis or ischaemia.[47]

 Attempts to remove the mesenteric tumour should be undertaken as early as possible, when growth in the mesentery is less extensive.[38,45] If a mesenteric tumour remains, our experience is that the patients will survive with medical treatment but more or less invariably reach a stage where abdominal complications represent a major threat.

Prophylactic removal of the mesenterico-intestinal tumour is strongly recommended even in the absence of abdominal symptoms, as this may prevent intestinal complications. Tardy surgical consultation will make the disease increasingly difficult or impossible to manage surgically.[45]

Liver metastases

The treatment of liver metastases requires many modalities: medical treatment, surgery, radiofrequency (RF) ablation, liver embolisation, transplantation, radiolabelled octreotide therapy and [131I]meta-iodobenzylguanidine (131I-MIBG) therapy.[5,29,38] An initial period of medical treatment with somatostatin analogues and interferon can help alleviate symptoms and slow disease progression.

It also allows some time for observation and makes surgery or ablation of liver disease safer. Liver surgery is more likely to be beneficial in patients with classical midgut carcinoids with high differentiation and low proliferation rate demonstrated by Ki67 staining.[5]

Liver surgery

The majority of patients with advanced midgut carcinoids have multiple and bilaterally disseminated liver metastases, and are mainly considered for medical therapy.

In 5–10% of cases, solitary and unilateral or grossly dominant liver metastases occur (**Fig. 6.9**). Liver surgery consisting of formal hepatic lobectomy or parenchyma-saving liver resections should be undertaken, and this may be combined with wedge resections or simple enucleations of superficially located additional, and even bilateral lesions.[1,38,48–50] Recent developments of surgical and anaesthetic techniques allow safe multiple wedge resections for bilobar hepatic metastases. Two-stage surgical resection may reduce the risk of liver insufficiency, with initial resection of one lobe and removal of additional tumour after some months of liver regeneration. Preoperative portal embolisation may help induce regeneration of a hepatic lobe (without metastases)

that is planned to remain after hepatic lobectomy for removal of metastatic tumour.

Debulking liver surgery may be increasingly important in patients who no longer respond to medical therapy, and larger metastases may represent cloned tumour cells that have ceased to be affected by medical therapy. Outcome is poorer in patients with more than 50% liver involvement or with more rapidly proliferating lesions.[49] Since liver surgery may considerably relieve symptoms associated with the carcinoid syndrome, it may also be indicated in the presence of concomitant or bilateral smaller metastases.

A number of reports have described series of patients who have undergone successful liver surgery with long survival and no evidence of disease,[48–50] and with significant symptom alleviation after palliative surgery.

The indications for liver surgery may be widened by the combination with other treatment modalities, especially RF ablation.[51–53]

Substantial and sustained palliation of the carcinoid syndrome and reduction of tumour markers can be expected, especially after removal of large (>10 cm) dominant lesions, or if around 90% of the tumour volume can be excised or ablated (Fig. 6.9).[48,49] A 5-year survival of 70% or more has been reported after apparently 'curative' surgery, and symptom palliation has also been obtained with non-curative resections.[48–50]

However, virtually every patient will recur with new tumour after liver resection or ablative therapy, if follow-up time is long enough. Reflecting slow progression of the carcinoid tumours, clinical symptoms (e.g. carcinoid syndrome) have reappeared 4–5 years after apparently 'curative' liver resection, but the patient may have been efficiently palliated until then.[44–48]

Radiofrequency ablation

Radiofrequency (RF) ablation has recently been introduced as an efficient and safe method for ablation of moderately large liver metastases.[51–53] Using a needle introduced with ultrasound guidance into the tumour, the application of current with alternating radiowave-length frequency induces

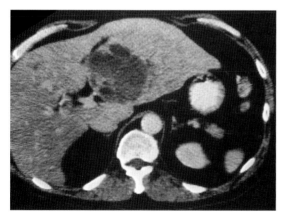

Figure 6.9 • Computed tomography image of large midgut carcinoid metastasis within the left liver lobe. The patient had smaller metastases in contralateral liver but remained free from carcinoid syndrome 4 years after resection of the larger lesion. Reproduced with permission from Åkerström G, Hellman P, Öhrvall U. Midgut and hindgut carcinoid tumors. In: Doherty GM, Skogseid B (eds) Surgical endocrinology, 1st edn. Philadelphia: Lippincott Williams & Wilkins, 2001; pp. 448–52. With permission from Lippincott Williams & Wilkins.

ionic oscillation, with production of heat around the needle leading to tissue necrosis within a range of around 5 cm. RF ablation can be performed intra-operatively, laparoscopically or repeatedly as a per-cutaneous ultrasound-guided procedure. Somewhat larger tumours may be coagulated by overlapping treatment or by reduction of hepatic circulation during ablation, with hepatic artery clamping during surgery, or concomitant embolisation during percutaneous RF ablation. However, tumours larger than 4 cm and tumours close to major vessels may be inefficiently treated (due to heat loss through the perfusing vessels). Although survival advantage after RF treatment remains to be verified, the treatment has been demonstrated to provide symptom relief for patients with liver metastases from midgut carcinoids.[53]

We use RF ablation and surgery as complementary therapies, and have found that the possibility of ablation has broadened indications for surgery of bilateral tumours with the aim of cytoreduction.[51,53] However, the number of lesions needs to be limited and the method is of less value in patients with numerous small metastases. Although methods for visualisation of liver metastases have improved, our experience from operations confirms that many patients have multiple small liver metastases, often not accurately visualised before surgery. A correct estimate of the spread is therefore often best achieved at laparotomy, where availability for surgical resection or RF ablation can be appropriately evaluated. Our own series has shown local recurrence after RF ablation in 10% and a complication rate of ≈5%.[51,53] Since large vessels reduce the efficiency and bile ducts seem to be the most vulnerable structures, we try to avoid RF treatment of tumours located in the hepatic hilum. We have utilised liver surgery combined with RF ablation in a number of patients, and demonstrated reduction of tumour markers and symptom alleviation, but prospective, randomised studies are needed to further evaluate RF ablation and other treatment modalities for liver metastases.[53]

Liver embolisation

Liver tumours are generally fed mainly by arterial supply, and obstruction of the blood flow will cause tumour ischaemia. As a consequence liver metastases may be efficiently treated by selective liver artery embolisation. Embolisation with gel foam powder, sometimes performed as a repeated procedure, has provided tumour regression and symptomatic control in approximately 50% of patients during median follow-up of 7–14 months, and with resulting reduced need for somatostatin analogues and improved effects of interferon treatment.[5,29,54,55]

Patent portal blood flow is crucial for perfusion of the normal liver parenchyma, and angiography is performed prior to embolisation to verify a patent portal vein and to characterise the vascular anatomy.[29] Embolisation is generally contraindicated if tumour burden relative to normal liver parenchyma exceeds 50%, and in patients with raised bilirubin and liver enzymes as signs of hepatic insufficiency. Superselective and repeated embolisations with some months interval has been performed in cases with large tumours, and in patients with recurrent tumour after previous hemihepatectomy.

The procedure is associated with complications and even mortality rates around 5%, and may cause liver insufficiency of variable degree.[29] Most common is transient elevation of liver enzymes, and 2 or 3 days of fever, nausea and abdominal pain, with disappearance of symptoms within a week.

Complications are reduced in the hands of an experienced interventional radiologist, by prophylactic octreotide infusion during the procedure, and the use of forced diuresis and haemodynamic monitoring during and after the procedure. Special caution is needed in cases where the right hepatic artery originates from the superior mesenteric artery, since mesenteric artery embolism may occur. Patients who have undergone hepatico-jejunostomy or papillotomy are more prone to develop cholangitis or hepatic abscesses afterwards.

The results of embolisation are good, although not every patient will respond as expected. Effects may be of short duration and survival benefits still remain unclear. The success rate is lower and risks higher with extensive liver metastases. Embolisation may be used in cases of multiple unresectable metastases, but it is crucial to carefully consider if the remaining healthy liver parenchyma is sufficient to prevent liver failure in the post-embolisation period.

Chemoembolisation is arterial embolisation combined with intra-arterial infusion of chemotherapy, and may be more effective than embolisation alone with possibly more pronounced tumour reduction in some cases.[55] The treatment may have severe side-effects and may be less efficient in midgut carcinoids with their typically low proliferation than in tumours with lower differentiation and higher proliferation rates.

Liver transplantation

Liver transplantation may be considered for patients with liver metastases from midgut carcinoids, because of generally slow disease progression.[38,56–59] Meta-analysis of patients with endocrine tumours subjected to liver transplantation revealed a nearly 50% 1-year survival but varying 5-year survival (24–48%), possibly due to different selection procedures between centres.[56] Carcinoids have been reported with more favourable survival (69% at 5 years) than endocrine pancreatic tumours. Recent results indicate reduced operative risks and improved results after transplantation in neuroendocrine tumours, with up to 77% 1-year tumour-free survival, 90% overall 5-year survival, but only around 20% 5-year tumour-free survival.[57–59] Ki67 proliferation index <5% and absence of markers for aggressive tumours have generally been required.[59] Patients should have extra-abdominal metastases excluded by biochemical markers and sensitive imaging with specific tracers, but distant disease is not invariably detected. The new liver will often become the site for new metastases, emphasising that carcinoid tumours are tenacious, with high recurrence rate also after apparently radical removal of primary and regionally localised lesions.[44] Indications for transplantation must be balanced against favourable results of medical treatment and the possibility that immunosuppression can promote tumour growth. Cases considered for liver transplantation therefore have to be carefully selected, and perhaps chosen from patients in whom liver metastases cannot be removed, are markedly space occupying or threaten to cause liver failure, although limited tumour burden (<50% of liver volume) has also been favourable for transplantation.

Prophylaxis against carcinoid crisis

Operation and embolisation in patients with the carcinoid syndrome always entails the risk of inducing a carcinoid crisis, with hyperthermia, shock, arrhythmia, excessive flush or bronchial obstruction.

As prophylaxis to prevent crisis during surgery or intervention, patients with midgut carcinoids should preferably be pretreated with octreotide (patient's regular dose or daily 100 µg × 3, s.c.). Adrenergic drugs should generally be avoided if hypotension were to occur during surgery.[1,38] Patients with foregut carcinoids and atypical carcinoid syndrome are treated with octreotide, histamine blockade and cortisone, and avoidance of histamine-releasing agents (morphine and tubocurarine). In patients with carcinoid flush syndrome we routinely provide i.v. octreotide (500 µg in 500 mL saline, 50 µg/h) during surgery or embolisation procedures, and the same treatment or increased dose (100 µg/h) is given if carcinoid crisis should occur.[38]

Medical treatment

Biotherapy, including somatostatin analogues and interferon, has been shown to improve clinical symptoms in 50–70% of patients with midgut carcinoids, often with significant reduction of tumour markers and stabilisation of the disease for several years, but less often with significant tumour reduction.[1,5,29,60] Chemotherapy has been of little benefit in midgut carcinoids with typical low proliferation.[5,29]

Somatostatin analogues (octreotide, lanreotide) have been a breakthrough in the treatment of carcinoid tumours.[5,29,60] By binding to specific somatostatin receptors (types 2 and 5) the analogues reduce the release of bioactive peptides from tumour cells, and may also block peripheral responses of target cells. They may also inhibit tumour growth, induce apoptosis and counteract angiogenesis.

The analogues have induced subjective and biochemical responses in up to 70% of patients with carcinoid syndrome, caused moderate tumour reduction in around 5%, and stabilisation of disease for an average of 3 years in approximately half of the patients.[60]

The analogues are usually given in daily doses of 50–150 µg × 3 s.c. Higher doses (>3000 µg/day) have resulted in slightly greater tumour reduction but otherwise no greater response rate. Tachyphylaxis often occurs after 9–12 months of treatment and may often indicate a requirement for increased dosage. Long-acting formulations have become available (octreotide-LAR, lanreotide-PR, Somatuline Autogel), offering the possibility of monthly administration, and therefore are much easier to use. Side-effects of all analogues include gallstone formation, pancreatic enzyme deficiency and symptoms relating to biliary colic, sometimes necessitating cholecystectomy.

Interferon-α (IFN-α) reduces hormone secretion and stimulates natural killer cells with effects on cell growth in tumours with slow progression.[5,29,60] Clinically, IFN-α administration induces biochemical and subjective responses in about 50% of patients, while antitumour effects may be seen in around 15% with doses of $15-25 \times 10^6$ U/week; the duration of response is around 3 years, and stabilisation of the disease occurs in 35%.[60] Recently a pegylated form has become available (PegIntron®) for subcutaneous administration once a week, with possible improved tolerance. Combinations of somatostatin analogue and interferon therapy may increase response rate. Interferon is associated with more adverse effects than somatostatin analogues, mainly flu-like symptoms initially, and later on chronic fatigue and sometimes depression. Autoimmune phenomena may be induced with antithyroid antibodies, causing thyroid dysfunction and occasionally other complications. Neutralising interferon antibodies may develop and interfere with the effects.[29,60] Some patients have to discontinue treatment, and the rather high risk of side-effects has somewhat limited the use of interferon.

Radiotherapy

External radiotherapy is generally not efficient in treating carcinoid tumours but it can be used for long-term palliation of brain metastases, and especially for alleviation of pain due to bone metastases.[5]

Internal or tumour-targeted radiation has been developed during recent years, using ^{131}I-MIBG and radioactive somatostatin analogues.[61,62]

Effects of ^{131}I-MIBG therapy have been limited, with subjective responses in 30–40% of patients and biochemical responses in less than 10%.[61] Predosing with non-labelled MIBG has resulted in prolonged biochemical and clinical responses.

Neuroendocrine tumours, including carcinoids, express somatostatin receptor subtypes 2 and 5, which become internalised in tumour cells after binding of radiolabelled octreotide.[29,62] Remission has been seen after treating neuroendocrine tumours with [^{111}In]DTPA-octreotide used for OctreoScan® examinations.[29,62] New compounds with beta- and gamma-emitting isotopes linked to somatostatin analogues have been developed ([^{90}Y-DOTA]-octreotide, [^{90}Y-DOTA]-lanreotide and [^{177}Lu-DOTA, Tyr[3]]-octreotate), with affinity for different somatostatin receptors and better tumour penetration.[29,62] Some of these compounds have shown very promising responses and mild side-effects, and combinations may become of special value for this developing type of therapy.[29,62]

Survival

Age-adjusted overall 5-year survival for all midgut carcinoids in Sweden between 1960 and 2000 was 67%, which was similar to the series from the SEER Program of the National Cancer Institute (NCI), 1973–1999.[1,63]

Survival has been improved during recent years, probably by active management, but remains largely dependent on the extent of disease, with the presence of liver metastases and carcinoid heart disease identified as the most significant adverse prognostic factors.[7] The importance of surgery has also been documented by survival analyses.[44,46,48–50] Among 314 patients treated in Uppsala, Sweden, median survival was 12.4 years and 5-year survival rate was 91% in patients who underwent apparently grossly radical resections of mesenteric metastases, without having liver metastases.[46] The value of mesenteric resection remained, but with shorter expected survival in patients with liver metastases.[46] Patients undergoing successful surgery for mesenteric ischaemia had favourable survival prospects, with a median of 8 years.[44] The value of surgical removal of dominant or large liver metastases has also been demonstrated, with extended survival and prolonged symptom palliation.[44,47,48,64]

Patients with inoperable liver metastases in the Uppsala series had 50% 5-year survival (similar to the results in the NCI series), and survival was 42% with inoperable liver and mesenteric lymph node metastases.[46] Survival was better for younger age groups (<50 years) and for patients who had received biotherapy.[46] Other negative factors for survival (except for liver metastases and heart disease) have been lymph gland metastases, high 5-HIAA values, old age (>75 years), tumour discovered during emergency surgery, significant weight loss, and presence of extra-abdominal metastases.[44,46]

Appendiceal carcinoids

Appendiceal carcinoids belong to midgut carcinoids and constitute ≈8% of gastrointestinal carcinoids, having apparently decreased in frequency.[1,65,66] Carcinoid is one of the most common tumours of the appendix. The majority of appendiceal carcinoids are argentaffin and originate from serotonin-producing EC cells; a few are non-argentaffin and produce other peptides.[1] The tumours appear to have a neuroectodermal origin and more benign features than other carcinoids.[65] Appendiceal carcinoids are prevalent at autopsy, and rarely attain clinical significance. Many of these carcinoids may perhaps undergo spontaneous involution, since the prevalence is reported as higher in children than in adults.[65]

Appendiceal carcinoids are often an incidental finding at surgery, and are expected to occur in 1 in 200 appendectomies,[65] but have probably frequently been overlooked. Approximately 75% of the carcinoids are located in the tip of the appendix (**Fig. 6.10**), and therefore only a few cases have had appendicitis due to an occluded appendix lumen.[65] Patients with appendiceal carcinoids are generally younger than those with other carcinoids, having a mean age ≈40 years, with a slight female predominance, and even children may be affected. The overall metastasis rate has been determined as 3.8%, with distant metastases in 0.7%.[1] Patients with larger tumours and metastases tend to be younger (29 years) than patients with smaller benign lesions (42 years).

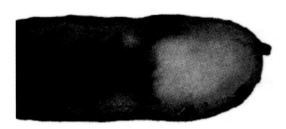

Figure 6.10 • Appendiceal carcinoid, with the typical yellow colour and location in tip of the appendix. Reproduced With permission from Capella C, Solcia E, Sobin L et al. Endocrine tumours of the appendix. In: Hamilton SR, Aaltonen LA (eds) WHO Classification of Tumours. Pathology and genetics of tumours of the digestive system. Lyon: IARC Press, 2000; pp. 99–101.

 The majority (≈90%) of appendiceal carcinoids are <1 cm in diameter and have minimal risk of presenting with metastases, which implies that these lesions may be treated by simple appendectomy.[65,66] This treatment is also apparently safe for most lesions measuring 1–2 cm, although rare cases in this group have presented with lymph node metastases.[65,66] Lesions >2 cm, as well as cases with residual tumour at resectional margins or with lymph gland metastases, should be treated by right hemicolectomy. Tumours in the base of the appendix require a similar aggressive approach since they may represent colon- rather than appendix-derived tumours. Although a strict evidence base is lacking, hemicolectomy may also be recommended if operative specimens show signs of angioinvasion, high Ki67 index or high mitotic index.[65,66]

The prognosis for appendiceal carcinoids is favourable overall, with a 5-year survival rate of 84% for patients with local disease, 81% for those with regional metastases and 28% for the few patients with distant metastases.[1,65,66]

Atypical goblet-cell carcinoid

Adenocarcinoid or goblet-cell carcinoid represents a more malignant variant, with elements of carcinoid tumours and mucinous adenocarcinomas, the most common origin being in the appendix.[65–67] This type has also been named 'atypical' or 'intermediate' carcinoid. The tumours do not express somatostatin receptors and cannot be visualised by OtreoScan®. Special histological markers may be used to identify the lesions. Although many goblet-cell carcinoids may be localised, some have aggressive spread in the mesoappendix and intraperitoneally. Treatment for this tumour has mainly included extended ileocolic and mesenteric resection, often performed as re-operation, and additionally chemotherapy.[65–67] The goblet-cell carcinoids have had unpredictable and generally less favourable survival, with a 60% 10-year survival rate.[65–67] Recently a much more aggressive therapy has been proposed, adding cytoreductive surgery and intraperitoneal heated chemotherapy.[68] The cytoreductive therapy has included omentectomy, splenectomy and peritonectomy.

Colon carcinoids

Carcinoids of the colon are rare and constitute only about 8% of gastrointestinal carcinoid tumours and 1–5% of colorectal neoplasms.[1,69,70] These tumours develop preferentially in older individuals, with a mean age of ≈65 years, but have also occasionally been reported in children. Tumours of the proximal colon (caecum) are most common, and may infrequently (5%) be associated with the carcinoid syndrome, which does not occur in association with more distally located colonic lesions.[69] The majority of colon carcinoids have less well-differentiated histological features and are generally large and exophytic rather than ulcerating, apparently slow growing, and may reach conspicuous size before diagnosis. These tumours have higher proliferation rate, commonly regional metastases and high incidence of liver metastases.[69] Patients then generally present with typical malignant symptoms, pain, palpable abdominal mass and more occasionally occult rectal bleeding. Tumours of the right colon may be larger when detected than those of the left colon, which may cause obstruction. Occasional tumours have been encountered in patients with colitis or Crohn's disease.[69] Although some authors have recommended limited resection for colon carcinoids <2 cm in diameter, it is probably wise to treat all patients with hemicolectomy. Due to their slow growth rate, palliative tumour debulking may also be undertaken if possible. The 5-year survival rate for colon carcinoids has averaged 37%, slightly better than the survival for adenocarcinoma.[69]

Rectal carcinoids

Rectal carcinoids have previously been regarded as uncommon, but the incidence is increasing, and they constitute ≈11% of gastrointestinal carcinoids and 1–2% of all rectal tumours.[1,68,70] Genetic predisposition may be noted in the different annual incidence of approximately 0.35 per 100 000 in whites and 1.2 in black people, as well as a roughly fivefold higher incidence in the Asian compared with the non-Asian North American population. The increased incidence compared with earlier reports may be due to increased awareness of the diagnosis and use of recently developed diagnostic methods, such as endosonography, as well as more accurate histopathology. The majority of rectal carcinoids are small and discovered accidentally at early stages. The overall prognosis is favourable, with up to 88.3% 5-year survival,[1,69] although a more thorough classification of different variants of rectal carcinoids is needed.

Presentation

The development of the tumour usually occurs in the sixth decade, about 10 years earlier than non-carcinoid rectal tumours. The majority – up to about 60% – are small, less than 1.0 cm in greatest dimension (**Fig. 6.11**), and may be discovered after presenting symptoms such as perianal pain, pruritus ani or haematochezia leading to endoscopic procedures. However, most patients are asymptomatic and the tumours are found incidentally, which is prognostically beneficial compared with symptomatic presentation. The smaller tumours usually present as submucosal yellowish nodules, and up to 75% may be within reach of digital examination at 8 cm from the anal verge. The findings at digital palpation can be variable and described as firm, smooth or rubbery in consistency. Diagnosis is made after histopathological evaluation of biopsies or after removal

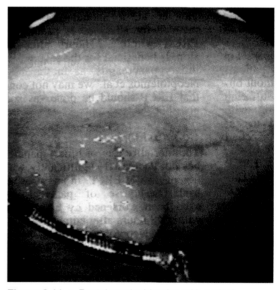

Figure 6.11 • Rectal carcinoid polyp with typical yellowish colour and submucosal location. Reproduced from McNevin MS, Read TE. Diagnosis and treatment of carcinoid tumors of the rectum. Chir Int 1998; 5:10–12.

of the whole nodule. Patients with tumours <1 cm exhibit a low risk for metastases (<2%).[69–71]

Patients with larger tumours generally have more symptoms, and those with metastatic disease may present with generalised symptoms such as weight loss and even cachexia. The carcinoid syndrome is extremely rare among these patients and only exceptionally present in cases with liver metastases. Occasional large tumours can be fixed to perirectal tissues and may initially be difficult to distinguish from rectal adenocarcinoma. Previous reports have proposed an increased incidence of concurrent colonic adenocarcinoma.

Tumours exceeding 1.0 cm in greatest dimension are much more prone to dissemination. Thus, patients with tumours between 1.0 and 1.9 cm have an intermediate incidence of metastatic spread (10–15%), while patients with larger tumours (>2 cm) exhibit a 60–80% incidence of distant metastases. The main sites for tumour spread are regional lymph nodes and the liver, and less commonly lung and bone.[69]

Rectal carcinoids may prognostically and in terms of management be divided up according to their size.[69–71] Patients with tumours <1 cm seldom demonstrate symptoms, have a favourable outcome, are generally cured by local excision and almost never have metastases. Patients with tumours >2 cm usually present with symptoms and the majority have metastases to regional lymph nodes, lung or liver. Thus, the smaller (<1 cm) and the larger (>2 cm) tumours have a predictable outcome, whereas the tumours measuring 1.0–1.9 cm in diameter are unpredictable.[69] Although the patients with smaller, non-invasive tumours generally may be considered as cured after tumour excision, patients with tumours measuring 1.0–1.9 cm need to be thoroughly examined for the presence of local infiltration and metastatic disease, and should also be closely surveyed. Transrectal endosonography should be used for more precise assessment of tumour extension, possible infiltration in the muscularis propria, and to reveal regional lymph node metastases. Computed tomography (CT) or magnetic resonance tomography (MRT) can clarify local tumour growth in the pelvis, and also the presence of lymph node and liver metastases. Octreotide scintigraphy (OctreoScan®) is most often negative in patients with rectal carcinoids due to lack of or few somatostatin receptors, regardless of tumour size.

Diagnosis and immunohistochemistry

The diagnosis is usually made after histopathological examination. Rectal carcinoids are derived from enterochromaffin cells of neuroendocrine origin, and display cells arranged in rosettes, ribbons or in a glandular pattern, surrounded by a dense fibrous stroma. The cells contain acidophilic granules and demonstrate argentaffin silver reaction (Masson staining) in 8–30%. However, by addition of an exogenous reducing agent, a positive argyrophil reaction may occur in up to 70% of rectal carcinoids.[72] Cells with positive silver staining are generally also reactive with serotonin and chromogranin A antisera.[72] The most sensitive markers, however, seem to be neurone-specific enolase (NSE), being positive in 87%, and, interestingly, prostate-specific acid phosphatase (in 80–100%), which makes differentiation from prostatic carcinoma difficult.[59] A limited fraction of cells generally are positive for chromogranin A.[72] Several studies have concluded that there is a correlation between Ki67 expression, tumour size and risk for metastases, although the Ki67 expression generally is low.[73] Classical tumour markers like CA19-9, CA50 and α-fetoprotein are poorly expressed or absent, while carcinoembryonic antigen (CEA) has been demonstated in up to 25% of cells. The CEA expression is possibly related to the occasional rectal carcinoid tumour that exhibits histopathological signs of both adenocarcinoma and carcinoids, referred to as adenocarcinoids. Rectal carcinoids generally show multihormonal expression, in which glucagon, somatostatin, pancreatic polypeptide, substance P and β-endorphins may be detected. The immunoreactivity for the different markers is generally unevenly distributed in groups of cells exhibiting focal and patchy distribution. This may indicate development of multiclonal lesions, where additional genetic derangements are prone to occur, causing more aggressive disease in fractions of tumour cells as well as in individual patients.

The tumours measuring <1 cm in diameter are only occasionally locally infiltrative, whereas tumours >2 cm almost invariably show signs of atypical histopathology, including infiltration of muscularis propria, invasion of lymphovascular and perineural structures, and a high number of mitotic figures. These tumours are frequently associated with distant metastases, local invasion and reduced survival.

It is rare that release of measurable peptides occurs in the circulation, implying that s-chromogranin A or urinary 5-HIAA are less useful diagnostic or surveillance tools for rectal carcinoids. Similarly, OctreoScan® is of minor importance due to lack of or minimal expression of somatostatin receptors.

Treatment

Smaller, non-invasive rectal carcinoids are safely treated by local excision. In patients with tumours between 1.0 and 1.9 cm in size, minimally invasive surgical techniques using transanal endoscopic microsurgery have been reported to provide excellent survival in the absence of local invasion or regional metastases.[69–74] Incompletely removed polyps that are found to be carcinoids after removal may be re-excised using such techniques.

The presence of local invasion or regional metastases favours an aggressive approach with abdominoperineal or anterior resection and total mesorectal excision. Mucosal invasion can be expected, especially in cases with larger, ulcerated, fibrotic or bleeding tumours. Most patients with tumours >2.0 cm have locally infiltrative disease and already suffer from lymph node or distant metastases to liver, lung or bone, leading some authors to suggest palliative treatment only. However, recent results have documented more favourable survival rates than previously depicted, and local tumour removal may also be advocated in the presence of metastases.[1] Five-year survival for rectal carcinoids with distant metastases is about 32%, which favours an aggressive approach for this group of patients, even in the face of local invasion in the pelvis or distant lymph node, liver, lung or skeletal metastases.

Our experience of individual patients with large tumours and distant metastases supports this view. Thus we suggest surgery in these patients, in combination with chemotherapy, which can be effective in some patients. However, patients with atypical histopathological features are less likely to benefit from the aggressive surgical treatment.

Although most reports demonstrate poor results of chemotherapy in rectal carcinoids, there are occasional patients who respond. To date there is no prognostic indicator selecting these patients from non-responders, which has led to wide indications for the initiation of such therapy. IFN-α and paclitaxel have in some patients resulted in reduced disease progression and also regression of metastases, and in the few patients with a positive OctreoScan®, somatostatin receptor analogues may be useful.[75] Moreover, reports of success with such analogues in the absence of positive imaging may indicate a wider role for these agents.[75] Occasional patients with liver metastases may benefit from hepatic artery chemoembolisation. In carefully selected cases liver resection may be indicated, with the understanding, however, that these patients generally have a poor outcome and short survival.

Outcome

Prediction of outcome in rectal carcinoids should rely on several factors such as tumour size, histology (typical or atypical features), microinvasiveness as well as presence of symptoms at presentation, but no study has yet evaluated all of these factors systematically. Nevertheless, tumour size and microinvasiveness have generally been accepted as the clinically most important factors.[69,71] Overall 5-year survival for patients with rectal carcinoids is about 88%, ranging from 20–30% for patients with distant metastases to 91% for patients with localised disease.[1,69] Patients with deeply invasive tumours had a median survival of 6–7 months in one study.[71] Patients with a carcinoid tumour confined to the submucosa and smaller than 1 cm will rarely die from the disease.[69–71]

Recommendations

Patients with rectal carcinoid tumours measuring 1.0–1.9 cm and those >2 cm should be thoroughly investigated (MRT, CT, transrectal endosonography) for evidence of spread of disease, e.g. local or distant metastases. These patients should generally undergo surgery with the aim of achieving total tumour clearance, and the specimens should be thoroughly investigated for signs of atypical histopathology. The larger the tumour, the higher the risk for metastatic disease. There are no studies demonstrating benefit of preoperative medical or irradiation treatment. Patients with rectal carcinoids >1 cm, including those with infiltrative or disseminated disease, need follow-up, and if not removed may require palliation against pelvic pain. Selected individuals may be offered more aggressive medical (and surgical) treatment for distant metastases.

Key points

- Carcinoids are rare tumours derived from neuroendocrine cells with wide distribution in the body. One-third occur in the lungs, bronchi and thymus, and around 70% in the gastrointestinal tract.
- Lung, thymic and occasional metastasising gastric carcinoids of sporadic type may cause an atypical carcinoid syndrome due to production of histamine.
- Carcinoids of the small intestine (midgut) with liver metastases and serotonin production are the most common cause of a classical carcinoid syndrome, with often severe and incapacitating symptoms of flush, diarrhoea and fibrotic valvular heart disease.
- Carcinoid tumours may be histologically identified with chromogranin A, synaptophysin, and for some tumours NSE stainings.
- The Ki67 antibody stain is increasingly used as a marker for tumour cell proliferation and can help predict prognosis, and also support decisions about therapy.
- The various types of carcinoid tumour require different treatment, dependent on histological type, location and proliferation rate.
- Most carcinoid tumours are well differentiated and slow growing, and should be surgically excised when this is possible. Occasional tumours have low differentiation and a higher proliferation rate, and may respond better to chemotherapy.
- Specific tumour markers, urinary 5-HIAA excretion and especially serum chromogranin A measurements can be used for clinical diagnosis and to monitor effects of therapy, and are also important predictors of prognosis.
- Multiple gastric carcinoids occur most commonly as a result of gastrin excess in patients with hypergastrinaemia due to chronic atrophic gastritis. These carcinoids are generally benign and can often be safely removed and controlled by endoscopy. A minority are associated with the MEN 1/Zollinger–Ellison syndrome.
- Sporadic, solitary gastric carcinoids are markedly more malignant and require more extensive surgery.
- For the midgut carcinoids surgical treatment is important and should include efforts to remove mesenteric metastases, which may cause severe long-term abdominal complications with obstruction and ischaemia of the small bowel. Attempts can also be made to surgically remove or ablate liver metastases, since this may provide considerable palliation of the carcinoid syndrome.
- For patients with the carcinoid syndrome surgery is also combined with continous medical treatment by somatostatin analogues (in long-acting release forms) and interferon, both of which may markedly alleviate symptoms, and seem to stabilise disease and slow its progression.
- Small, non-invasive rectal carcinoids can be removed by endoscopy, whereas larger lesions are more malignant and need wider resection, and in addition often chemotherapy.
- The diagnosis and treatment of carcinoid tumours have progressed markedly and should now include close cooperation between surgeons and internists with special interest in endocrine oncology. This collaboration is important to ensure that patients with carcinoids receive adequate surgery, and can help individualise therapy, utilising various treatment modalities. These include liver resection and radiofrequency (RF) ablation of liver metastases, and radioactively targeted somatostatin analogues.

References

1. Modlin IM, Lye K, Kidd M. Carcinoid tumors. In: Schwartz AE, Persemlidis D, Gagner M (eds) Endocrine surgery, Chap. 51. New York: Marcel Dekker, 2004; pp. 613–41.

   Excellent presentation of epidemiology and treatment of carcinoid tumours.

2. Rindi G, Azzoni C, La Rosa S et al. ECL cell tumor and poorly differentiated endocrine carcinoma of the stomach: prognostic evaluation by pathological analysis. Gastroenterology 1999; 116:532–42.

3. Solcia E, Klöppel G, Sobin LA et al. Histological typing of endocrine tumors. In: WHO classification of endocrine tumors. New York: Springer-Verlag, 2000.

4. Van Eeden S, Qaedvlieg PF, Taal BG et al. Classification of low-grade neuroendocrine tumors

of midgut and unknown origin. Hum Pathol 2002; 33:1126–33.

5. Öberg K. Carcinoid tumors: current concepts in diagnosis and treatment. Oncologist 1998; 3: 339–45.

6. Solcia E, Fiocca R, Villani L et al. Hyperplastic, dysplastic, and neoplastic enterochromaffin-like-cell proliferations of the gastric mucosa. Classification and histogenesis. Am J Surg Pathol 1995; 19(Suppl 1):S1–7.

7. Modlin IM, Kidd M, Lye KD. Biology and management of gastric carcinoid tumours: a review. Eur J Surg 2002; 168:669–83.

   Excellent review article about the different varieties of gastric carcinoids and their management.

8. Rindi G, Paolotti D, Fiocca R et al. Vesicular monoamine transporter 2 as a marker of gastric enterochromaffin-like cell tumors. Virchows Arch 2000; 436:217–23.

9. Åkerström G. Management of carcinoid tumors of the stomach, duodenum, and pancreas. World J Surg 1996; 20:173–82.

10. Borch K. Atrophic gastritis and gastric carcinoid tumours. Ann Med 1989; 21:291–7.

11. Lehy T, Roucayrol AM, Miignon M. Histomorphological characteristics of gastric mucosa in patients with Zollinger–Ellison syndrome or autoimmune gastric atrophy: role of gastrin and atrophying gastritis. Microsc Res Tech 2000; 48: 327–38.

12. Jensen RT. Management of the Zollinger–Ellison syndrome in patients with multiple endocrine neoplasia type 1. J Intern Med 1998; 243:477–88.

13. Debelenko LV, Emmert-Buck MR, Zhuang Z et al. The multiple endocrine neoplasia type I gene locus is involved in the pathogenesis of type II gastric carcinoids. Gastroenterology 1997; 113:773–81.

14. Bordi C, Falchetti A, Azzoni C et al. Aggressive forms of gastric neuroendocrine tumors in multiple endocrine neoplasia type I. Am J Surg Pathol 1997; 21:1075–82.

15. Sjöblom SM, Sipponen P, Jarvinen H. Gastroscopic follow up of pernicious anaemia patients. Gut 1993; 34:28–32.

16. Gough DB, Thompson GB, Crotty TB et al. Diverse clinical and pathologic features of gastric carcinoid and the relevance of hypergastrinemia. World J Surg 1994; 18:473–9.

17. Wilander E, El-Salhy M, Pitkänen P. Histopathology of gastric carcinoids: a survey of 42 cases. Histopathology 1984; 8:183–93.

18. Matsui K, Jin XM, Kitagawa M et al. Clinicopathologic features of neuroendocrine carcinomas of the stomach: appraisal of small cell and large cell variants. Arch Pathol Lab Med 1998; 122:1010–17.

19. Yoshikane H, Tsukamoto Y, Niwa Y et al. Carcinoid tumors of the gastrointestinal tract: evaluation with endoscopic ultrasonography. Gastrointest Endosc 1993; 39:375–83.

20. Granberg D, Wilander E, Stridsberg M et al. Clinical symptoms, hormone profiles, treatment, and prognosis in patients with gastric carcinoids. Gut 1998; 43:223–28.

21. Krenning EP, Kooij PP, Pauwels S et al. Somatostatin receptor: scintigraphy and radionuclide therapy. Digestion 1996; 57(Suppl 1):57–61.

22. Borch K, Ahren B, Ahlman H et al. Gastric carcinoids: biologic behavior and prognosis after differentiated treatment in relation to type. Ann Surg 2005; 242:64–73.

23. Ichikawa J, Tanabe S, Koizumi W et al. Endoscopic mucosal resection in the management of gastric carcinoid tumors. Endoscopy 2003; 35:203–6.

24. Delle Fave G, Capurso G, Milione M et al. Endocrine tumours of the stomach. Best Pract Res Clin Gastroenterol 2005; 19:659–73.

25. ENETS Consensus Guidelines for the Management of Patients with Digestive Neuroendocrine Tumors. Part 1 – Stomach, Duodenum and Pancreas. Neuroendocrinology 2006; 84.

    Updated review on treatment of neuroendocrine tumours.

26. Hirschowitz BI, Griffith J, Pellegrin D et al. Rapid regression of enterochromaffin-like cell gastric carcinoids in pernicious anemia after antrectomy. Gastroenterology 1992; 102:1409–18.

27. Ahlman H, Kölby L, Lundell L et al. Clinical management of gastric carcinoid tumors. Digestion 1994; 55(Suppl 3):77–85.

28. Richards ML, Gauger P, Thompson NW et al. Regression of type II gastric carcinoid in multiple endocrine neoplasia type 1 patients with Zollinger–Ellison syndrome after surgical excision of all gastrinomas. World J Surg 2004; 28:652–8.

29. Öberg K, Ahlman H. Medical management of neuroendocrine gastrointestinal tumors. In: Schwartz AE, Persemlidis D, Gagner M (eds) Endocrine surgery. New York: Marcel Dekker, 2004; pp. 685–96.

    Excellent review on medical treatment of neuroendocrine gastrointestinal tumours.

30. Burke AP, Sobin LH, Federspiel BH et al. Carcinoid tumors of the duodenum. A clinicopathologic study of 99 cases. Arch Pathol Lab Med 1990; 114:700–4.

31. Pipeleers-Marichal M, Somers G, Willems G et al. Gastrinomas in the duodenums of patients with multiple endocrine neoplasia type 1 and the Zollinger–Ellison syndrome. N Engl J Med 1990; 322:723–7.

32. Cisco RM, Norton JA. Surgery for gastrinoma. Adv Surg 2007; 41:165–76.

    Updated review on surgery for gastrinoma.

33. Thompson NW, Bondeson AG, Bondeson L et al. The surgical management of gastrinoma in MEN I syndrome patients. Surgery 1989; 106:1081–5.

34. Pipeleers-Marichal M, Donow C, Heitz PU et al. Pathologic aspects of gastrinomas in patients with Zollinger–Ellison syndrome with and without multiple endocrine neoplasia type 1. World J Surg 1993; 17:481–8.

   Important article emphasising high incidence of tiny duodenal gastrinomas as a cause of sporadic and MEN 1-related Zollinger–Ellison syndrome.

35. Wheeler MH, Curley IR, Williams ED. The association of neurofibromatosis pheochromocytoma, and somatostatin-rich duodenal carcinoid tumor. Surgery 1986; 100:1163–9.

36. Ricci JL. Carcinoid of the ampulla of Vater: local resection or pancreaticoduodenectomy. Cancer 1993; 71:686–90.

37. Zyromski NJ, Kendrick ML, Nagomey DM et al. Duodenal carcinoid tumors: how aggressive should we be? J Gastrointest Surg 2001; 5:588–93.

38. Åkerström G, Hellman P, Öhrvall U. Midgut and hindgut carcinoid tumors. In: Doherty GM, Skogseid B (eds) Surgical endocrinology. Philadelphia: Lippincott Williams & Wilkins, 2001; pp. 447–59.

39. Funa K, Papanicolaou V, Juhlin C et al. Expression of platelet-derived growth factor β-receptors on stromal tissue cells in human carcinoid tumors. Cancer Res 1990; 50:748–53.

40. Eckhauser FE, Argenta LC, Strodel WE et al. Mesenteric angiopathy, intestinal gangrene and midgut carcinoids. Surgery 1981; 90:720–8.

41. Knowlessar OD, Law DH, Sleisinger MH. Malabsorption syndrome associated with metastatic carcinoid tumor. Am J Med 1959; 27:673–7.

42. Westberg G, Wängberg B, Ahlman H et al. Prediction of prognosis by echocardiography in patients with midgut carcinoid syndrome. Br J Surg 2001; 88:865–72.

43. Öhrlefors H, Sundin A, Ahlström H et al. Positron emission tomography with 5-hydroxytryptophan in neuroendocrine tumors. J Clin Oncol 1998; 16: 2534–41.

44. Makridis C, Ekbom A, Bring J et al. Survival and daily physical activity in patients treated for advanced midgut carcinoid tumors. Surgery 1997; 122:1075–82.

   Survival and life-quality analyses in patients with advanced midgut carcinoids.

45. Öhrvall U, Eriksson B, Juhlin C et al. Method of dissection of mesenteric metastases in mid-gut carcinoid tumors. World J Surg 2000; 24:1402–8.

   Emphasises the importance of surgery for removal of mesenteric tumours in patients with midgut carcinoids. Describes technical aspects of a surgical procedure with low rate of complications.

46. Hellman P, Lundström T, Öhrvall U et al. Effect of surgery on the outcome of midgut carcinoid disease with lymph node and liver metastases. World J Surg 2002; 26:991–7.

   Demonstrates clear effect and benefit of surgery of primary tumour as well as carcinoid metastases.

47. Makridis C, Rastad J, Öberg K et al. Progression of metastases and symptom improvement from laparotomy in midgut carcinoid tumors. World J Surg 1996; 20:900–7.

48. Wängberg B, Westberg G, Tylén U et al. Survival of patients with disseminated midgut carcinoid tumors after aggressive tumor reduction. World J Surg 1996; 20:892–9.

   Provides survival data substantiating the importance of surgical resection of liver metastases in patients with midgut carcinoids.

49. Touzios JG, Kiely JM, Pitt SC et al. Neuroendocrine hepatic metastases. Does aggressive management improve survival?. Ann Surg 2005; 241:776–85.

50. Que FG, Sarmiento JM, Nagorney DM. Hepatic surgery for metastatic gastrointestinal endocrine tumors. Adv Exp Med Biol 2006; 574:43–56.

51. Hellman P, Ladjevardi S, Skogseid B et al. Radiofrequency tissue ablation using cooled tip for liver metastases of endocrine tumors. World J Surg 2002; 26:1052–6.

52. Mazzaglia PJ, Berber E, Milas M et al. Laparoscopic radiofrequency ablation of neuroendocrine liver metastases: a 10-year experience evaluating predictors of survival. Surgery 2007; 142:10–19.

53. Eriksson J, Stålberg P, Eriksson B et al. Surgery and radiofrequency ablation for treatment of liver metastases from midgut and foregut carcinoids and endocrine pancreatic tumors. World J Surg, in press.

   Demonstrates promising results of RF ablation for treatment of liver metastases.

54. Strosberg RJ, Choi J, Cantor AB et al. Selective hepatic artery embolization for treatment of patients with metastatic carcinoid and pancreatic endocrine tumors. Cancer Control 2006; 13:72–8.

55. Bloomston M, Al-Saif O, Klemanski D et al. Hepatic artery chemoembolization in 122 patients with metastatic carcinoid tumor: lessons learned. J Gastrointest Surg 2007; 11:264–71.

56. Lehnert T. Liver transplantation for metastatic neuroendocrine carcinoma: an analysis of 103 patients. Transplantation 1998; 66:1307–12.

57. Pascher A, Klupp J, Neuhaus P. Transplantation in the management of metastatic endocrine tumors. Best Pract Res Clin Gastroenterol 2005; 19:637–48.

58. Olausson M, Friman S, Herlenius G et al. Orthotopic liver or multivisceral transplantation as treatment of metastatic neuroendocrine tumors. Liver Transpl 2007; 13:327–33.

59. Rosenau J, Bahr MJ, von Wasielewski R et al. Ki67, E-cadherin, and p53 as prognostic indicators of long-term outcome after liver transplantation for metastatic neuroendocrine tumors. Transplantation 2002; 73:386–94.

60. Öberg K. Carcinoid tumors: molecular genetics, tumor biology, and update of diagnosis and treatment. Curr Opin Oncol 2002; 14:38–45.

61. Taal BG, Zuetenhorst H, Valdes Olmos RA et al. [131I]MIBG radionuclide therapy in carcinoid syndrome. Eur J Surg Oncol 2002; 28:243.

62. Forrer F, Valkema R, Kvekkebom DJ et al. Peptide receptor radionuclide therapy. Best Pract Res Clin Endocrinol Metab 2007; 21:111–29.

63. Zar N, Garmo H, Holmberg L et al. Long-term survival in small intestinal carcinoid. World J Surg 2004; 28:1163–8.

64. Musunuru S, Chen H, Rajpal S et al. Metastatic neuroendocrine hepatic tumors: resection improves survival. Arch Surg 2006; 141:1000–4.

65. Goede AC, Caplin ME, Winslet MC. Carcinoid tumour of the appendix. Br J Surg 2003; 90:1317–22.

    Succinct and comprehensive review on appendiceal carcinoids.

66. Donnel ME, Carson J, Garstin WIH. Surgical treatment of malignant carcinoids of the appendix. Int J Clin Pract 2007; 61:431–7.

67. Bucher P, Gervaz P, Ris F et al. Surgical treatment of appendiceal adenocarcinoid (goblet cell carcinoid). World J Surg 2005; 29:1436–9.

68. Sugarbaker PH. Peritonectomy procedures. Surg Oncol Clin North Am 2003; 12:703–27.

69. Vogelsang H, Siewert R. Endocrine tumours of the hindgut. Best Pract Res Clin Gastroenterol 2005; 128:1717–51.

    Excellent review on colorectal neuroendocrine tumours and their management.

70. Kang H, O'Connell JB, Leonard MJ et al. Rare tumors of the colon and rectum: a national review. Int J Colorectal Dis 2007; 22:183–9.

71. Naunheim KS, Zeitels J, Kaplan LE et al. Rectal carcinoid tumors – treatment and prognosis. Surgery 1983; 94:670–6.

72. Kimura N, Sasano N. Prostate-specific acid phosphatase in carcinoid tumors. Virchows Arch 1986; 410:247–51.

73. Hotta K, Shimoda T, Nakanishi Y et al. Usefulness of Ki-67 for predicting the metastatic potential of rectal carcinoids. Pathol Int 2006; 56:591–6.

74. Maeda K, Maruta M, Utsumi T et al. Minimally invasive surgery for carcinoid tumors in the rectum. Biomed Pharmacother 2002; 56(Suppl 1): 222s–6s.

75. Hillman N, Herranz L, Alvarez C et al. Efficacy of octreotide in the regression of a metastatic carcinoid tumour despite negative imaging with In-111-pentetreotide (Octreoscan). Exp Clin Endocrinol Diabetes 1998; 106:226–30.

7

Clinical governance, audit and medico-legal aspects of endocrine surgery

Barnard J. Harrison
Anthony E. Young

Clinical governance

"Thou wilt learn one piece of Humility, viz. not to trust too much on thine own judgement."

Richard Wiseman
(*Severall Chirurgicall Treatises*, **1676**)

We are now in the third health revolution. The first was the arrival of technology to improve care, the second the impact of financial constraints and the third the era of accountability.[1] The measurement and regulation of clinical activity is here to stay.

The key points of clinical governance are to improve clinical care, avoid risk and detect adverse events rapidly. We can influence these by continued professional development, quality improvement, risk management and clinical effectiveness.

At a national level in the UK the following agencies are involved in the improvement of clinical care:

- The Department of Health (www.doh.gov.uk) sets appropriate targets and structures the service so that they can be delivered.
- NICE, the National Institute of Clinical Excellence (www.nice.org.uk), is an independent organisation charged with defining best practice from the welter of available evidence. To date in relation to endocrine surgery it has issued guidance on the use of cinacalcet for patients with secondary hyperparathyroidism, on thoracoscopic excision of mediastinal parathyroid tumours, laparoscopic distal pancreatectomy and

it will report on the use of intraoperative nerve monitoring in thyroid surgery.
- The Healthcare Commission (www.healthcare-commission.org.uk) is the inspection body in England for the NHS and the independent sector in terms of quality and value for money. Its duties in England are to:
  - assess the management, provision and quality of NHS healthcare and public health services;
  - review the performance of each NHS trust and award an annual performance rating;
  - regulate the independent healthcare sector through registration, annual inspection, monitoring complaints and enforcement;
  - publish information about the state of healthcare;
  - consider complaints about NHS organisations that the organisations themselves have not resolved;
  - promote the coordination of reviews and assessments carried out by ourselves and others;
  - carry out investigations of serious failures in the provision of healthcare.

The Healthcare Commission also has certain duties in respect to Wales, mainly relating to national reviews and an annual 'State of Healthcare' report.

- The NCAS, the National Clinical Assessment Service (www.ncaa.nhs.uk), is an advisory body that can be called on by an employing organisation, manager or practitioner to intervene if a doctor's practice is below standard up to the level of an assessment of a practitioner's performance. The General Medical Council acts when that practice falls so far from accepted standards that a doctor's licence to practice is called into question.

- The Royal Colleges and professional organisations also have central roles to play in ensuring that practice is of high quality, and they have a special role in relation to education. For endocrine surgery, the British Association of Endocrine and Thyroid Surgeons (BAETS) within the UK is the relevant professional body and advises on training.
- At a local level, hospital trusts should facilitate clinical governance with audit and risk management.

More information about the practical workings of these local and national bodies can be found in *The Medical Manager*.[2]

"Expert knowledge is often incomplete and influenced by strongly held beliefs and personal interest."

There is ample evidence that doctors left to their own devices are not as effective as they would like to think they are, and never have been. Most surgeons would agree that unacceptable variations in standards of care and outcomes must be made to disappear yet, despite good intentions, therapeutic activity that is ineffective or unsubstantiated may take many years to disappear from clinical practice. In addition, our individual practice and the interventions that we use inevitably reflect the current fashion, albeit in the absence of any evidence base. We should not lose sight of the fact that the 'evidence base' and systematic reviews may be adversely affected by subjective analysis, interpretations of variations in the results from previous studies, publication bias and missing data. Changes in clinical practice can be exciting but surgeons should be wary of advancing through errors. From an idea and hypothesis through to a technical development there should be systematic progression that ends in development and assessment of appropriate outcome measures.[3] This certainly applies to the development of minimally invasive surgery of the thyroid and parathyroid glands.[4] Are mortality and readmission rates, complications and duration of hospital stay suffi-

cient to show that the new is an improvement on what has gone before?

Examination of new and old controversies in endocrine surgery as shown below tells us that there is currently little evidence to support a rigid approach to how we advise our patients. For example:

Thyroid disease

- Do all patients with retrosternal goitre require surgery?
- Radioiodine or surgery for patients with thyrotoxicosis?
- The extent of surgery for differentiated thyroid cancer?
- The extent of lymph node surgery in differentiated and medullary thyroid cancer?
- When to complete primary surgery/re-operate in patients with medullary thyroid cancer?

Parathyroid

- The indications for surgery in patients with mild hypercalcaemia?
- What are the indications for re-operative parathyroid surgery?
- Which imaging studies are appropriate prior to re-operative surgery?
- What is the role of minimally invasive surgery?

Adrenal

- Transperitoneal or retroperitoneal laparoscopic surgery?
- What size of incidentaloma should be removed?
- Partial adrenalectomy in familial disease?

Pancreas

- Which preoperative localisation/regionalisation studies are required in patients with insulinoma/gastrinoma?
- When to operate on the pancreas in patients with multiple endocrine neoplasia type 1 (MEN 1)?

In endocrine surgery there will never be evidence based on prospective randomised controlled trials to support much of what we do, yet should we practise our craft in the manner that our peers have demonstrated to be the most effective? Critical review of our current practice will benefit our patients prior to, during and after surgery.

Guidelines should help us make decisions about what is appropriate and, in association with a review of whatever evidence there is, lead to change and improvement in patient care. It should be remembered that guidelines are 'explicit' information that help us to make decisions, but the art of medicine needs as much 'tacit' as 'explicit' input.[5]

For the moment we need to stick to guidelines while remembering that they should be part of an iterative process of regular criticism and review, and that they will often need to be adapted to local circumstances. Guidelines available for the treatment of adult and paediatric endocrine surgical disease were constructed to avoid a dogmatic approach as to what are 'appropriate' treatments. These include those produced by the BAETS,[6] the British Thyroid Association[7] and the British Society of Paediatric Endocrinology and Diabetes.[8]

What is good practice?

Clinical governance and quality are synonymous with achieving and maintaining good practice. As there are few if any emergencies in endocrine surgery, endocrine surgeons have ample time before any elective intervention to ask:

- Which biochemical/cytological tests and imaging studies are necessary prior to surgery, and will their results alter the management of the patient?
- Is an operation required? What is the purpose and aim of the procedure? How will this benefit the patient?
- Which operation is appropriate in this specific case?
- Does the patient understand the indications, implications and risks of surgery in order to give informed consent?

Who should perform surgery on the endocrine glands?

In the USA, thyroid operations comprise fewer than 5% of an average general surgeon's practice. This figure justifies the 1996 consensus statement on thyroid disease by the Royal College of Physicians of London and Society of Endocrinology,[9] which stated: 'each District General Hospital should have access to an experienced thyroid surgeon'. Although surgery of the endocrine glands is currently the scene of dispute between general surgeons (endocrine/upper gastrointestinal/hepatobiliary), head and neck, oromaxillofacial, ENT surgeons and urologists, no individual group has an unassailable

right to care for and treat the patients. The needs of the patient must come first. The introduction to the BAETS guidelines states:

> "[the guidelines do] not define an endocrine surgeon or specify who should practice endocrine surgery … Elective endocrine surgery will not be in the portfolio of every District General Hospital, but where it is, based on experience and caseload, it should be in the hands of a nominated surgeon with an endocrine interest. Those patients requiring more complex investigation and care as detailed in the guidelines should be referred to an appropriate centre. These rare and complex diseases will only be managed effectively by multidisciplinary teams in Units familiar with these disorders … this category includes patients with endocrine pancreatic tumours, adrenal tumours, thyroid malignancy especially medullary thyroid carcinoma, familial syndromes and those requiring reoperative thyroid and parathyroid surgery."

The advantages of subspecialisation

It is all too easy to lose sight of the important issues:

1. **The surgeon should have been appropriately trained.**

In the UK, the higher surgical trainee who declares an interest in endocrine surgery should spend at least 1 year in an approved unit, which should consist of:

- one or more surgeons with a declared interest in endocrine surgery;
- an annual operative workload in excess of 50 cases (verified by BAETS audit);
- on-site cytology and histopathology services;
- at least one consultant endocrinologist on site, holding one or more dedicated endocrinology clinics per week, with joint clinics or formal meetings held not less than once per month;
- a Department of Nuclear Medicine on site;
- on-site magnetic resonance imaging (MRI) and computed tomography (CT) scanning.

In practical terms flexible rotations between regions may be required for more specialised areas of endocrine practice, such as adrenal surgery.

The current syllabus (www.iscp.ac.uk/Documents/Syllabus_GS.pdf) and curriculum (www.baes.info/Pages/BAETS%20Guidelines.pdf) for endocrine surgical training in the UK are well defined. Examples of how endocrine surgical operative experience and competence for an individual trainee can be identified and rated (www.nthst.org.uk/Assets/Files/RITA_forms/NTHST_OpComp_Endocrine_v_1.doc) are available, and in future will help define what constitutes 'appropriately trained'.

2. **The surgeon must be part of an experienced multidisciplinary team.**

Complication rates of thyroid and parathyroid procedures are higher in patients treated by non-specialists,[10,11] and lower when 'high-volume' surgeons operate[12] or patients are treated in high-volume centres.[13] Supervised trainees and newly established endocrine surgeons can perform thyroid surgery safely.[14-16]

The care of patients with thyroid cancer should be the responsibility of a specialist multidisciplinary team (MDT) that comprises surgeon(s), endocrinologist and oncologist (or nuclear medicine physician) with support from pathologist, medical physicist, biochemist, radiologist and clinical nurse specialist. All should have expertise and interest in the management of thyroid cancers and show commitment to continuing education in the field.

There is evidence from the UK and the USA to support a continued need for subspecialisation in endocrine surgery and adherence to good practice, e.g. total thyroidectomy and lymph node dissection is the standard of care in patients with medullary thyroid cancer (MTC) yet 10–15% of patients with MTC undergo less than total thyroidectomy and 40% of patients have no cervical node dissection.[17,18] MTC is rare; all patients should be referred for surgical treatment to a cancer centre.

3. **As the quality of the care received by the patient is paramount it should be subject to assessment by audit and benchmarking against agreed standards.**

In 1998 a retrospective study from a single district hospital identified that only 42% of patients with thyroid cancer presenting with a thyroid nodule had preoperative fine-needle aspiration cytology (FNAC).[19] The situation has improved; BAETS audit data from 2007 reported that 62% of solid thyroid lesions had undergone fine-needle aspiration (FNA) prior to surgery and 80% of treated patients, confirmed at histology to have a neoplastic lesion, underwent FNA prior to the operation.[17] The collection of such prospective information on endocrine surgical activity in the UK is crucial, not only for issues of surgical subspecialisation but for education and training. For UK surgeons, continuing membership of the BAETS is conditional upon the submission of their clinical activity to the audit. It is likely in the future that General Medical Council (GMC) revalidation will require confirmation that surgeons take part in comparative national audit. The following standards and outcome measures are suggested as being applicable to current endocrine surgical practice.

Thyroid surgery
Standards

- The indications for operation, risks and complications should be discussed with patients prior to surgery.
- FNAC should be performed routinely in the investigation of solitary thyroid nodules.
- The recurrent laryngeal nerve should be routinely identified in patients undergoing thyroid surgery.
- All patients scheduled for re-operative thyroid surgery should undergo preoperative examination of their vocal cords by an ENT surgeon. All patients reporting voice change after thyroid surgery should undergo examination of their vocal cords. Permanent vocal cord palsy should not occur in more than 1% of patients.
- A return to theatre to control postoperative haemorrhage should occur in less than 5% of patients.
- All patients with thyroid cancer should be reviewed by the Cancer Centre designated specialist multidisciplinary team.

Outcome measures

There should be documented evidence to support that:

- The patient was informed of the indications for surgery and its risks and complications.
- FNAC was performed in at least 90% of patients prior to operation for solitary/dominant nodule.
- The recurrent laryngeal nerve(s) were identified during a surgical procedure.
- The permanent postoperative vocal cord palsy rate is not more than 1%.

- All patients scheduled for re-operative thyroid surgery have undergone preoperative examination of their vocal cords.
- The re-operation rate for postoperative haemorrhage after thyroidectomy is less than 5%.
- Patients with thyroid malignancy have been reviewed by the specialist multidisciplinary team.

Parathyroid surgery
Standards

In patients who undergo first-time operation for primary hyperparathyroidism:

- The indications for operation, risks and complications should be discussed with patients prior to surgery.
- The surgeon should identify and cure the cause of the disease in at least 95% of cases.
- All patients reporting voice change after parathyroid surgery should undergo examination of their vocal cords. Permanent vocal cord palsy should not occur in more than 1% of patients.
- All patients scheduled for re-operative parathyroid surgery should undergo preoperative examination of their vocal cords.
- Permanent hypocalcaemia should not occur in more than 5% of patients.

Outcome measures

There should be documented evidence to support that:

- The patient was informed of the indications for surgery and its risks and complications.
- After first-time parathyroid surgery, at least 90% of patients are normocalcaemic without calcium or vitamin D supplements.
- The permanent postoperative vocal cord palsy rate is not more than 1%.
- All patients scheduled for re-operative parathyroid surgery have undergone preoperative examination of their vocal cords.

Adrenal surgery
Standards

There should be multidisciplinary working to agreed diagnostic and therapeutic protocols to ensure that an appropriate strategy is developed for patients. This should include the management of the preoperative, peroperative and postoperative metabolic syndrome.

Outcome measures

There should be documented evidence to demonstrate that all patients have been discussed with the multidisciplinary team.

Biochemical cure should be evident in at least:

- 95% of patients with phaeochromocytoma;
- 95% of patients with Conn's syndrome;
- 95% of patients with Cushing's syndrome.

Pancreatic surgery
Standards

- There should be multidisciplinary working to agreed diagnostic and therapeutic protocols to ensure that an appropriate strategy is developed for patients. This should include management of the preoperative, perioperative and postoperative metabolic syndrome.
- Patients with familial endocrine disease should be identified prior to surgery.
- The aims of any surgical procedure must be clearly defined prior to surgery.

Outcome measures

There should be documented evidence to demonstrate that all patients have been discussed with the multidisciplinary team.

- Insulinoma: surgery should result in biochemical cure in at least 90% of cases.
- Gastrinoma: surgery should result in biochemical cure or clinically useful response in at least 60% of cases.

Risk management

Risk management encapsulates the notion that all surgical activity involves some degree of risk and that the risk must be managed so as to achieve the best outcome for the patient. In the past it was sufficient merely to be properly trained, caring and conscientious; today, this does not suffice.

Medical care should be given effectively and carefully; in addition it must be seen to be given effectively and carefully. However cynical one might be about the mechanics of clinical governance and however self-confident one may feel as a professional, there is now a need to take public and documented steps to ensure that risk is being managed. There is evidence that the risk management process has positive advantages in terms of delivering a high quality of care, measured as an improved process of care with better outcome. Whether or not the current bureaucratic process of clinical governance can measurably improve clinical outcome to justify its considerable expense and disruption remains to be seen.[20] We will probably never know.

Staff issues

Are the consultants properly trained and up to date with their postgraduate education in endocrine surgery? Are other consultants undertaking endocrine surgery on an occasional basis because they enjoy it rather than because they are trained in it? When appropriate, are complex patients referred to a specialist centre? The endocrine surgeon must be part of a team that includes endocrine physicians, oncologist, radiologists, cytopathologist and histopathologist, chemical pathologist and clinical/molecular geneticists.

Are trainees appropriately engaged in the process? Are surgical procedures delegated by an appropriate person in the full knowledge of the trainee's competence? Is their supervision appropriate? It is not acceptable to let a new specialist registrar undertake a thyroidectomy prior to supervised assessment of their operative competence.

Communication issues

Are patients properly informed about proposed surgery, particularly the various therapeutic options open to them, in addition to the risks and implications of any choice they make (see 'Consent' below)? Are there information sheets available and in use?

Protocol issues

Are there written protocols in use such as the BAETS Guidelines to aid clinical decision-taking, as well as local protocols for the care of patients with postoperative airway obstruction, hypocalcaemia and steroid replacement after adrenalectomy?

Record-keeping

Clear and contemporaneous evidence must be available in the notes, to show that patients were properly counselled prior to operation and warned about the risks of surgery. The operation notes should be contemporaneous, written by the operating surgeons (or at the very least countersigned by them) and should confirm that, for example, at thyroidectomy the recurrent laryngeal nerves were seen and protected and that parathyroid tissue was retained with its blood supply intact.

Support services

An increasingly common issue in litigation is delay in diagnosis or incorrect diagnosis. In this context it is imperative that the pathologists with whom you work should be competent in the specific and often difficult area of thyroid cytology and histology.

Audit

Remember that simply keeping audit records and having regular audit meetings is not sufficient. The audit cycle must be seen to be occurring such that what has been learned from audit is applied and the whole cycle repeated. Sadly this does not consistently happen. A National Audit Office report has found that only one formal audit study in six had gone round the whole audit cycle and was being repeated.[21]

Medico-legal aspects of endocrine surgery

Even if Trusts, teams and individual clinicians adhere conscientiously to all the requirements of good clinical governance, errors may still occur or will be thought by the patient to have occurred. In this section we cover the specific steps needed to avoid complaint and litigation in endocrine surgery, and suggest some responses should it occur, with an outline of the processes involved. In legal actions the jurisdiction that applies is that of the country in which injury occurred, and we have based our views on an interpretation of English law.

Consent

A formal process of consent in surgery is essential as it is that consent that renders surgical intervention legal. Consent requires that the patient has the **capacity** to understand the process,[22] has the **information** about the nature and the purpose of the surgery to allow informed consent, and provides consent **voluntarily**. Failure to respect these principles means that there was effectively no consent, and the doctor is therefore open to charges of battery or to a claim of negligence. 'Battery' is the unlawful infliction of force on another person; negligence is the failure to take reasonable care. The courts have shown no enthusiasm for pursuing medical cases as battery; most cases that concern the adequacy of information given are brought under the tort of negligence.

In the hallmark UK case of Sidaway, Lord Justice Dunn said that 'the concept of informed consent forms no part of English law'.[23] There is no explicit legal meaning to the term 'informed consent' used by doctors. The case of Sidaway involved a patient who experienced spinal cord complications after an operation on a cervical vertebra as treatment for nerve root pain. She had not been informed about this particular rare complication when she gave her consent, and she claimed that she would not have had the operation if more information had been available. In this case, the patient was not warned because the neurosurgeon judged the risk to be remote, i.e. less than 1%. The problem highlights the potential gap between the 'patient standard', which is what the patient might wish to know, and the 'professional standard', which is what the doctor thinks the patient ought to or needs to know. Patients who experience a complication from an operation will, with the wisdom of hindsight, wish they had been told about a rare but damaging complication, whereas surgeons might reasonably not tell patients of all potential risks that could occur.

In the matter of consent (as in most other medico-legal issues), case law in England and Scotland tends to reflect the application of the 'Bolam test' (see below), namely that the information that the surgeon needs to give is the information that a reasonable and responsible member of the medical profession would think it proper to give in the circumstances. The amount of information that is given to validate 'informed' consent is not defined in law. The rule of thumb is that it should be any risk that is likely to occur in more than 1–2% of cases, but it is important to remember that the quality of information given for consent in medical care is an ethical not a legal requirement of a doctor and is to do with the respect for the autonomy of the patient.[24] Sidaway puts the onus on doctors to decide what information to give; the ethical requirement is merely to give what the doctors' best judgement of each patient defines as the patient's need, and to give it in terms appropriate to the patient's understanding and their education. This trend is also likely to be encouraged by the Council of Europe's Convention on Human Rights: Biomedicine, 1997, which explicitly notes the 'need to restrain the paternalist approaches which might ignore the wishes of the patient'.[25] It is better to look at the process of 'informed' consent as part of a shared decision-making process, founded in adult debate with patients about the management

---

Box 7.1 • Key issues in risk reduction on matters of consent

- Obtain consent well before the operation
- Do not obtain consent after sedation has been given
- The doctor obtaining consent should be knowledgeable about the procedure and its potential complications
- Explain 'material risks'
- Answer questions in an open and honest manner
- Do not alter the consent form after the patient has signed it
- Do not exceed the authority given by the consent form

---

of their disease. The risks and consequences of various treatment options should be discussed in sufficient detail to be understood so that patients can make informed decisions. In practical terms the surgeon, or somebody who is familiar with the disease and its treatment, must sign the consent form together with the patient. We recommend the use of patients' information sheets (as illustrated in the BAETS Guidelines), but remember that their use does not obviate the need for detailed personal discussions between patients and surgeons (Box 7.1).

When things do not go smoothly

Only a tiny percentage of problems and errors mature into a complaint. It is clear that if complaints are handled effectively and promptly and if there is good and honest communication of facts, the number of complaints that mature into litigations are few. One of the virtues of proper handling of complaints is that they often show that although things did not turn out for the best, the problems that occurred were within the boundaries of those experienced in medical care and were not a sign of negligence. It is much more common for complaints to reflect a sequence of unsatisfactory events in the patient's care and in 72% of instances a perception of staff insensitivity or a communication breakdown is the element that precipitates the complaint.[26] Of the other factors at work in precipitating a complaint, 25% relate to failure to investigate or treat and 20% claim a failure of clinical competence.[27]

Handling complaints

Informal complaints should be dealt with as promptly and as honestly as possible in the context of normal communication. It is important to remember that if there has been a degree of error then admit to it and apologise early. An apology does not represent an admission of liability. However, we believe that if the surgeon or the person to whom the complaint has been made makes an honest and insightful assessment of the problem and considers that there has **not** been an error, there is no requirement to apologise. A verbal complaint that is dealt with orally should be recorded as a written or typed note and placed in the clinical record.

Nothing should be sent out in writing without first checking the text with the Trust's complaints officer and/or your defence organisation. This is invaluable if an informal complaint subsequently turns into a formal one.

Local resolution of complaints

Procedures that came into force in April 1996 have defined in detail how and in what timeframe hospitals must respond to complaints. These processes have some key objectives:

- Ease of access to the complaints system.
- A simple, rapid, open process.
- Fairness for complainants and staff alike.
- Lessons from complaints to be used to improve patient services.
- Investigation of complaints to be entirely separate from any subsequent disciplinary proceedings.

Complaints must be made within 6 months of the event complained about or from the moment that a patient realised that there had been a problem. The complaint can go through consecutive stages:

1. Local resolution.
2. Independent review.
3. Appeal to the health service ombudsman.

An early review of the workings of the complaints system noted that it was perceived as 'biased, closed and inadequate' and that 'patients feel suspicious, frustrated and let down' and clinicians 'undervalued and beset'.[28] The same survey characterised the processes as tending 'to investigate superficially, to analyse defensively, and to jump to conclusions about the remedy, if any action is taken at all'. Attempts have been made to improve the process and there is now an 'Independent Complaints Advocacy Service' (www.carersfederation.co.uk) which has attempted to ease the process. The NHS last modified its complaints procedures in 2007 and regulations in 2006 (www.dh.gov.uk/en/Policyandguidance/Organisationpolicy/Complaintspolicy/NHScomplaintsprocedure/index.

htm). The surgeon can find more practical guidance in the paper by Cave and Dacre.[29]

However skilfully they are handled, complaints can still turn into litigation, although in fact this occurs relatively rarely. Of the NHS Litigation Authority (NHSLA) cases, 96% are settled out of court through a variety of methods of 'alternative dispute resolution' (ADR). An analysis of all clinical claims handled by the NHSLA over the past 10 years shows that 41% were abandoned by the claimant, 41% settled out of court, 4% settled in court (mainly court approvals of negotiated settlements) and 14% remain outstanding. Fewer than 50 clinical negligence cases a year are contested in court.[30]

Complaints that turn into litigation

As far as endocrine surgeons are concerned cases will be based in personal injury owing to an alleged breach of duty by them or their team. A complication of surgery or a delay in diagnosis will be the probable reason. There are no published figures to indicate how often endocrine surgery in the UK has led to litigation in the past and how successful that has been. The best data, although incomplete, come from the USA. In a paper presented at the annual meeting of the American Association of Endocrine Surgeons in 1993, Kern identified 62 cases of malpractice from 21 states between 1985 and 1991, for analysis. In 54% of instances the problem arose from a surgical complication, almost all during thyroid surgery; 35% arose from delayed diagnosis, equally of thyroid and adrenal disease; and 11% were from morbidity attributed to radioiodine or propylthiouracil. It is sobering to see that even 10 years ago mean payouts for successful litigation for a recurrent nerve injury approached $1 million and the maximum was $2.5 million.[31] The number of endocrine cases currently passing through the system in the USA or the UK is not known.

The first intimation of litigation will usually be a letter from the solicitor to the hospital, and this may come without patients having troubled to go through a formal complaint process first, or patients may have been through some sort of formal or informal process and not been satisfied with the outcome. Once a problem turns into a formal process of litigation it is protracted, time-consuming, distressing for all concerned and, from the NHS's point of view, expensive. It is important that clinicians handle complaints in as dispassionate and efficient a way as possible, however distressed they may feel by the complaint itself and by the process of dealing with it.

The solicitor's letter

The first manifestation will normally be a solicitor's letter asking for release of copies of all the notes, X-ray films, pathology reports, etc. In NHS practice the hospital complaints or litigation officer should receive this, together with an indication that the request for release signifies or does not signify an impending action against the Trust.

At this stage you may be asked by the hospital to confirm that you are happy for copies of the notes to be released. In effect you have no choice about this, but the solicitor requesting them must give sufficient detail, setting out the expected case against the doctor, to comply with the requirements of section 33 of the Supreme Court Act, 1981. Before the release of the notes you need to make sure that they are in sensible order, that copies of all the originals are retained by the hospital and that you have reviewed any part that you or your team had in the incident that has led to the litigation. You also need to check that it is the patient who indirectly is asking for release of the files. If it is not, then you will need the patient's permission to release the file. When reviewing the notes it is in order to ensure that the filing of the notes is logical, but you must not add anything, change anything or remove anything from the notes. Do, however, refresh your memory, as it may be several years since the events occurred. If you receive a request for notes in your capacity as a private practitioner, check the notes and photocopy them, but only release them to the patient's solicitors through your medical defence organisation.

The solicitors acting for the patient will now be finding an expert and getting an initial opinion. Additionally, experience shows that they will often be applying to the Legal Aid board for a certificate to confirm that this client's costs will be covered if they are eligible. It is a sad reflection on access to justice that medical negligence litigation is not realistically affordable by any but the very rich and those receiving legal aid. There will, in any event, be a lull, the extent of which is governed only by the limitation period of 3 years from the time that the plaintiff could reasonably have known that he or she had a cause for action. There are, however, situations where this time may be extended, but this requires a formal plea in court to disbar a defence plea that a claimant's action is disbarred by lapse of time.[32]

The next communication will probably be a writ and a statement of claim from the claimant's solicitors, outlining in detail the allegations and often enclosing the expert's report in the details of which the claim is usually grounded. The writ formally indicates the beginning of a legal action.

Most doctors become depressed, distressed, angry or all three of these at this point, and fortunately the handling of the process from here on is not in their hands but in those of the solicitors acting for the hospital, or the medical defence organisation if the matter relates to a private patient.

If you believe that the allegation of negligence is completely unfounded, it is important at this stage to ensure that the hospital is aware of the strength of your feelings and is prepared to defend the claim rather than simply settle to reduce costs (particularly in relation to claimants receiving legal aid). You may want to liaise with your medical defence organisation about this, even if it is an NHS case. Many textbooks describe the detail of the legal processes and the details of the underlying laws, principles and customs. Currently, the most readable of these is *Medicine, Patients and the Law* by Brazier and Cave.[33]

Essentially the case will revolve around the fact that you, the surgeon, are claimed to have been negligent. Although negligence has lay meanings as a word, it has very specific legal meanings.

Medical negligence

Surgical cases come to court almost invariably as a result of patients suing in an action for negligence. This is a civil prosecution.

Negligence is an area considered under the civil law called tort, i.e. civil wrongs. Any formal legal action in this area only succeeds if a particular legal formula is fulfilled. The components of this formula are:

1. A relationship must exist between the parties (the surgeon and the patient), which gives rise to a **duty of care**.
2. The duty of care must have been **breached** in some way due to an unreasonable act or omission by one of the parties. This breach of the duty of care is the negligence.
3. In addition to the negligence the injured party must have experienced some **damage**, loss or injury of a type recognised by the law.

4. The damage must have been caused **by the other party**, in this case the surgeon.

5. The action must be brought within a specified time after the injury has occurred (this is known as the **period of limitation**; see above).

Duty of care

As the NHS surgical patient will already have come under the care of a hospital, either as an outpatient or inpatient, the plaintiff will have no difficulty in establishing that the hospital Trust has a duty of care. In private practice (and this includes patients admitted to NHS pay beds) the relationship is primarily directly with the surgeon and separately with the other providers, such as the hospital, anaesthetist, pathology laboratory, etc. The duty of care in this latter situation arises through the 'contract' that arises implicitly between the surgeon and patient.

Breaching of duty of care

A successful negligence claim requires that the patient claimant demonstrates that the defendant (Trust or surgeon) was in breach of its duty of care. In English law the breach or lack of it is determined by judging what an equivalent body of other doctors would have done in similar circumstances. This is known as the 'Bolam test'.

Bolam[34] is the legal case cited in England. In Scotland it is *Hunter v. Hanley*.[35] Essentially these cases have the same conclusion, which is generally favourable to the surgeon.

The more recent case of *Bolitho v. City and Hackney Health Authority* slightly changed the principles behind the Bolam judgement. Medical evidence from eight experts was divided. The judge accepted that both bodies of evidence were respectable and concluded that he was in no position to 'prefer' one view. This was in line with Lord Scarman's view in another case that: 'a judge's preference for one body of distinguished opinion over another, also professionally distinguished, is not sufficient to establish negligence in a practitioner'.[36]

The case was appealed eventually to the House of Lords, who supported the trial judge's conclusion but added an important rider to the 'Bolam test' in that it was no longer sufficient for experts to claim that something was acceptable practice but they needed to show that in 'forming their view, they, the experts, have directed their minds to the question of comparative risks and benefits and have reached a defensible conclusion on the matter'.[37] Courts in the Republic of Ireland have in general also accepted the Bolam test but have spelled out the same limitations, that the treatment supported must be logical. Experts supporting or rejecting a particular course of action must therefore ground their views in a defensible clinical assessment of the pros and cons of any particular course of action.

A recent twist to this has been the position of guidelines and protocols. Many surgeons are apprehensive that they may not, on the basis of their own experience and reading, agree with protocols that are promulgated either nationally or within their own organisation, and therefore they might feel particularly threatened if they departed from those guidelines. Guidelines and protocols hold no special status legally and they should merely be regarded as an extension of the Bolam principle, as defining the views of other reputable practitioners. A guideline should not be published unless the authors can justify their joint view with reference to normal good clinical practice and the literature. Similarly, surgeons who depart from guidelines must be able logically and clinically to defend their departure from those guidelines. It is the courts who retain the right to decide whether a particular clinical practice is acceptable or not. Expert evidence of professional habits will carry the day in most cases, but surgeons cannot rely on this with complete certainty. There seem to be only a tiny number of cases where the court has chosen not to accept the expert medical evidence.

It is hardly surprising that doctors have a duty to keep themselves informed of major developments such as might be encompassed by guidelines. That duty cannot extend to a requirement that they know everything there is to know. For example, in the case of *Crawford v. The Board of Governors of Charing Cross Hospital*, the plaintiff had developed a brachial palsy because of his position on the operating table. Six months prior to the event, an article had appeared in the *Lancet* warning of this danger, but the anaesthetist involved in the case had not read the article. The Court of Appeal found in favour of the anaesthetist, Lord Denning stating that:

"It would I think be putting too high a burden on a medical man to say he has read every article appearing in the current medical press; and it would be quite wrong to suggest

a medical man is negligent because he does not at once put into operation a suggestion which some contributor or other might make in a medical journal. The time may come in a particular case where a new recommendation may be so well proved, and so well known, and so well accepted that it should be adopted; this was not so in this case."[38]

A widely promulgated guideline could, however, in Lord Denning's terms fall into a recommendation 'so well proved and so well known and so well accepted that it should be adopted'.

Damage

Damage cited by plaintiffs must have been caused directly by the defendants' negligence, not, for example, simply by progression of underlying disease. Damages subsequently awarded in the UK simply aim to place defendants in the position they were in before the damage was sustained, plus an element for pain and suffering. The situation in the UK is totally different from that pertaining in the USA, where juries, not judges, decide damages and a strong punitive element is often included.

Causation

Letters from solicitors will often use the term 'causation', a term not immediately understood by doctors (Box 7.2). In the legal setting 'causation' is merely the establishment of a factual and legal link between the breach of duty and the damage caused. This is often difficult to prove. Normally the 'but for' test is used. For example, 'but for the failure to take a fine-needle biopsy at the first outpatient visit the patient's thyroid carcinoma would have been diagnosed 6 months earlier'. Note that in negligence cases guilt or innocence is decided on grounds of 'balance of probability' rather than 'beyond reasonable doubt', as applies in criminal cases.

Expert opinions

Although it is for the court to decide on matters put before it – right or wrong, true or false, negligent or not negligent – it can only do so in medical cases by drawing on expert advice from clinicians and others. More importantly – and more commonly – expert advice is also used to determine whether a case needs to be put before the court or should be abandoned or settled out of court. Anyone asked to provide an expert report will usually receive with that request guidance notes advising that the expert's duty is to the court and not to the plaintiff, the defendant or the solicitor that has instructed him. Therefore:

- The report is addressed to the court.
- It contains a statement that experts understand that their duty is to the court.
- Experts may if they wish file a written request to the court for directions to assist them in carrying out their function as an expert. They do not need to give the claimant, defendant or the instructing solicitor any notice of such a request.

Box 7.2 • Examples illustrating the legal meaning of causation

Causation

A patient comes into hospital for thyroidectomy. The cords are checked preoperatively and both move. After the operation the patient is hoarse and laryngoscopy shows one cord is not moving.

The plaintiff's barrister could readily show that there was a duty of care, that there was damage and could prove causation. But it would be hard to prove negligence. Laryngeal nerve palsy ipso facto is not evidence of negligence.

No causation

A patient comes to the outpatient department with a long-standing mass in the neck. The mass is fixed to the surrounding structures. The surgeon neither biopsies the mass nor operates. Two weeks later the patient dies and the post-mortem shows an anaplastic carcinoma obstructing the airway.

There was a duty of care but there was no causation in that on a balance of probability failure to biopsy the mass or arrange treatment did not alter the outcome.

Reforms

The surgeon should be aware of several changes that will affect medical litigation over the next 10 years:

1. Conditional/contingency fees ('no win, no fee').
2. The recommendations of the Woolf report.
3. Attempts to control the cost of legal aid.

No win, no fee

The legislation to allow lawyers and their clients to come to conditional agreements about fees – the fee being conditional on the outcome of the case – came into effect in July 1995. In the UK the loser must pay the other party's costs. The option, therefore, of not having to pay your lawyer if you lose does not guarantee a risk-free exercise for the plaintiff. The 'no win, no fee' arrangement also puts greater pressure on the claimant's solicitor to check that the case is worth pursuing, and that pressure is much greater than it is in cases supported by legal aid. Overall, the system tends to reduce rather than increase the number of vexatious and speculative claims.[39]

The Woolf report

The Woolf report of 1996[40] reviewed the whole of the civil justice system in England and Wales and recommended radical change. Medical negligence litigation did not escape Lord Woolf's attentions because he considered most cases currently to be unduly long, complex and expensive. The recommendations of the report have been summarised as follows:

1. Greater effort at prevention and early resolution of disputes. As steps towards this, Lord Woolf recommended that medical record keeping should be better, the procedures for local resolution of problems should be clearer, and that there should be more use of mediation with jointly instructed experts where possible and a greater use of experts' meetings. Overall though, he recommended a more sparing use of experts.
2. An improved summary disposal procedure to weed out weak claims and weak defences.
3. The introduction of a system of plaintiff 'offers to settle', with sanctions where a defendant unreasonably refused to cooperate.
4. Claims of £10 000 or less to be handled by a slimmed down procedure with a limited range of legal processes conforming to tightly controlled timetables and costs.
5. Large and complex claims to be handled by a 'multitrack' process, where the management of each case legally is decided by the courts themselves rather than by lawyers.

Changes to legal aid legislation

The costs of legal aid are rising annually, and this is a cause of concern for the Government. Recent changes to the rules to reduce access to legal aid excluded medical negligence cases. Subsequently there have been more definite steps to limit the management of medical negligence cases to legal practices with proven expertise.

Conclusions

The endocrine surgeon is not simply a technician; he or she must be both self-regulator and a knowledgeable member of the endocrine team.

Effective clinical governance will help define:

- the appropriateness and effectiveness of our interventions;
- the lack of evidence that supports some of our current practice;
- the needs for further research.

There is a clear need to improve the standards of care for patients with endocrine surgical disorders in the UK. Guidelines and audit will help surgeons pass the 'shadow line' to achieve:

"... gains not only to oneself, but to the whole practice of surgery ... not at the expense of overlooking how much there must always be to learn; the confidence and pride in one's own abilities that allows criticism from both within and without ... a view of medicine as a whole that can allow all its surprises and uncertainties to be one's companions throughout one's career not as spectres reflecting inadequacy, but as impartial guides who point out the way forward."

R. Hayward[41]

Complaint and litigation will not go away. An increase in individualism, loss of respect for professionals, more mechanical medical processes and a good supply of well-trained, proficient lawyers is going to ensure that whatever the changes in legislation and clinical practice, litigation will continue. Risk reduction activity by surgeons should include the routine practice of documenting that an appropriate consent process has occurred and the use of patient information material. Adherence to protocols, competence-based training and career-long postgraduate education should aim to reduce the incidence of harm to the unavoidable minimum. Complaints that are not satisfactorily resolved may be better handled by processes of arbitration or mediation rather than the traditional confrontationalism of the legal process. The legal aid process is already attempting to weed out such cases.

It is the placement of that fine boundary between misadventure and negligence that is behind most medical litigation in endocrine surgery as in all other branches of medicine.

References

1. Relman AS. Assessment and accountability. N Engl J Med 1988; 319:1220–2.

2. Young AE. The medical manager, 2nd edn. London: BMJ Books, 2003.

3. Lorenz W, Troidl H, Solomkin JS et al Second step: testing outcome measurements. World J Surg 1999; 23:768–80.

4. Miccoli P. Minimally invasive surgery for thyroid and parathyroid diseases. Surg Endosc 2002; 16:3–6.

5. Wyatt JC. Management of explicit and tacit knowledge. J R Soc Med 2001; 94:6–9.

6. British Association of Endocrine and Thyroid Surgeons. Guidelines for the surgical management of endocrine disease and training requirements for endocrine surgery (www.baes.info/Pages/guidelines.php), 2004.

7. Perros P (ed.) British Thyroid Association, Royal College of Physicians – Guidelines for the management of thyroid cancer. Report of the Thyroid Cancer Guidelines Update Group, 2nd edn. London: Royal College of Physicians, 2007.

8. Spoudeas H (ed.) Paediatric endocrine tumours. A multi-disciplinary consensus statement of best practice from a working group convened under the auspices of the British Society of Paediatric Endocrinology and Diabetes and the United Kingdom Children's Cancer Study Group (www.bsped.org.uk/professional/guidelines/index.htm), 2005.

9. Vanderpump MP, Ahlquist JA, Franklyn JA et al. Consensus statement for good practice in the management of hypothyroidism and hyperthyroidism. The Research Unit of the Royal College of Physicians of London, the Endocrinology and Diabetes Committee of the Royal College of Physicians of London, and the Society for Endocrinology. Br Med J 1996; 313:539–44.

10. Harness JK, van Heerden JA, Lennquist S et al. Future of thyroid surgery and training surgeons to meet the expectations of 2000 and beyond. World J Surg 2000; 24:976–82.

11. Sosa JA, Bowman HM, Tielsch JM et al. The importance of surgeon experience for clinical and economic outcomes from thyroidectomy. Ann Surg 1998; 228:320–30.

12. Stavrakis AI, Ituarte PH, Ko CY et al. Surgeon volume as a predictor of outcomes in inpatient and outpatient endocrine surgery. Surgery 2007; 142: 887–99.

13. Pieracci FM, Fahey TJ 3rd. Effect of hospital volume of thyroidectomies on outcomes following substernal thyroidectomy. World J Surg 2008; (Epub ahead of print).

14. Hassan I, Koller M, Kluge C et al. Supervised surgical trainees perform thyroid surgery for Graves' disease safely. Langenbecks Arch Surg 2006; 391:597–602.

15. Sywak MS, Yeh MW, Sidhu SB et al. New surgical consultants: is there a learning curve? Aust NZ J Surg 2006;76:1081–4.

16. Erbil Y, Barbaros U, Issever H et al. Predictive factors for recurrent laryngeal nerve palsy and hypoparathyroidism after thyroid surgery. Clin Otolaryngol 2007; 32:32–37.

17. British Association of Endocrine Surgeons second national audit report, 2nd edn. Henley on Thames: Dendrite Clinical Systems, 2007.

18. Kebebew E, Greenspan FS, Clark OH et al. Extent of disease and practice patterns for medullary thyroid cancer. J Am Coll Surg 2005; 200:890–6.

19. Vanderpump MP, Alexander L, Scarpello JH et al. An audit of the management of thyroid cancer in a district general hospital. Clin Endocrinol (Oxf) 1998; 48:419–24.

20. Goodman NW. Accountability, clinical governance and the acceptance of imperfection. J R Soc Med 2000; 93:59–61.

21. National Audit Office. Clinical audit in England. London: Stationery Office, 1995.

22. Nicholson TR, Cutter W, Hotopf M. Assessing mental capacity: the Mental Capacity Act. Br Med J 2008; 336:322–5.

23. *Sidaway* v. *Board of Governors of the Bethlehem Royal Hospital* [1984] QB493 at 517, [1984] 1 All ER 1018 at 1030, CA.

24. Davies M. Textbook on medical law. London: Blackstone Press, 1996; pp. 166–74.

25. Medical Law Monitor 1997; 4(10):6.

26. Bark P, Vincent C, Jones A et al. Clinical complaints: a means of improving quality of care. Qual Health Care 1994; 3:123–32.

27. Donaldson LJ, Cavanagh J. Clinical complaints and their handling: a time for change? Qual Health Care 1992; 1:21–5.

28. Hill AP, Baeza J. Dealing with things that go wrong. Lancet 1999; 354:2099–100.

29. Cave J, Dacre J. Dealing with complaints Br Med J 2008; 336:326–8.

30. NHS Litigation Authority. Factsheet 3: Information on claims; www.nhsla.com/NR/rdonlyres/C1B3F310-E13D-4C71-B248-C5384438E603/0/NHSLAFactsheet320062007.doc, 2007.

31. Kern KA. Medicolegal analysis of errors in diagnosis and treatment of surgical endocrine disease. Surgery 1993; 114:1167–74.

32. Finch J. Speller's law relating to hospitals, 7th edn, section 5.2. London: Chapman & Hall Medical, 1993.

33. Brazier M, Cave F. Medicine, patients and the law, 4th edn. London: Penguin, 2007.

34. *Bolam* v. *Friern Hospital Management Committee* [1957] 2 All ER 118, [1957] 1 WLR 582.

35. *Hunter v. Hanley*. 1955 SC 200.

36. *Maynard v. West Midlands Regional Health Authority* [1984] 1 WLR 634 at 639.

37. *Bolitho* [1997] 4 All ER 771.

38. Mason JK, McCall Smith RA. Law and medical ethics. London: Butterworths, 1994; p. 202.

39. Barton A. Conditional fees: access to justice for all. Clin Risk 1997; 3:130–1.

40. Lord Woolf. Access to justice. London: Stationery Office, 1996.

41. Hayward R. The shadow-line in surgery. Lancet 1987; 1:375–6.

8

The salivary glands

Steven J. Thomas
Zenon Rayter

Introduction

Salivary glands are exocrine glands which produce and excrete saliva. The major glands consist of three pairs of glands: the parotid, the submandibular and the sublingual. Diseases of the salivary glands are relatively uncommon, but the pathology is diverse. Most lesions of the parotid gland are inflammatory, although there is also a wide spectrum of neoplastic conditions, some of which are unique to the parotid gland. The differential diagnosis of a parotid mass in particular remains an important aspect of a surgeon's training.

Anatomy

The parotid gland is predominantly serous producing. It occupies an irregular space with the external auditory meatus, the mastoid process and the sternomastoid muscle at its posterior border, the mandible and its attached muscles at the anterior border, and the styloid process and its attached muscles medially. It extends upwards as far as the zygomatic arch and forwards, both deep and superficial to the ramus of the mandible. The gland is separated from the skin by the general investing layer of the deep fascia of the neck, which above the angle of the mandible passes over the gland and fuses with the masseter muscle on the outer aspect of the ramus of the mandible. The fascia is attached to the zygomatic arch

and becomes continuous with the temporal fascia. There is no true capsule to the parotid gland, and the lobules of gland substance fill the available space and conform to the shape of the surrounding structures. The duct of the gland (Stensen's duct) follows the masseter muscle to its anterior edge, where it turns medially through buccinator to open on to the mucous membrane of the cheek opposite the crown of the upper second molar tooth. As Stensen's duct passes over the masseter, it may receive the duct of an accessory parotid gland, which is found overlying the masseter muscle in approximately 20% of people, usually just above Stensen's duct.

The facial nerve emerges from the stylomastoid foramen lateral to the styloid process and enters the parotid. Before entering the parotid gland, the facial nerve gives off branches to the stylohyoid, the posterior belly of the diagastric muscle, and posterior auricular and occipitalis muscles. The main trunk of the nerve then usually divides (the pes anserinus, or goose's foot) into its upper and lower divisions two-thirds of the way to the mandible. The two divisions are the temporozygomatic and cervicofacial branches, which pass through the parotid gland superficial to the retromandibular vein.[1] The two divisions divide into peripheral branches. The nerves to the forehead muscles and the upper and lower eyelids arise from the temporozygomatic branch, and the buccal branch and nerves to the upper and lower lips arise from the cervicofacial branch (**Fig. 8.1**). Variations to this pattern are

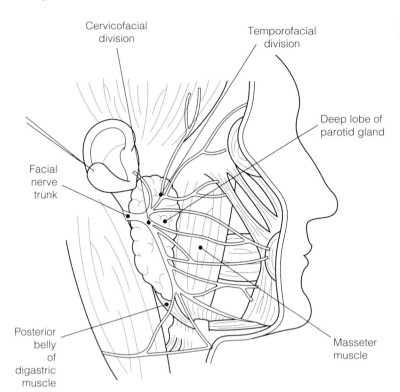

Cervicofacial division

Temporofacial division

Figure 8.1 • Surgical anatomy of the parotid salivary gland.

Deep lobe of parotid gland

Facial nerve trunk

Masseter muscle

Posterior belly of digastric muscle

common. This division of the parotid gland by the facial nerve into superficial and deep lobes is important when operating on parotid lesions.

The external carotid artery enters the deep surface of the parotid and divides at about the level of the neck of the mandible into the superficial temporal artery, which emerges from the upper edge of the gland, and the maxillary artery, which passes medially out of the gland. In the substance of the gland are numerous lymph nodes. The anterior surface of the gland is in contact with the mandible and the masseter and medial pterygoid muscles. The posterior surface is in contact below with the mastoid process and the sternomastoid and digastric muscles, and above with the external auditory meatus. Medially, the gland is separated by the digastric muscle from the internal jugular vein and the styloid process, and by the stylohyoid muscle from the internal carotid artery. Above, the gland overlies the capsule of the temperomandibular joint. The postganglionic nerve supply of the gland runs in the auriculotemporal nerve from the otic ganglion. The preganglionic fibres arise in the inferior salivary nucleus, run in the glossopharyngeal nerve and its tympanic branch to the lesser petrosal nerve and so enter the otic ganglion and then to the gland via

the auriculotemporal nerve. The parotid and periparotid lymph glands drain primarily into the internal jugular chain nodes, with some drainage going to the upper spinal accessory chain of nodes.

The submandibular glands secrete mixed serous and mucinous saliva. The gland extends around the posterior margin of the mylohyoid muscle which defines the larger superficial lobe and the smaller deep lobe. The submandibular duct extends from the deep lobe of the gland forwards from the posterior margin of the mylohyoid to the floor of the mouth mucosa, passing between the mylohyoid and hyoglossus and then the sublingual gland and the genioglossus. It emerges in the mouth at the sublingual papilla. The secretory fibres for the submandibular and sublingual glands run from the inferior salivary nucleus via the facial nerve, chorda tympani and lingual nerves, the submandibular ganglion then to the glands via the lingual nerve.

Developmental abnormalities

Developmental abnormalities of the parotid glands are rare. When they do occur, other facial abnormalities may be present and are associated with xerostomia, sialadenitis and dental caries. Parotid gland agenesis has been reported with hemifacial microsomia, mandibulofacial dysostosis, cleft palate and anophthalmia.[2]

Ectopic location of salivary gland tissue can occur in many sites, including the external auditory canal and middle ear cleft, the anterior mandible, the inner-posterior mandible (Stafne cyst), the pituitary gland and even the cerebellopontine angle.[3]

Investigation

Clinical evaluation

Most lesions of the parotid gland are either due to inflammatory conditions, the obstruction of Stensen's duct or tumours. The commonest presentations of parotid pathology are therefore swelling of the whole gland (in inflammatory conditions and obstructions of the duct) or a solitary mass (tumour) in the parotid region. It should be possible for the clinician to make this distinction,[4] which is important as a mass nearly always implies a neoplasm. In the assessment of a parotid mass, particular attention should be paid to the presence or absence of facial palsy, as its presence strongly suggests malignancy.[5] Other important aspects of the clinical examination are fixity and site of the lesion within the parotid. Thus, a recent study concluded that 96% of tumours in the tail of the gland (that region lying inferiorly) were benign if there was no facial palsy, pain, trismus or fixation.[5] This may be useful in the assessment of frail elderly patients in whom fine-needle aspiration may not be performed.

In assessing any parotid mass, the patient should be asked to clench teeth to contract the masseter muscles; this allows the examiner to assess if the swelling is due to hypertrophy of the masseter or whether the mass is in the substance of the muscle (haemangioma or myxoma). Complete examination of all the other salivary glands should be performed to ascertain whether multiple masses are present or whether other glands are involved in a systemic disease (as in Sjögren's syndrome). All glands should be examined bimanually and each duct orifice inspected and palpated. No examination is complete without examination of the pharynx to ascertain the presence of a parapharyngeal tumour, which may be shaped like a dumb-bell and present as a parotid mass. The diagnosis of a parotid mass is not usually difficult,

Box 8.1 • Differential diagnosis of a parotid mass not caused by a parotid tumour

- Epidermoid cyst
- Enlarged lymph node
- Lipoma
- Lymphangioma
- Hypertrophic masseter
- Mandibular tumour
- Branchial cyst

but clinicians should bear in mind the rarer causes of an apparent parotid mass (Box 8.1). The most common reason for excision of the submandibular gland is when a calculus is present within the gland or when the gland is chronically infected.

Radiology

The choice of imaging modalities has increased and the emphasis is now on ultrasonography, computed tomography (CT) and magnetic resonance imaging (MRI). As a general rule, CT is most useful for inflammatory lesions, whereas tumours are identified well using MRI. Ultrasonography is typically used to identify solid and cystic masses; it is also useful for identifying sialoliths and assessing chronic inflammatory conditions.[6]

Sialography

This remains a detailed method of visualising the fine duct system but is now rarely used except in the assessment of suspected sialectasis. Magnetic resonance imaging sialography is now able to examine the major and secondary intraglandular ducts, and the finer detail is rarely required to aid clinical decisions.

Computed tomography

If the patient's history is suggestive of inflammatory disease, CT will identify the site of the disease and may also identify the calculi responsible.[7] It can distinguish between cellulitis and abscess formation, submassateric and parotid disease, and submandibular gland sialadenitis and lymph node disease. Although CT is able to detect salivary tumours MRI is even more sensitive. Usually, little extra information is obtained with the use of contrast.[8]

Magnetic resonance imaging

This is probably the preferred method of imaging a mass suspected of being a tumour (**Figs 8.2 and 8.3**).

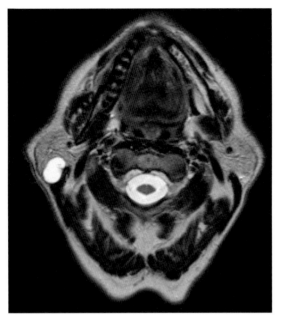

Figure 8.2 • MRI scan of a pleomorphic adenoma of the parotid gland.

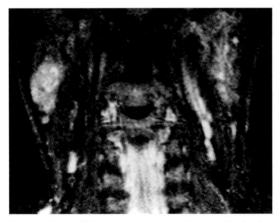

Figure 8.3 • MRI scan of maltoma of the parotid gland.

This is sometimes combined with contrast and is useful in assessing perineural tumour spread in parotid malignancies.[9] MRI studies are usually performed as 3-mm-thick slices with a 1-mm interslice gap. Non-contrast T1- and T2-weighted sequences and then T1-weighted, postcontrast, fat-suppressed images are obtained. Axial views are obtained for all sequences and sagittal and coronal views obtained as required.[7,10] Normally, the facial nerve is not imaged. The recent use of high-resolution three-dimensional Fourier-transformed MRI has allowed the facial nerve to be consistently visualised on contiguous

scans.[11] MRI is also particularly useful in lesions situated within the deep lobe of the parotid.

MR sialography is undertaken without the introduction of any intraductal contrast material. It has shown very good results in the investigation of suspected ductal salivary gland disease as it is able to depict not only the main duct system and first- and second-order branches, but also third-order branches. In a recent study, digital subtraction sialography had a sensitivity and specificity of 96% and 100% respectively in the diagnosis of chronic sialadenitis, and a sensitivity and specificity of 90% and 98% in the diagnosis of sialolithiasis.[12]

Ultrasonography

This technique identifies solid and cystic masses in the salivary glands and sialoliths. It can also be used to identify the more advanced stages of autoimmune disease (Sjögren's syndrome) and to differentiate between lymphomatous and non-lymphomatous nodes,[13] although not with sufficient accuracy to avoid biopsy. Ultrasonography is particularly useful in children, in whom exposure to radiation is to be avoided. For lesions that have spread beyond the capsule, it does not provide the detailed anatomical information obtained with CT and MRI.[6]

Other radiological techniques

Radionuclide salivary gland scans are based on the fact that salivary glands normally concentrate technetium pertechnetate (^{99m}Tc) and some masses excessively accumulate the radionuclide, especially Warthin's tumours and oncocytomas.[14,15] Radionuclide scans are rarely used now that CT and MRI are freely available. Angiography was useful in the investigation of tumours situated in the parapharyngeal space to differentiate salivary gland tumours from chemodectoma of the carotid or from a nerve sheath tumour. Its use has also been superseded by CT and MRI. Positron emission tomography (PET) scanning may have a role in combination with other salivary imaging techniques. It can be used for detecting recurrent disease and is potentially useful for staging at the initial presentation of salivary gland tumours.[16]

Fine-needle aspiration cytology

Fine-needle aspiration cytology (FNAC) of a discrete parotid mass remains controversial.[17,18] Its proponents argue that it has a high diagnostic accuracy, may influence the decision to operate, may allow planning of the most appropriate operative procedure and allows better-informed preoperative counselling.[19-22] Its detractors argue that it is not sufficiently accurate at diagnosing low-grade malignant lesions, and that the decision to operate is clinically based and the extent of the surgery is not influenced by the cytology, since in the parotid gland more radical surgery for a malignant lesion does not influence outcome.[17] However, all authorities are agreed that FNAC does not cause tumour seeding and that it is free of any major morbidity. A recent survey of 34 institutions with a major interest in salivary gland tumours concluded that approximately one-third of surgical oncologists did not employ FNAC, one-third always employed it and one-third employed it selectively.[17]

 Numerous series now attest to the accuracy of FNAC.[18] FNAC is particularly accurate in the diagnosis of pleomorphic adenoma,[19] and a study highlighting the features of infarction and squamoid metaplasia achieved an accuracy of up to 88% for adenolymphoma.[22]

A typical example of a cytological smear obtained by fine-needle aspiration of a pleomorphic adenoma is shown in **Fig. 8.4**.

Proponents of the technique have emphasised the pitfalls in diagnosis. In selected populations it is predictive of the histological diagnosis in neoplastic disease; however, the negative predictive value

is low and clinical suspicion remains an important factor in diagnosis. In particular a lymphocyte-predominant aspirate is highly indicative of lymphoma.[20] FNAC is useful if lymphadenopathy is suspected due to sarcoid, tuberculosis[21] and lymphoma.[20] It may assist in distinguishing a parotid lesion from other local structures such as a branchial cyst or lymph node. It can often confirm a benign neoplasm in an elderly, unfit patient for whom surgery would carry significant risk. It is essential to discriminate between a parotid lesion and a secondary deposit from a melanoma or squamous cell lesion. In the current climate of informed consent, the most useful role of FNAC may be in preoperative counselling of the patient.

Sialoendoscopy

Advances in technology have enabled the development of mini-endoscopes to view the distal portions of the ducts of the major salivary glands. There are three types of mini-endoscope: flexible, rigid and semi-rigid. The rigid endoscope provides a better image than the flexible endoscope, but its main disadvantage is the inability to negotiate sharp corners. The semi-rigid endoscope combines properties of both rigid and flexible endoscopes and also has the advantage of allowing the passage of miniaturised surgical tools. The semi-rigid endoscope is only 1 mm in diameter and can be used with two types of outer sleeve: an exploration unit (1.3 mm in diameter) and a treatment unit (2.3 mm in diameter). The latter has three channels, one for the endoscope, one that will accept a surgical device up to 1 mm in diameter, and a third that is an irrigation port. Indications for sialoendoscopy are:

- calculi in the proximal portion of the major salivary gland duct;
- screening the ductal system for residual calculi;
- to confirm evidence of ductal dilatation or stenosis seen on sialography or ultrasound scanning;
- to investigate recurrent episodes of major salivary gland swelling without obvious cause.

The sialoendoscope can be used in conjunction with an intracorporeal lithotripter for stone fragmentation and balloon dilatation to resolve strictures. It also reduces duct stenosis. In their series of 1078 salivary gland endoscopies, Nahieli et al[23]

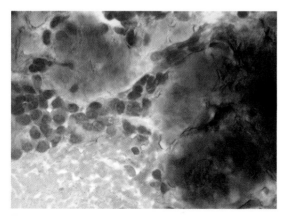

Figure 8.4 • Fine-needle aspiration cytology of a pleomorphic adenoma showing epithelial and mucinous components.

were unable to perform the technique in 4.4% of cases and failed to resolve symptoms in 4.7%. Complications following sialoendoscopy include swelling of the salivary gland, which subsides spontaneously after a few hours, and ductal stricture in 2.5% of cases.

Infections of the salivary glands

Bacterial infections

Bacteria usually reach the gland by retrograde infection from the mouth, although occasionally infection may be blood borne. The commonest causative organisms are *Staphylococcus aureus*, *Streptococcus viridans*, *Streptococcus pyogenes*, *Haemophilus influenzae*, *Escherichia coli* and *Streptococcus pneumoniae*.[24] Infection is usually unilateral and may involve intraparotid and periparotid lymph nodes. The aetiology of acute parotitis is usually due to debility and dehydration, but may be idiopathic, secondary to Sjögren's syndrome, obstruction of Stensen's duct (usually due to calculi) or a complication of septicaemia.

The clinical features are painful swelling of the side of the face in parotid disease and fever. Pus or purulent fluid may be expressed from the duct. Untreated, the condition may progress to a parotid abscess, which may subsequently extend to the upper neck or to the parapharyngeal space. The treatment of acute bacterial parotitis consists of oral hygiene, correction of dehydration and appropriate antibiotics. Signs of improvement are usually evident within 48 hours. If no improvement after this time has occurred, a parotid abscess should be suspected. CT[25] not only confirms the diagnosis but helps to plan the best site to incise and drain the abscess. If no abscess is present and fulminating parotitis is suspected, decompression of the parotid gland should be considered.[26] Recurrent subacute and chronic parotitis is more common than an acute infection and is usually due to parotid calculi (see below).

Bacterial and viral infections are much less common in the submandibular glands than in the parotid. Even primary tuberculosis of a salivary gland seems to occur less frequently in the submandibular gland compared with the parotid (27% vs. 70%).[27] The principles of diagnosis and treatment are the same as those outlined for the parotid gland.

Viral infections

The commonest viral infection of the parotid glands is mumps.[28] It can also occur in the submandibular and sublingual glands. Mumps is most reliably diagnosed during epidemics or by measuring serum antibody titres. It usually affects children between the ages of 4 and 12 years. Common manifestations of active disease include bilateral or occasionally unilateral parotid swelling, fever, chills, joint pain and myalgia. Uncommon manifestations include epididymitis, orchitis, pancreatitis, thyroiditis, meningo-encephalitis and unilateral sensorineural hearing loss. The treatment relies on isolation of the patient, adequate hydration and nutrition, and measures to relieve symptoms.

Other viruses that can cause acute viral parotitis include Coxsackie viruses, parainfluenza viruses (types 1 and 3), influenza virus type A, herpesvirus, echovirus and choriomeningitis virus.[24,29] Two large studies of human immunodeficiency virus (HIV)-positive women have concluded that xerostomia is more common in these patients, and their salivary glands may be enlarged (in 4.3%) and tender (in 6.9%). These clinical findings are positively associated with viral load.[30,31] Histologically, HIV-associated salivary gland disease is similar to Sjögren's syndrome and there is an increased risk of lymphomatous change. However, in addition large lymphoepithelial cysts may be present in HIV salivary disease.

Granulomatous and other diseases

These diseases may affect the intraparotid and extraparotid lymph nodes, and the parenchyma of the parotid gland can also be affected. The chief granulomatous diseases affecting the major salivary glands include sarcoidosis, tuberculosis, atypical mycobacterial infection, syphilis, cat-scratch fever, toxoplasmosis and actinomycosis.[27,32] In practice, not all of these diseases produce histologically recognisable granulomata.

Sarcoidosis is a systemic disease characterised by non-caseating granulomas involving many organs. Its presumed aetiology is infectious. The parotid glands are affected in 10–30% of patients and occasionally may be the only manifestation of the disease. It usually presents as a non-tender, painless, chronic enlargement of the gland, which may mimic malignancy. CT and MRI reveal multiple, benign, non-cavitating masses. The major differential diagnosis is lymphoma, although if the lesion is solitary it may be difficult to distinguish between other benign lesions. If FNAC excludes a neoplasm, incisional biopsy may be performed and will confirm the diagnosis.[32] Most cases resolve with treatment of the generalised condition.

Primary involvement of the salivary glands is rare in tuberculosis. Usually, the salivary gland disease arises from a focus in the tonsils and spreads to the salivary gland via the regional lymph nodes. FNAC is often a helpful diagnostic procedure. Treatment is with appropriate antituberculous chemotherapy, and surgery is rarely necessary.

Sjögren's syndrome

Autoimmune disease affecting the salivary glands is best considered as Sjögren's syndrome. This is a systemic disorder of the exocrine glands that occurs either alone (primary Sjögren's syndrome) or combined with other connective tissue disease (secondary Sjögren's syndrome). The diagnosis is suspected when two or more of the following clinical features are present: keratoconjunctivitis sicca, xerostomia and a connective tissue disease, which is usually rheumatoid arthritis.[33] Usually the lacrimal and salivary glands are affected but other exocrine glands can also be involved.[34]

The incidence of Sjögren's syndrome is difficult to establish, but among the autoimmune diseases it is probably second in frequency only to rheumatoid arthritis.[34] The adult form of the disease is 10 times more common than the childhood form, and children are less likely to develop the advanced features.[35] It is important to establish the diagnosis early in children because many cases may spontaneously resolve by puberty, and this knowledge may avoid unnecessary surgery.

The adult form of the disease is most common between the ages of 40 and 60 years, with a male to female ratio of 1:9. It tends to be progressive. The incidence of parotid enlargement varies from 25% to 55% of cases, and either parotid or submandibular gland enlargement occurs in 80% of all cases of Sjögren's syndrome. The risk of developing non-Hodgkin's lymphoma is greater than in normal controls and this risk is higher in primary Sjögren's syndrome. Local radiotherapy or immunosuppression may further increase this risk.

Two types of pathological appearance are evident in the salivary glands: the benign lymphoepithelial lesion, occurring primarily in the parotid glands, and focal lymphocytic sialadenitis, occurring in the other major and minor salivary glands.[36]

The diagnosis is most reliably made by labial salivary gland biopsy, and usually biopsy of the parotid gland is not required unless this is the only gland affected.[32,36] The possibility of malignant lymphoma should be considered in this subset of patients. Sialography is the most useful radiological adjunct to diagnosis, initially showing a normal central duct system and numerous peripheral punctate collections of contrast material uniformly scattered throughout the gland. Eventually, larger globular collections of contrast material may also be seen scattered uniformly throughout the gland, and MRI findings of these globular changes are diagnostic.[25]

The management of patients with Sjögren's syndrome centres on preventing irreversible damage to the teeth and eyes. Thus, attention should be paid to treating and preventing dental caries, treating oral candidiasis, stimulating the remaining salivary glands to produce more saliva and selectively using saliva substitutes.[36] Stimulation of the salivary glands may be accomplished by local gustatory stimuli, or by systemic sialagogues. Dryness of the eyes can be managed by artificial tears.

Obstructive salivary gland disease

Sialolithiasis

Stone formation in the submandibular gland is much more common than in the parotid gland. It may be primary or secondary. Stasis or slow clearance of salivary gland secretions occurs with one or more predisposing factors, including anatomical alterations in the duct, damaged duct epithelium from infection or trauma, stricture and alteration of the physicochemical composition of salivary secretions. A history of recurrent progressive glandular swelling, initially associated with meals, is common; this may be accompanied by pain and infection. The stone may occasionally be palpated along the course of the duct. Diagnosis is best made by sialography. Treatment depends on the location of the stone. If located in the distal portion of the duct, the stone may be removed via the oral cavity. If located in the proximal duct or in the hilum of the gland, the stone may be removed by removal of the gland. Multiple small stones may be dealt with by irrigation, stenting and ductoplasty.

 Advances in technology have enabled the development of minimally invasive techniques for the treatment of salivary gland stones. The techniques include intraoral surgery and similar protocols that have been adapted from experience with renal calculi, namely basket retrieval and extracorporeal shock-wave lithotripsy. The development of an extracorporeal shock-wave lithotripsy machine with a smaller shock-wave focus has reduced the need for analgesia. Complete success in stone clearance was achieved in 38.5% of patients and partial success in 45.4%. Intraoral surgery was used as primary treatment or followed attempted basket retrieval or extracorporeal shock-wave lithotripsy and was successful in 95.8% of cases.[37]

Stricture of the parotid duct

This may be caused by repeated infection, iatrogenic injury, congenital abnormality, trauma or through compression by a tumour. The clinical features are of pain and swelling of the parotid gland associated with eating. The diagnosis is established by sialography, which may also establish whether calculi are present. Distal duct or orifice stricture can now be treated by repeated duct dilatation, and surgery is seldom indicated. In patients who fail to respond, a formal stenotomy or marsupialisation of the duct orifice may be required. Duct reimplantation or excision of the gland is rarely required. Proximal duct stricture is more difficult to deal with, and alternative forms of treatment may be duct ligation (usually leading to atrophy of the gland) or, rarely, radiotherapy.

Sialectasis

This is a disease of unknown aetiology in which progressive destruction of the alveoli and parenchyma of the gland is accompanied by duct stenosis and cyst formation as the alveoli coalesce. Most patients are thought to have congenital sialectasis and in children it may mimic mumps, although mumps seldom recurs. Approximately 50% of children have no symptoms by the time they reach adulthood,

and only a small proportion require treatment.[38] The typical presentation is painful enlargement of one salivary gland after eating. The attack regresses after a few hours but is made worse by eating again. Attacks vary in frequency and are due to the main ducts being blocked by stones or epithelial debris. The diagnosis may be confirmed by sialography. Surgery to remove stones may be necessary, and occasionally the gland may require excision.

Cysts in the parotid gland

Salivary gland cysts can be divided into congenital and acquired cysts. Developmental cysts are usually unilateral, painless swellings unless infected. Lymphoepithelial cysts of the parotid are more common in females in the fifth decade. Other types are rare and include true branchial cysts and dermoid cysts in the salivary glands and congenital sialectasis. Many acquired cysts develop as a result of obstruction of the salivary duct, usually affecting the parotid. When seen in the sublingual gland the sialocyst is called a ranula. AIDS-related parotid cysts present as unilateral or bilateral painless masses. Cervical lymphadenopathy may be present, although this is less common with better medical control of HIV patients.[6] Cystic lesions may be solitary or multiple. Multiple cysts most often occur in Warthin's tumour and in HIV infection when they are associated with multiple cervical lymphadenopathy.[25]

Sialadenosis

Sialadenosis is a soft symmetrical painless swelling, usually of both parotid glands. The aetiology is neither inflammatory nor neoplastic. It is most commonly seen in alcoholism in the presence of liver damage and diabetes. It is associated with other endocrine disorders as well as malnutrition. The treatment is by management of the predisposing condition.[39]

Post-irradiation sialadenitis

This is due to irradiation of the gland as part of the planned treatment for head and neck malignancy. After 40 Gy, the gland atrophies and xerostomia results. The use of intensity-modulated radiotherapy as a parotid sparing technique reduces the likelihood of irradiation damage.

Tumours of the salivary glands

Classification and staging

There have been a variety of classifications of salivary gland tumours but the most widely used is the World Health Organisation's (WHO) classification. This has been comprehensively reviewed[40] (Table 8.1). The TNM staging of salivary gland tumours is illustrated in Table 8.2.

Aetiology

The strongest evidence implicating high-dose ionising radiation in the development of salivary gland tumours has been provided by studies of the survivors of the atomic bombs in Hiroshima and Nagasaki in 1945. The most recent study, which had a follow-up of 37 years, confirmed an increased incidence of benign and malignant neoplasms of the salivary glands. This was especially so for Warthin's tumour and mucoepidermoid carcinoma.[41] Therapeutic head and neck radiation, ultraviolet radiation and iodine-131 therapy have also been implicated.[42,43]

A recent review of salivary gland tumours[40] commented that several viruses have been implicated in the aetiology of salivary gland tumours, including Epstein–Barr virus HPV 16 and 18, polyomavirus and HIV type 1 infection. An increased risk of salivary gland tumours has also been found with second primary breast cancers. Only Warthin's tumour seems to be commoner in smokers (see 'Warthin's tumour' below). A wide variety of occupational exposures have been linked with the development of salivary gland neoplasms, including rubber manufacturing, nickel and asbestos.[40]

Table 8.1 • WHO histological classification of tumours of the salivary glands

Malignant epithelial tumours		Benign epithelial tumours	
Acinic cell carcinoma	8550/3	Pleomorphic adenoma	8940/0
Mucoepidermoid carcinoma	8430/3	Myoepithelioma	8982/0
Adenoid cystic carcinoma	8200/3	Basal cell adenoma	8147/0
Polymorphous low-grade adenocarcinoma	8525/3	Warthin's tumour	8561/0
Epithelial–myoepithelial carcinoma	8562/3	Oncocytoma	8290/0
Clear cell carcinoma, not otherwise specified	8310/3	Canalicular adenoma	8149/0
Basal cell adenocarcinoma	8147/3	Sebaceous adenoma	8410/0
Sebaceous carcinoma	8410/3	Lymphadenoma	
Sebaceous lymphadenocarcinoma	8410/3	Sebaceous	8410/0
Cystadenocarcinoma	8440/3	Non-sebaceous	8410/0
Low-grade cribriform cystadenocarcinoma		Ductal papillomas	
Mucinous adenocarcinoma	8480/3	Inverted ductal papilloma	8503/0
Oncocytic carcinoma	8290/3	Intraductal papilloma	8503/0
Salivary duct carcinoma	8500/3	Sialadenoma papilliferum	8406/0
Adenocarcinoma, not otherwise specified	8140/3	Cystadenoma	8440/0
Myoepithelial carcinoma	8982/3		
Carcinoma ex-pleomorphic adenoma	8941/3	**Soft tissue tumours**	
Carcinosarcoma	8980/3	Haemangioma	9120/0
Metastasising pleomorphic adenoma	8940/1	**Haematolymphoid tumours**	
Squamous cell carcinoma	8070/3	Hodgkin's lymphoma	
Small cell carcinoma	8041/3	Diffuse large B-cell lymphoma	9680/3
Large cell carcinoma	8012/3	Extranodal marginal zone	9699/3
Lymphoepithelial carcinoma	8082/3	B-cell lymphoma	
Sialoblastoma	8974/l	**Secondary tumours**	

Morphology code of the International Classification of Diseases for Oncology (ICD-O) {821} and the Systematised Nomenclature of Medicine (http://snomed.org). Behaviour is coded /0 for benign tumours, /3 for malignant tumours and /1 for borderline or uncertain behaviour.

Table 8.2 • TNM classification of carcinomas of the salivary glands

TNM classification[*][†]	
T	Primary tumour
TX	Primary tumour cannot be assessed
T0	No evidence of primary tumour
T1	Tumour 2 cm or less in greatest dimension without extraparenchymal extension[‡]
T2	Tumour more than 2 cm but not more than 4 cm in greatest dimension without extraparenchymal extension
T3	Tumour more than 4 cm and/or tumour with extraparenchymal extension[‡]
T4a	Tumour invades skin, mandible, ear canal or facial nerve
T4b	Tumour invades base of skull, pterygoid plates or encases carotid artery
N	Regional lymph nodes[§]
NX	Regional lymph nodes cannot be assessed
N0	No regional lymph node metastasis
N1	Metastasis in a single ipsilateral lymph node, 3 cm or less in greatest dimension
N2	Metastasis as specified in N2a, N2b, N2c below
N2a	Metastasis in a single ipsilateral lymph node, more than 3 cm but not more than 6 cm in greatest dimension
N2b	Metastasis in multiple ipsilateral lymph nodes, none more than 6 cm in greatest dimension
N2c	Metastasis in bilateral or contralateral lymph nodes, none more than 6 cm in greatest dimension
N3	Metastasis in a lymph node more than 6 cm in greatest dimension
M	Distant metastasis
MX	Distant metastasis cannot be assessed
M0	No distant metastasis
M1	Distant metastasis

Stage grouping			
Stage I	T1	N0	M0
Stage II	T2	N0	M0
Stage III	T3	N0	M0
	T1, T2, T3	N1	M0
Stage IV A	T1, T2, T13	N2	M0
	T4a	N0, N1, N2	M0
Stage IV B	T4b	Any N	M0
	Any T	N3	M0
Stage IV C	Any T	Any N	M1

[*] (947, 2418).

[†] A help desk for specific questions about the TNM classification is available at http://uicc.org/index.php?id=508.

[‡] Extraparenchymal extension is clinical or macroscopic evidence of invasion of soft tissues or nerve, except those listed under T4a and T4b. Microscopic evidence alone does not constitute extraparenchymal extension for classification purposes.

[§] The regional lymph nodes are cervical nodes. Midline nodes are considered ipsilateral nodes.

Molecular biology of salivary gland tumours

A variety of chromosomal and molecular changes have been described in benign and malignant tumours that may help to identify markers, which in turn assist in diagnosis, prognosis and management. However, there are still few data on the genetic mechanisms responsible for the development of salivary gland tumours.

 Some of the more consistent findings have been summarised by Cheuk and Chan in a recent comprehensive review.[44] They drew attention to evidence for specific chromosomal translocations involving *PLAG1* or *HMGA2* gene in pleomorphic adenomas and fusion of *MECT1–MAML2* genes in mucoepidermoid carcinomas. A variety of new pathological entities were documented. In regard to prognosis the Ki67 index is considered an important imunohistochemical marker. Poor survival in mucoepidermoid carcinoma, adenoid cystic carcinoma and acinic cell carcinoma are associated with a high Ki67 index. On the contrary, altered *p53* expression is not convincingly associated with survival. Reduced expression or overexpression of NM23 protein is correlated with tumour metastasis. In particular nuclear expression of NM23 in salivary gland tumours is used to predict metastases. The membrane-bound mucin MUC1 expression is of importance in mucoepidermoid carcinomas predicting high-grade as well as high rates of recurrence and metastasis. In contrast, MUC4 is a marker of low-grade, low-recurrence tumours. The marker CD43 may be useful in identifying adenoid cystic carcinomas. Loss of heterozygosity, amplification and overexpression of genes in chromosome 12q may be important and a possible role in transformation for *p53* has been cited. Immunopositivity for *c-erbB2* may identify carcinoma ex-pleomorphic adenoma. The putative mechanisms for dedifferentiation include *p53* mutation, increased cyclin D1 expression and *c-erbB2* overexpression.

Lalami et al[45] reviewed possible candidate genes associated with salivary gland tumours, including *p53*, *p21*, *myc* and vascular endothelial growth factor (VEGF); they also commented on the role of epigenetic events which may be important in salivary gland carcinogenesis such as the methylation status of RB1. While identification of these mechanisms may offer a therapeutic approach at a molecular level, these techniques remain under development.

Benign epithelial parotid neoplasms

Pleomorphic adenoma

This is the most common salivary gland tumour, accounting for 60% of all salivary gland tumours and approximately 80% of parotid tumours, and so called because of its mixed epithelial and mesenchymal elements. A study has suggested that epithelial–mesenchymal transition occurs within this tumour.[46]

 The annual incidence of parotid pleomorphic adenoma in the UK is approximately 1.4 per 100 000 people.[47,48] The peak age of incidence is in the fifth decade, and women are more commonly affected than men. The commonest site within the parotid gland is in the tail,[5,47] with most tumours lying superficial to the facial nerve.

The history is usually that of a slowly growing painless mass in the parotid, and pain and facial palsy are rare. The latter should prompt consideration of a malignant lesion. Fortunately, malignant transformation of a previously benign pleomorphic adenoma is rare.[47]

The diagnosis is primarily clinical, and it has been argued that radiological and cytological investigations are unnecessary,[17,47] although FNAC is useful in distinguishing between benign and malignant neoplasms and in determining pleomorphic adenoma from Warthin's tumour.[22] Radiological confirmation of a truly single lesion may be accomplished using ultrasonography or MRI and may show the depth of the neoplasm. The value of this is in preoperative counselling of the patient in the likelihood of a neuropraxia. Treatment is usually by some form of superficial or total conservative parotidectomy, with identification of the facial nerve during surgery (see 'Surgery of the parotid gland' below). An example of an excised parotid tumour is shown in **Fig. 8.5**.

Pleomorphic adenoma recurs locally, and the reasons for this have been hotly debated. When the

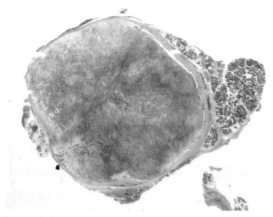

Figure 8.5 • Pathological specimen showing the cut surface of a pleomorphic adenoma of the parotid gland.

surgical management in the early 20th century was local excision (for fear of damaging the facial nerve), local recurrence was of the order of 20–45%.[47] By the 1940s, superficial parotidectomy with dissection of the facial nerve was being advocated, and this reduced local recurrence. In 1957, Patey and Thackray demonstrated that small tumour buds protrude from the tumour surface into the surrounding tumour capsule.[49] This came to be accepted as the cause for local recurrence but was disproved by Nicholson and Gleave, who practised the technique of 'extracapsular dissection' for 45 years with results that were equally as good as those for superficial parotidectomy.[50] It is therefore clear that the main factor regarding recurrence was incomplete surgical excision, and the same group confirmed a recurrence rate of only 1.6% after a median follow-up of 12.5 years. This low rate of local recurrence has also been achieved by other groups.[51] This also explains the paradox that preserving the facial nerve did not increase the risk of tumour recurrence despite the observation that, in 50% of patients, a branch of the nerve was in direct contact with the tumour capsule.[47] Other factors said to contribute to local recurrence are young age at presentation[52] and inadequate surgical margins.[53,54] Rupture of the capsule as a cause of local recurrence has recently been disputed. Tumour spillage due to simple rupture of the capsule is associated with a recurrence rate of 8% and it has been argued that radiotherapy in such patients is unhelpful.[54]

Most pleomorphic adenomas are probably best treated by superficial parotidectomy with identification and preservation of the facial nerve. However,

the case for capsular surgery for benign parotid disease has been advocated as having similar results to superficial parotidectomy in respect of recurrence with less surgical morbidity.[55]

 The authors analysed 821 patients with parotid tumours classified as clinically 'simple' if they were discrete, mobile and <4 cm. Outcomes for these clinically benign tumours (662) were examined for those patients who underwent superficial parotidectomy (159) and those who had extracapsular dissection (503). Five percent of these lesions proved to be malignant histologically. Cancer-specific survival and recurrence rates were similar; however, morbidity was less in the extracapsular dissection group.[55]

A review of retrospective studies of pathological specimens of parotid pleomorphic adenomas were correlated to outcomes to compare three surgical techniques, partial superficial parotidectomy, total parotidectomy and extracapsular dissection.[56]

 The author concluded that for smaller (<4 cm) pleomorphic adenomas, the surgical technique does not alter the outcome in terms of capsular exposure, capsular rupture recurrence, tumour–facial nerve interface and facial nerve dysfunction. Dissecting pleomorphic adenoma from the facial nerve results in cases with positive margins due to incomplete capsule resection or perforating pseudopodia, and it was concluded that minimal margin parotid surgery with extracapsular dissection should be discouraged. However, if larger amounts of parotid tissue are removed then the risk of transient facial nerve dysfunction and Frey's syndrome are increased.[56]

Whichever surgical technique is used the most important determinant of success in removing the tumour with minimal adverse affect is careful dissection.

Warthin's tumour

It is apparent that its incidence has been increasing since its description, and it may now constitute 18% of all salivary gland neoplasms and up to 33% of all parotid neoplasms.[57,58] The highest incidence of tumours confined almost entirely to the parotid gland occurs in the sixth and seventh decades, with a male:female ratio of 1.6:1.[58] Smoking has been noted to be a strong aetiological factor and may explain the increasing incidence of this tumour and the change in its sex distribution over the past 70 years.[58,59]

Clinically, this tumour presents as an ovoid, smooth lump containing cystic spaces filled with fluid and lined by papillary epithelium set in a lymphoid stroma. The epithelium develops from parotid duct cells as a result of metaplasia, forming two layers. Lining the cysts, the inner layer of epithelium is formed largely by tall columnar cells called oncocytes, whereas the basal layer of epithelium is formed by small, elongated irregular cells containing oval vesicular nuclei.[58] The most satisfactory explanation for the inclusion of lymphoid stroma lies in the embryological development of the parotid gland and that the tumour is due to a cellular response to the epithelium by the included residual lymphatic tissue. Cigarette smoking is a risk factor for Warthin's tumour. Irritants in smoke may cause metaplasia. Radiation exposure may have an aetological role and autoimmune diseases are more common in people with Warthin's tumour.[60] In up to 10% of patients, the lesions are multiple and occasionally bilateral, either synchronously or asynchronously.

Preoperative diagnosis has recently been improved by attention to specific cytological features of squamoid metaplasia and infarction.[17] Ultrasonography allows the detection of previously unsuspected multiple lesions within the same gland and occasionally identifies occult contralateral lesions. A correct preoperative diagnosis allows the correct surgical procedure to be planned. Because these tumours are benign and do not recur locally, a conservative surgical approach to their excision has been advocated in the form of 'controlled enucleation'.[58,61] This allowed a reduction in temporary facial neuropraxia from 43% for superficial parotidectomy to 8% for controlled enucleation.[58] This procedure is unsuitable for multiple lesions and identification of the facial nerve is then required, especially for lesions in the deep portion of the gland.

Other benign tumours of the salivary glands

Other benign salivary gland tumours are rare. Cystadenomas are characterised by multicystic growth in which epithelial elements demonstrate adenomatous proliferation. The majority of these tumours are found in the minor salivary glands.[62] Oncocytoma usually affects elderly people and may originate in the salivary glands. It presents as a slow-growing painless lump that is well circumscribed

and soft. It most commonly affects the parotid. Histologically, this tumour is characterised by epithelial cells with eosinophilic cytoplasm.[63] Treatment of adenomas should ensure a complete excision.

Malignant epithelial parotid neoplasms

Tumours of variable malignancy
Mucoepidermoid tumours

This is the most common salivary gland malignancy. It is usually a firm, fixed and painless swelling, most commonly in the parotid. Most patients have a good outcome. Survival is related to histological grade, with poorer survival among people with high-grade tumours in the parotid but not in submandibular glands.[64]

The age range of presentation is wide and these tumours may even occur in childhood, although the peak incidence lies in the fourth decade. The sex distribution is equal. These tumours may also be subdivided according to grade, which has a bearing on survival.[65–67] Thus, if all grades of tumour are included, mortality may be as low as 8.7%.[65] Spiro has shown that the overall survival of 434 patients with mucoepidermoid tumours was of the order of 70%.[66] For intermediate- and high-grade tumours, survival may fall to as little as 22.5%.[67]

Acinic cell tumour

This accounts for approximately 2% of all parotid tumours; it may be bilateral in 3% of patients. It is uncommon outside the parotid gland. It occurs in childhood, but its peak age of incidence is in the fifth decade. It may also occur in intraparotid lymph nodes. Although its biological behaviour is variable, in general it has a better prognosis than mucoepidermoid tumours, and survival over 20 years has been reported to be between 75% and 84%.[65,66] Approximately 10% metastasise.

Carcinomas of the parotid gland
Adenoid cystic carcinoma

This histological type of cancer accounts for only 10% of salivary neoplasms. Only about 20% arise within the parotid, and they form only 2% of all parotid tumours.[68] The median age of presentation for patients with tumours arising in the parotid gland is 43 years, 10 years younger than for patients whose tumours arise in other salivary glands.[68]

Histologically, these tumours contain round or oval cells forming strands or clusters in a myxomatous connective tissue matrix. The islands or strands of tumour cells interconnect to enclose characteristic cystic spaces, presenting a cribriform, cylindromatous pattern of growth. Classification into three grades is feasible but has not been found to be clinically useful.[69,70]

This tumour has a predilection for neural spread, and this may account for the high proportion of patients (18%) who present with some degree of facial weakness. The incidence of lymph node spread is relatively low (6–10%)[68,69] and the incidence of distant metastases is high (40%).[70]

Survival from adenoid cystic carcinoma tends to be better for parotid sites compared with other salivary gland sites, with 5- and 10-year survival of the order of 42% and 25% respectively. Local recurrence seems to be improved with the addition of postoperative radiotherapy but overall survival is apparently unaffected.[68]

The most important factor influencing survival seems to be stage at presentation,[68,70] and the previously reported finding that grade of tumour is an important determinant of survival of adenoid cystic carcinoma[71] has not been confirmed by later studies.[68,70]

Carcinoma ex-pleomorphic adenoma

This is sometimes described as a malignant mixed parotid tumour,[69] because the histological features show some characteristics of a benign mixed tumour (pleomorphic adenoma) with other areas containing carcinoma cells. These tumours comprise 18% of parotid cancers[69] and may arise as either malignant transformation in a long-standing pleomorphic adenoma (occurring in 10% after 15 years) or as a carcinoma arising in a mixed cell tumour. Lymph node metastases occur in approximately 20% of patients, and survival at 5 and 10 years has been reported to be 63% and 39% respectively.[69]

Adenocarcinoma

This comprises 10% of malignant tumours of the parotid and approximately 3% of all salivary gland tumours. The sex incidence is equal and this tumour occasionally occurs in children. The histological pattern varies from trabecular to tubular, solid, papillary or mucus-secreting varieties without epidermoid differentiation. They may be low, intermediate or high grade and this, along with stage at presentation, influences survival, which may be as low as 19% at 10 years with high-grade lesions.[69]

Squamous cell carcinoma

This is rare, occurring in only 3% of malignant parotid tumours, and is characterised by exhibiting epidermoid or squamous differentiation. It may be difficult to differentiate from squamous cell carcinoma arising in other sites.[69] It is an aggressive tumour, presenting clinically with pain, skin fixation, ulceration, facial nerve palsy and metastatic spread to lymph nodes in 50% of patients.[69] Survival is poor and depends on grade of tumour and stage at presentation.

Undifferentiated (anaplastic) carcinoma

This is a rare tumour, invariably of high grade and with a poor prognosis.

Benign non-epithelial parotid neoplasms

Within the parotid gland, these tumours are rare. **Haemangiomas** of the parotid may present as soft swellings usually in the first two decades, involving the parotid from a primary site nearby, such as the skin overlying the gland or the infratemporal fossa. Some tumours may spontaneously regress, and treatment by embolisation is preferable to surgery.[72] **Lipomas** usually lie lateral to the parotid gland and are unilateral. They need to be distinguished from fatty infiltration of the parotid, which is usually bilateral. There are three types of **lymphangiomas**: simple lymphangioma, cavernous lymphangioma and cystic hygroma. Cavernous lymphangiomas and cystic hygromas are prone to recur after excision because they are almost impossible to remove completely.

Lymphomas of the salivary glands

Hodgkin's lymphoma and non-Hodgkin's lymphoma are rare in salivary glands. Extranodal marginal zone B-cell lymphoma (EMZBCL) arises in mucosa-associated lymphoid tissue (MALT) lymphomas, which histologically exhibit centrocyte-like cell proliferation surrounding B-cell-reactive follicles. These tumours may develop in patients with Sjögren's syndrome.

Submandibular gland tumours

Submandibular gland tumours are classified as illustrated in Table 8.1, and according to the TNM classification as used for parotid tumours (Table 8.2). It should be emphasised that tumours of the submandibular gland are uncommon. They comprise 4–8% of all salivary tumours; also, 57–66% of all submandibular neoplasms are benign.[48,65,66] The commonest tumour is a pleomorphic adenoma. Diagnosis is confirmed by FNAC. Imaging of the gland with ultrasonography and MRI may be useful if malignancy is suspected due to local fixity, especially to the mandible.

Management of patients with a parotid neoplasm

Since most benign tumours occur in the superficial lobe of the parotid, the standard operation since the 1950s has been superficial parotidectomy with dissection and preservation of the facial nerve. This is also true for low-grade parotid carcinomas such as the mucoepidermoid tumours and acinic cell tumours, which uncommonly present with lymph node metastases.[47] Total conservative parotidectomy (with facial nerve preservation) may be indicated for these tumours depending on the size of the tumour and its position within the parotid gland, especially if located in the deep lobe. The aim of the surgery is to achieve a clear margin of excision around the tumour to minimise the risk of local recurrence. A variation on this procedure is subtotal parotidectomy, which has been described as a conservative resection of the superficial lobe with less than a full facial nerve dissection.[74] The merit of this procedure is that for benign and low-grade malignant lesions, surgical clearance is achieved with fewer postoperative complications, especially that of facial nerve paresis.

Postoperative radiotherapy may be given after excision of a low-grade carcinoma if the surgical margin is involved by tumour,[47] but its use after surgery for pleomorphic adenoma is controversial.[75] Postoperative radiotherapy may have a place in the management of patients with recurrent pleomorphic adenoma, especially in patients in whom recurrences are multinodular. In this situation, the addition of postoperative radiotherapy is associated with a significantly improved rate of local control.[52]

The treatment of Warthin's tumour has hitherto also been by superficial parotidectomy, but increasingly some authorities have advocated an even more conservative approach and have recommended enucleation.[59,61] The rationale for this approach has been the zero recurrence rate after complete excision and the greatly reduced incidence of facial nerve paresis compared with superficial parotidectomy (8% vs. 43% respectively).[58]

The management of patients with overtly malignant tumours is primarily surgical, the extent of surgery depending on the stage at presentation. Facial nerve paresis and clinically detectable lymphadenopathy both occur in approximately 20% of patients,[66,68,69] and careful clinical staging is essential. An accurate preoperative diagnosis using either FNAC or even a Tru-cut biopsy is desirable.[76] Imaging of the head and neck, as well as the chest, with CT scanning has been advocated,[76] although MRI is probably better for evaluating the primary tumour.[25] This allows better visualisation of the tumour – notably any deep-lobe extension – and may identify fixity to surrounding structures. It is also useful in identifying clinically occult lymph node metastases. Finally, MRI allows for better preoperative counselling of the patient, especially if the extent of the surgery is likely to sacrifice the facial nerve or if immediate reconstructive surgery is contemplated. While the need for a cervical lymph node dissection is clear if positive nodes are present, prophylactic cervical lymph node dissection remains controversial.[77] Indicators of increased risk include high histological grade and large tumour size. Postoperative radiotherapy may be required, and an oncologist should be involved early in the management of these patients.

Surgery of the parotid gland

A classification of approaches to parotidectomy has been proposed. These are a formal parotidectomy, which may be either superficial or total, a limited parotidectomy, which can be either a partial superficial lobectomy or a deep lobe resection, or an extracapsular dissection.[78]

For any of these procedures informed consent should describe the risk to the facial nerve including temporary or permanent weakness, as well as numbness of the pinna and cheek skin and the possibility of Frey's syndrome.

Chapter 8

Superficial parotidectomy

Superficial conservative parotidectomy is indicated for benign tumours and low-grade malignant tumours confined to the superficial lobe of the parotid.

The patient is positioned in the supine position with the neck slightly extended and the head turned away from the surgeon. The table is inclined in a slightly head-up position to reduce venous congestion, and a small swab can be placed in the external auditory canal to protect the tympanic membrane. The towels are arranged so that the ipsilateral eye and corner of the mouth can be viewed when necessary during stimulation of the facial nerve.

The incision begins near the top of the pinna in the preauricular crease, runs inferiorly until the point at which the ear lobe joins the face, and then sweeps posteriorly and upwards beneath and behind the ear lobe. The incision is then extended inferiorly along a suitable skin crease. The incision is then deepened into the underlying fat and the anterior skin flap is mobilised superficial to the parotid gland as far as its anterior border. The skin flap and the ear lobe may then be retracted out of the operative field with sutures. The great auricular nerve is identified lying on the deep cervical fascia investing the sternomastoid muscle. The sternomastoid muscle is separated from the posterior border of the parotid gland. The posterior border of the parotid gland is then separated from the mastoid process and the cartilaginous external meatus, opening up a sulcus between the parotid gland and these structures, which is extended inferiorly between the gland and the sternomastoid muscle. This sulcus can be further deepened to expose the posterior belly of the digastric muscle, which is then followed upwards to a point where it dips beneath the mastoid process. The stylomastoid foramen is just anterior to the insertion of digastric. A number of methods have been described to identify the facial nerve:

- The tympanomastoid groove between the bony external auditory meatus and the mastoid process leads to the main trunk of the facial nerve.
- Exposing the tragal cartilage to its pointed tip, the main trunk lies just deep and medial to the tip.
- Identification of peripheral branches of the nerve can be identified at the anterior margin of the gland and traced back (described below).

The sulcus between the posterior border of the parotid and the external meatus and mastoid process is deepened by carefully dividing the fibrous septa bridging it, and the main trunk of the facial nerve is identified. Identification of the facial nerve can be facilitated by the use of a nerve stimulator but, even so, great caution must be maintained during this and the subsequent dissection. The nerve has a characteristic appearance and usually has a tiny blood vessel on its surface. The parotid gland is then retracted forwards, and the plane between the nerve and the superficial lobe is dissected forwards until the bifurcation of the nerve is identified. A haemostat is now slid over the nerve and the blades opened. Glandular tissue overlying the posterior blade is divided with scissors to divide the posterior border of the gland. Keeping the superficial lobe retracted, the plane between the nerve and the superficial lobe is gently dissected so as to eventually identify all the branches of the nerve. It is important to remember that the smaller branches of the facial nerve become more superficial as the dissection proceeds distally, and care is needed to ensure that none of the peripheral branches of the nerve are damaged as the superficial lobe is dissected away from the nerve. The superficial lobe can then be mobilised sufficiently to allow it to be pedicled anteriorly and the superficial lobe eventually severed. Small bleeding vessels may be tied off with a fine absorbable suture. It is usual to see the retromandibular vein lying vertically deep to the branches of the facial nerve and emerging from the tail of the remaining gland just posterior to the mandibular branch. If the vein is divided, care must be taken to avoid damage to branches of the nerve with vascular clamps.

A small suction drain is used to drain the cavity and the skin is sutured with a subcuticular absorbable suture. The drain may be removed on the first postoperative day and the patient discharged.

Total conservative parotidectomy

Total conservative parotidectomy is indicated for neoplasms arising in the deep lobe of the gland. The operation involves removal of the superficial and deep lobes of the gland, with preservation of the facial nerve. A superficial parotidectomy is first performed. The branches and main trunk of the facial nerve are dissected off the underlying deep lobe using small scissors to divide the fascial attachments of the nerve to the underlying gland. This manoeuvre is facilitated by lifting the branches with a nerve hook. The deep lobe is separated with scissors from the posterior border of the ascending ramus of the mandible and from the temporomandibular joint. The deep aspect of the gland is gently separated from its underlying bed with small scissors, which are introduced above and below the main trunk of the nerve. Any attachments of the gland to the styloid process are divided. The upper and lower ends of the retromandibular vein and any anterior branches are divided between ligatures. The more deeply placed external carotid artery may not have to be interrupted if it does not actually penetrate the gland but lies deep to it. However, it often perforates the deep lobe, and that portion may have to be excised with the specimen. If so, the artery is divided at the lower border of the gland above the posterior belly of digastric and stylohyoid muscles and superiorly where it becomes the superficial temporal artery. The internal maxillary and transverse facial branches of the external carotid artery are then also divided, enabling the deep lobe to be dissected off its bed in a downward direction. The wound is closed as described for superficial parotidectomy.

Retrograde parotidectomy

Although the antegrade approach has been described for identification of the facial nerve thus far, the retrograde approach is also of value. The retrograde technique can be quicker, reduces blood loss and removes less normal parotid tissue than the antegrade approach. The skin flap is raised to the anterior superior and inferior borders of the gland superficial to the periparotid fascia. The buccal branch is identified first by its consistent relationship to the parotid duct. The zygomatic branches are identified below the zygomatic arch. The marginal branch has the least consistent position but can be identified by tracing the posterior facial vein superiorly; the marginal branch crosses the vein. Each branch is dissected by tunnelling superficial to the nerve until the bifurcation of the main trunk is revealed. The posterior border of the gland is mobilised as described previously. This technique has several advantages, in particular when the tumour is large and the main trunk of the facial nerve is displaced by tumour and difficult to locate in the restricted preauricular area.[79]

Partial superficial parotidectomy

This operation is designed for small tumours of the superficial lobe. The limit of the superficial parotid surgery is determined once adequate margins are obtained around the tumour. In this case the tumour is removed without sacrificing more of the normal gland than is necessary. Limited superficial parotidectomy implies a conventional surgical approach with identification of the facial nerve using either retrograde or antegrade surgical dissection depending on the position of the tumour, rather than a simple tumour enucleation or extracapsular dissection.[74]

In a recent series of 363 limited superficial parotidectomies for benign parotid tumours, very low rates of morbidity and recurrence were reported; thus, complete superficial parotidectomy is not required for benign localised tumours of the parotid.[80]

Extended parotidectomy

Large tumours can extend between the posterior border of the mandible and the stylomandibular ligament into the parapharyngeal space, or pass posterior to the stylomandibular ligament. These tumours make access more difficult; however, the technique requires a superficial parotidectomy to be completed initially to expose and protect the facial nerve. The trunk and the main divisions of the nerve are retracted superiorly with a nerve hook. It may be possible to dissect the deep part free of the soft tissue easily. If there is insufficient space to mobilise the tumour, then division of the stylomandibular ligament allows the mandible to be displaced anteriorly, improving access. For larger tumours a mandibular osteotomy may be required. This can be achieved using an inverted 'L'-shaped osteotomy of the mandibular ramus to preserve the inferior alveolar nerve. The masseter muscle overlying the ramus is elevated to reveal the ascending ramus. Prior to the osteotomy cuts being made, mini-plates are placed over the site of the cuts to ensure accurate relocation of the mandibular fragments. The cuts are made above and behind the lingula. The fragments can now be displaced to allow access to the deep lobe.

Radical parotidectomy

If the tumour is known to be malignant and invading adjacent structures including the facial nerve, then a radical parotidectomy may be carried out. In some patients, radical parotidectomy may be accompanied by a neck dissection to remove regional lymph nodes also involved by tumour. An incision similar to that described for superficial parotidectomy is performed. This may need to be extended inferiorly to accommodate a neck dissection. The following description applies to the parotid gland and does not take into account neck dissection in continuity.

The posterior limits of the dissection are defined in the same way as for superficial parotidectomy, thus dissecting the posterior border free from the sternomastoid muscle to expose the posterior belly of the digastric muscle. The gland is freed superiorly from the mastoid process and external auditory meatus. The retromandibular vein is then ligated and divided at the tail of the parotid. The parotid gland is then elevated to reveal the posterior belly of the digastric and the stylohyoid muscles, and the external carotid artery is ligated and divided just before it enters the deep aspect of the gland above the stylohyoid muscle. The soft tissues at the tail of the parotid gland are further incised in a forward direction until the angle of the mandible is reached. Starting at the lower border of the mandible and dissecting upwards along a vertical line anterior to the parotid gland, the soft tissues overlying the ascending ramus are divided down to bone as far as the zygomatic arch. The structures divided during this dissection include subcutaneous fat, branches of the facial nerve, the transverse facial artery and veins, the parotid duct and the masseter muscle. The cut peripheral branches of the facial nerve may be tagged with a suture for ease of identification if a nerve graft is considered.

The ascending ramus of the mandible may be included in the resection if indicated, otherwise a periosteal elevator is used to push the soft tissues of the specimen backwards to the posterior border of the ascending ramus of the mandible. The soft tissues overlying the zygomatic arch are incised down to the bone as far back as the pinna. Branches of the upper division of the facial nerve are divided during this step and may also be tagged with a suture. The superficial temporal artery and vein are divided at the point where they cross the arch. The incision is now carried inferiorly between the parotid gland and the cartilage of the external auditory meatus to join the earlier line of separation of the posterior border of the parotid gland.

By retracting the tail of the specimen superiorly, the gland is dissected away from its bed with scissors, starting from below and working upwards. It is separated from the posterior border of the mandible, the styloid process and the anterior aspect of the bony external meatus. The facial nerve is divided as it emerges from the stylomastoid foramen and samples sent for frozen section. The specimen can now be retracted downwards and laterally sufficiently to expose the maxillary artery and veins so that they can be divided between ligatures or clamps. A nerve graft consisting of branches of the cervical plexus

derived from a common stem can now be inserted between the divided trunk and branches of the facial nerve and sutured in place. The wound is closed as described for superficial parotidectomy.

Locally advanced tumours may require resection of adjacent tissues such as muscle, bone or overlying skin and this will require soft tissue reconstruction, for example with a radial forearm free flap. Primary reconstruction of the facial nerve is possible and gives the best functional result. The cervical plexus branches can be used as interposition nerve grafts and microscopic epineural repair can be performed. In younger patients good functional outcomes can be achieved, whereas older patients frequently require further surgical procedures for eye rehabilitation.[81]

Postoperative complications

Facial nerve injury

After superficial parotidectomy, permanent nerve injury occurs in only 1% of patients.[50] Transient nerve paresis occurs much more commonly, in 30–43%.[50,58] After total conservative parotidectomy, permanent and transient nerve paresis increase to 6% and 60% respectively,[52] and 90% of transient injuries recover within 12 months.[47] Clearly, more limited resection of the parotid gland is associated with a marked reduction of transient facial paresis to approximately 8%.[58]

Several techniques have been described to repair a divided facial nerve and consist of faciohypoglossal transposition, end-to-end anastomosis and cable graft anastomosis. The comparison of the results of such surgery has been facilitated by the development of facial function scoring systems such as the House–Brackmann scale. Results of these techniques indicate an improvement in facial function.[81]

Frey's syndrome

This consists of discomfort, sweating and occasionally redness of the skin overlying the parotid area, which occurs during and after eating. It is due to the severed ends of the parasympathetic secretomotor fibres growing into the skin; the fibres are then stimulated by eating, causing vasodilatation and sweating. It may occur in up to 100% of patients postoperatively, but only 40% of patients will comment if questioned and 10% actually complain about it.[82] The frequency with which it occurs varies with the extent of resection of the parotid gland.[50,51] The condition usually resolves spontaneously but if persistent it may be treated by tympanic neurectomy, which divides the parasympathetic pathway. Topical anticholinergic medications such as glycopyrrolate roll-on lotion or cream have been found to be effective in controlling gustatory in the short term.[82] Intracutaneous injection of botulinum toxin A is effective treatment lasting more than 6 months and can be repeated. A minimal parotid dissection and a thick skin flap help to reduce the incidence of Frey's syndrome, as do interpositional barriers including temperoparietal fascial flaps and sternomastoid flaps.[82]

Salivary fistula

This is uncommon and due to the excessive production of saliva from the remaining deep lobe after superficial parotidectomy. In most patients it resolves spontaneously after a few weeks, but if it does persist, the deep lobe of the gland may be removed; an alternative to this is to irradiate the remaining parotid gland. The use of a fascial flap has been advocated to prevent this complication.[83]

Hypoaesthesia of the ear lobe

It is common for patients to experience some hypoaesthesia of the preauricular region and the lower half of the pinna due to division of the posterior branch of the great auricular nerve. This usually improves with time and does not require any specific treatment.

Neuroma

Occasionally a neuroma may arise from the cut end of the posterior branch of the great auricular nerve. This complication should be borne in mind before concluding that the swelling is a recurrence of a parotid tumour.

Surgery of the submandibular gland

Removal of duct calculus

This may be performed under general or local anaesthesia if the stone is near the duct orifice. The tissues immediately behind the stone are grasped with tissue forceps, which steadies the stone, elevates it and prevents inadvertent dislocation proximally down the duct. An incision in the floor of the mouth is made on to the stone in the long axis of the duct and the stone retrieved. Haemostasis is achieved if necessary and the wound can be left unsutured.

Excision of the submandibular gland

The most common indication for excision of the submandibular gland is recurrent swelling and pain due to stones in the gland or in the proximal portion of Wharton's duct (**Fig. 8.6**). Other indications are after chronic sialadenitis. Neoplasia is an absolute indication for excision and may need to be combined with a neck dissection for malignant disease. Consent for patients undergoing submandibular gland excision should include risk of damage to the mandibular branch of the facial nerve and also the potential risk to the hypoglossal and lingual nerves.

The patient is positioned in the supine position, with a small sandbag under the shoulders and the head turned in the opposite direction. A horizontal skin incision is made well below the mandible, preferably in a skin crease just above the hyoid bone to avoid the lowest branch of the facial nerve. The incision should overlap the sternomastoid posteriorly and extend to just beyond the limit of the gland anteriorly. The incision is deepened through the fat and platysma to the level of the deep cervical fascia, which is then incised along the anterior border of the sternomastoid and horizontally above the hyoid bone to expose the fascial condensation around the gland. This is incised horizontally at the lower border of the gland.

The upper flap, consisting of skin, subcutaneous fat, platysma, deep cervical fascia and the fascial

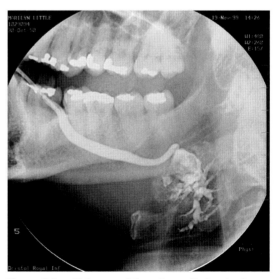

Figure 8.6 • Sialogram of the submandibular gland showing calculus obstruction.

capsule superficial to the gland, is now elevated by sharp dissection. The dissection proceeds from below and continues upwards and the tissues are retracted. The common facial or anterior facial vein is divided between ligatures, and the lower border of the gland is grasped by suitable traction forceps and lifted up. This reveals the common tendon of the digastric muscle and the hyoglossus muscle. The gland is separated from the muscular floor of the submandibular triangle using sharp dissection, and the hypoglossal nerve with its venae comitantes is identified on the hyoglossus muscle. The anterior segment of the gland is released from the mylohyoid muscle. Traction on the gland is applied forwards and upwards, and the stylohyoid and posterior belly of the digastric is retracted gently downwards and backwards. The facial artery is identified as it emerges from its position deep between these muscles and divided proximal to the gland between strong ligatures, freeing the gland posteriorly.

The gland is retracted downwards and its superior fascial attachments to the mandible divided. This exposes the facial artery and anterior facial vein, which are divided between ligatures as close to the gland as possible to avoid the mandibular branch of the facial nerve. A blunt retractor is inserted deep to the posterior free border of the mylohyoid, exposing the deep part of the gland. Traction on the gland drags down the lingual nerve, which should be separated from the gland. Traction in a downward and lateral direction exposes the duct, which is ligated and divided. Haemostasis is secured and the wound closed by suturing the platysma and skin. A suction drain may be employed if desired but is often unnecessary.

Postoperative complications

Paralysis of the depressor anguli oris due to damage of the mandibular branch of the facial nerve is the commonest complication. Hypoglossal nerve palsy leads to deviation of the tongue to the affected side and eventually fasciculation and wasting. It is uncommon and requires no action in a unilateral palsy. Lingual nerve damage is very uncommon and results in paraesthesiae in the homolateral half of the tongue.

Radiotherapy

Adjuvant radiotherapy has an import role in salivary gland malignancy. Postoperative radiotherapy has been recommended for all patients with malignant salivary tumours if there are positive or close margins or if the tumour is larger than 4 cm in diameter. Radiotherapy should also be considered in the presence of perineural or perilymphatic spread extension beyond the parotid and the presence of adenoidcystic carcinoma. Local recurrence is rare after complete excision of low-grade tumours, and radiotherapy is probably best reserved for those patients with high-grade tumours. More recent studies indicate that not only does radiotherapy improve local control of malignant salivary gland tumours, it also improves survival.[84]

Key points

- A wide range of investigational techniques are now available for the evaluation of the salivary glands. The biggest recent technological advance has been the development of the sialoendoscope. The quality of MRI and CT scans has continued to evolve.
- The majority of patients with infective and inflammatory conditions do not require surgery.
- Surgery for benign tumours of the parotid gland is increasingly conservative.

References

1. Davis RA, Anson BJ, Budinger JM et al. Surgical anatomy of the facial nerve and parotid gland based upon a study of 350 cervico-facial halves. Surg Gynecol Obstet 1956; 102:385–412.

2. Johns ME. The salivary glands: anatomy and embryology. Otolaryngol Clin North Am 1977; 10:261–71.

3. Mason DK, Chisholm DM. Salivary glands in health and disease. London: WB Saunders, 1975; pp. 37–69.

4. Hobsley M. Salivary tumours. Br J Hosp Med 1973; 10:555–62.

5. Phillps DE, Jones AS. Reliability of clinical examination in the diagnosis of parotid tumours. J R Coll Surg Edinb 1994; 39:100–2.

6. Sonn PM, Curtin HD. Head and neck imaging, 4th edition. Mosby, 2003; pp. 2006–133.

7. Bryan RN, Miller RH, Ferreyro RI et al. Computed tomography of the salivary glands. Am J Roentgenol 1982; 139:547–54.

8. Yousem DM. Head and neck imaging. Radiol Clin North Am 1998; 36:941–66.

9. Parker GD, Harnsberger HR. Clinical–radiologic issues in perineural tumour spread of malignant diseases of the extra-cranial head and neck. Radiographics 1991; 11:383–99.

10. Chaudhuri R, Bingham JB, Crossman JE et al. Magnetic resonance imaging of the parotid gland using the STIR sequence. Clin Otolaryngol 1992; 17:211–17.

11. McGhee RB Jr, Chakeres DW, Schmalkbrock P et al. The extra-cranial facial nerve: high resolution three-dimensional Fourier transform MR imaging. Am J Neuroradiol 1992; 14:465–72.

12. Kalinowski M, Heverhagen JT, Rehberg K et al. Comparative study of MR sialography and digital subtraction sialography for benign salivary gland disorders. Am J Neuroradiol 2002; 23:1485–92.

13. Ahuja A, Ying M, Yang WT et al. The use of sonography in differentiating cervical lymphomatous lymph nodes from cervical metastatic lymph nodes. Clin Radiol 1996; 51:186–90.

14. Brandwein MS, Huvos AG. Oncocytic tumours of major salivary glands: a study of 68 cases with follow-up of 44 patients. Am J Surg Pathol 1991; 15:514–28.

15. Cogan MI, Gill PS. Value of sialography and scintigraphy in diagnosis of salivary gland disorders. Int J Oral Surg 1981; 10:216–22.

16. Cernik TF, Mari A, Acikoz G et al. FDG PET in detecting primary and recurrent malignant salivary gland tumours. Clin Nuc Med 2007; 32(4):286–91.

17. McGurk M, Hussain K. Role of fine needle aspiration cytology in the management of the discrete parotid lump. Ann R Coll Surg Engl 1997; 79:198–202.

18. McGurk M, Drage N, Webb J. Investigation of salivary lumps. In: McGurk M, Renehan A (eds) Controversies in the management of salivary gland disease. Oxford: Oxford University Press, 2001; pp. 35–54.

19. Shaha A, Webber C, DiMaio T et al. Needle aspiration biopsy in salivary gland lesions. Am J Surg 1990; 160:373–6.

20. Cohen EG, Patel SG, Lin O et al. FNA biopsy of salivary gland lesions in a selected population. Arch Otolaryngol Head Neck Surg 2004; 130:773–8.

21. Rodriguez HP, Silver CE, Moisa II et al. Fine needle aspiration of parotid tumours. Am J Surg 1989; 158:342–3.

22. Lewis DR, Webb AJ, Lott MF et al. Improving cytological diagnosis and surgical management of parotid adenolymphoma. Br J Surg 1999; 86:1275–9.

23. Nahieli O, Nakar LH, Nazarian Y et al. Sialoendoscopy: a new approach to salivary gland obstructive pathology. JADA 2006; 137(10):1394–400.

24. Miglets AW. Infections, Part III. Clinical entities. In: Cummings CW, Fredrickson JM, Harker LA (eds) Otolaryngology – head and neck surgery, Vol. 2. St Louis: Mosby Year Book, 1986; pp. 999–1006.

25. Yousem DM. The radiologic clinics of North America; head and neck imaging, Vol. 36. Philadelphia: WB Saunders, 1998; pp. 949–50.

26. Harding Rains AJ, Ritchie HD (eds). Bailey and Love's short practice of surgery, 16th edn. London: HK Lewis, 1975; pp. 537–8.

27. Rabinov K, Weber AL. Radiology of the salivary glands. Boston: G Hall, 1985; pp. 153–66.

28. Moss-Salentijn L, Moss L. Development and functional anatomy. In: Rankow RM, Polayes IM (eds) Diseases of the salivary glands. Philadelphia: WB Saunders, 1976; pp. 17–31.

29. Al-Deeb SM. Herpes simplex encephalitis mimicking mumps. Clin Neurol Neurosurg 1993; 95: 49–53.

30. Navazesh M, Mulligan R, Barron Y et al. A 4-year longitudinal evaluation of xerostomia and salivary gland hypofunction in the Women's Interagency HIV Study participants. Oral Surg Oral Med Oral Pathol Oral Radiol Endod 2003; 95: 1079–2104.

31. Mulligan R, Navazesh M, Komaroff E et al. Salivary gland disease in human immunodeficiency virus-positive women from the WIHS study. Oral Surg Oral Med Oral Pathol Oral Radiol Endod 2000; 89:702–9.

32. Marx RE, Hartman KS, Rethman KV. A prospective study comparing incisional labial to incisional parotid biopsies in the detection and confirmation of sarcoidosis, Sjögren's disease, sialosis and lymphoma. J Rheumatol 1988; 15:621–9.

33. Mavragani CP, Moutsopoulos NM, Moutsopoulos HM. The management of Sjögren's syndrome. Nat Clin Pract Rhematol 2006; 2:252–61.

34. Hudson NP. Manifestations of systemic disease. In: Cummings CW, Fredrickson JM, Harker LA et al. (eds) Head and neck surgery, Vol. 2. St Louis: Mosby Year Book, 1986; pp. 1007–13.

35. Bloch KJ. Sjogren's syndrome. In: Stein JH (ed.) Internal medicine. Boston: Little Brown, 1983; pp. 1034–6.

36. Daniels TE, Whitcher JP. Association of patterns of labial salivary gland inflammation with keratoconjunctivitis sicca. Analysis of 618 patients with suspected Sjögren's syndrome. Arth Rheum 1994; 37:869–77.

37. McGurk M, Escudier MP, Brown JE. Modern management of salivary calculi. Br J Surg 2005; 92:107–12.

38. Thackray AC. Sialectasis. Arch Middlesex Hosp 1955; 5:151.

39. Mandel L, Hamele-Bena D. Alcoholic parotid sialadenosis. JADA 1997; 128:1411–15.

40. Barnes L., Eveson JW, Reichart P et al. (eds). World Health Organisation classification of tumours. Pathology and genetics of head and neck tumours. Lyon: IARC Press, 2005.

41. Saku T, Hayashi Y, Takahara O et al. Salivary gland tumours among atomic bomb survivors, 1950–1987. Cancer 1997; 79:1465–75.

42. Katz AD, Preston Martin S. Salivary gland tumours and previous radiotherapy to the head or neck. Am J Surg 1984; 147:345–8.

43. Hoffman DA, McConahey WM, Fraumeni JF Jr et al. Cancer incidence following treatment of hyperthyroidism. Int J Epidemiol 1982; 11: 218–24.

44. Cheuk W, Chan JKC. Advances in salivary gland pathology. Histopathology 2007; 51(1):1–20.

45. Lalami Y, Vereecken P, Dequanter D et al. Salivary glands carcinomas, paranasal sinus cancers and melanoma of the head and neck: an update about rare but challenging tumors. Curr Opin Oncol 2006; 18(3):258–65.

46. Eveson JW, Kusafuka K, Stenman G et al. Pleomorphic adenoma. In: Barnes L, Eveson JW, Reichart P et al. (eds) World Health Organisation classification of tumours. Pathology and genetics of head and neck tumours. Lyon: IARC Press, 2005; pp. 254–8.

47. McGurk M. Parotid pleomorphic adenoma. Br J Surg 1997; 84:1491–2.

48. Renehan A, Gleave FN, Hancock BD et al. Long-term follow-up of over 1000 patients with salivary gland tumours treated in a single centre. Br J Surg 1996; 83:1750–4.

49. Patey DH, Thackray AC. The treatment of parotid tumours in the light of pathological study of parotidectomy material. Br J Surg 1957; 45:477–87.

50. McGurk M, Renehan A, Gleave EN et al. Clinical significance of the tumour capsule in the treatment of parotid pleomorphic adenomas. Br J Surg 1996; 83:1747–9.

51. Leverstein H, van der Wal JE, Tiwari RM et al. Surgical management of 246 previously untreated pleomorphic adenomas of the parotid gland. Br J Surg 1997; 84:399–403.

52. Renehan A, Gleave EN, McGurk M. An analysis of the treatment of 114 patients with recurrent pleomorphic adenomas of the parotid gland. Am J Surg 1996; 172:710–14.

53. Buchanan C, Stringer SP, Mendenhall WM et al. Pleomorphic adenoma: effect of tumour spill and inadequate resection on tumour recurrence. Laryngoscope 1994; 104:1231–4.

54. Natvig K, Soberg R. Relationship of intraoperative rupture of pleomorphic adenomas to recurrence: an 11–25 year follow-up study. Head and Neck 1994; 16:213–17.

55. McGurk M, Thomas BL, Renehan AG. Extra capsular dissection for clinically benign parotid lumps: reduced morbidity without oncological compromise. Br J Cancer 2003; 89:1610–13.

56. Witt RL. The significance of the margin in parotid surgery for pleomorphic adenoma. Laryngoscope 2002; 112: 2141–54.

57. Kennedy TL. Warthin's tumour: a review indicating no male predominance. Laryngoscope 1983; 93:889–91.

58. Ebbs SR, Webb AJ. Adenolymphoma of the parotid: aetiology, diagnosis and treatment. Br J Surg 1986; 73:627–30.

59. Cadier M, Watkin G, Hobsley M. Smoking predisposes to parotid adenolymphoma. Br J Surg 1992; 79:929–30.

60. Simpson RHW, Eveson JW. Warthin tumour. In: Barnes L, Eveson JW, Reichart P et al. (eds) World Health Organisation classification of tumours. Pathology and genetics of head and neck tumours. Lyon: IARC Press, 2005; pp. 263–5.

61. Heller KS, Attie JN. Treatment of Warthin's tumour by enucleation. Am J Surg 1988; 156:294–6.

62. Skalova A, Michal M. Cystadenoma. In: Barnes L, Eveson JW, Reichart P et al. (eds) World Health Organisation classification of tumours. Pathology and genetics of head and neck tumours. Lyon: IARC Press, 2005; p. 273.

63. Huvos AG. Oncocytoma. In: Barnes L, Eveson JW, Reichart P et al. (eds) World Health Organisation classification of tumours. Pathology and genetics of head and neck tumours. Lyon: IARC Press, 2005; p. 266.

64. Goode RK, El-Naggar AK. Mucoepidermoid carcinoma. In: Barnes L, Eveson JW, Reichart P et al. (eds) World Health Organisation classification of tumours. Pathology and genetics of head and neck tumours. Lyon: IARC Press, 2005; pp. 219–20.

65. Gleave EN, Whittaker JS, Nicholson A. Salivary tumours – experience over thirty years. Clin Otolaryngol 1979; 4:247–57.

66. Spiro RH. Salivary neoplasms: overview of a 35-year experience with 2807 patients. Head Neck Surg 1986; 8:177–84.

67. Guzzo M, Andreola S, Sirizzotti G et al. Mucoepidermoid carcinoma of the salivary glands: clinicopathological review of 108 patients treated at the National Cancer Institute of Milan. Ann Surg Oncol 2002; 9:688–95.

68. Spiro RH, Huvos AG, Strong EW. Adenoid cystic carcinoma: factors influencing survival. Am J Surg 1979; 138:579–83.

69. Spiro RH, Huvos AG, Strong EW. Cancer of the parotid gland. Clinicopathological study of 288 primary cases. Am J Surg 1975; 130:452–9.

70. Spiro RH, Huvos AG. Stage means more than grade in adenoid cystic carcinoma. Am J Surg 1992; 164:623–8.

71. Perzin KH, Gullane PJ, Clairmont AA. Adenoid cystic carcinoma arising in salivary glands: a correlation of histological features and clinical course. Cancer 1978; 42:265–82.

72. Odell E. Haemangioma. In: Barnes L, Eveson JW, Reichart P et al. (eds) World Health Organisation classification of tumours. Pathology and genetics of

head and neck tumours. Lyon: IARC Press, 2005; p. 276.

73. Chan ACL, Chan JKC, Abbondanzo SL. Haematolymphoid tumours. In: Barnes L, Eveson JW, Reichart P et al. (eds) World Health Organisation classification of tumours. Pathology and genetics of head and neck tumours. Lyon: IARC Press, 2005; pp. 277–80.

74. Helmus C. Subtotal parotidectomy: a 10-year review (1985–1994). Laryngoscope 1997; 107:1024–7.

75. Slevin N, Natvig K. The treatment of spillage and residual pleomorphic adenoma. In: McGurk M, Renehan A (eds) Controversies in the management of salivary gland disease. Oxford: Oxford University Press, 2001; pp. 85–95.

76. Ball ABS, Thomas JM. Salivary glands. In: Allen-Mersh TG (ed.) Surgical oncology. London: Chapman & Hall Medical, 1996; pp. 93–9.

77. Frankenthalter R. Factors that predict for neck metastases and their treatment. In: McGurk M, Renehan A (eds) Controversies in the management of salivary gland disease. Oxford: Oxford University Press, 2001; pp. 173–82.

78. Snow G. The surgical approaches to the treatment of parotid pleomorphic adenomas. In: McGurk M, Renehan A (eds) Controversies in the management of salivary gland disease. Oxford: Oxford University Press, 2001; pp. 57–66.

79. O'Regan B, Bharadwaj G, Bhopal S et al. Facial nerve morbidity after retrograde nerve dissection in parotid surgery for benign disease: a 10-year prospective observational study of 136 cases. Br J Oral Maxillofac Surg 2007; 45(2):101–7.

80. O'Brien CJ. Current management of benign parotid tumours – the role of limited superficial parotidectomy. Head and Neck 2003; 25:946–52.

81. Reddy PG, Arden RL, Mathog RH. Facial nerve rehabilitation after radical parotidectomy. The Laryngoscope 1999: 109(6): 894–9.

82. de Bree R, van der Waal I, Leemans RC Management of Frey syndrome. Head and Neck 2007; 29:773–8.

83. Jianjun Y, Tong T, Wenzhu S et al. The use of a parotid fascia flap to prevent postoperative fistula. Oral Surg Oral Med Oral Pathol Oral Radiol Endod 1999; 87:673–5.

84. Slevin N, Frankenthaler R. The role of radiotherapy in the management of salivary gland cancer. In: McGurk M, Renehan A (eds) Controversies in the management of salivary gland disease. Oxford: Oxford University Press, 2001; pp. 163–72.

Index

abdominal pain, midgut carcinoids, 161
accountability, 177
achlorhydria, 105
    gastrinoma, 132
    pentagastrin-resistant, 150
acinic cell carcinoma, 201, 203
ACTH *see* adrenocorticotropic hormone (ACTH)
ACTH-dependent Cushing's syndrome, 78, 80–1
ACTH-independent adrenal hyperplasia, familial, 117
ACTH-independent Cushing's syndrome, 78–9, *79–80*, 79–80, 116
ACTH-independent macronodular adrenal hyperplasia, 117
ACTHoma, **122**, 139
actinomycosis, 196
acute suppurative thyroiditis, 63
Addisonian crisis, 92
Addison's disease, 92
adenocarcinoid, 169
adenocarcinoma
    colorectal, 159
    parotid gland, 204
adenoid cystic carcinoma, 201, 203–4
adenoma
    ACTH-secreting pituitary, 78
    adrenal, Cushing's syndrome, 78–9, *80*
    adrenal cortex, 88
    carcinoma ex-pleomorphic, 204
    double, 14, *14*
    ductal, of breast, 116
    growth hormone-secreting, 104
    intrathyroid parathyroid, 23
    mediastinal, 23
    parathyroid *see* parathyroid adenoma
    pituitary, 78
    pleomorphic, 201–2, *202*
    primary hyperparathyroidism *see* parathyroid adenoma
    solitary parathyroid, 24, *24*
adrenal adenoma, Cushing's syndrome, 78–9, *80*
adrenal carcinoma, Cushing's syndrome, 78–9, *79*
    see also adrenocortical carcinoma
adrenalectomy, 92–5
    bilateral, Cushing's syndrome, 81
    controversies, 178

laparoscopic, 93–5
    left, 94, *94*
    phaeochromocytoma, 87–8
    posterior retroperitoneal approach, 95
    retroperitoneal approach, 95
    right, 94–5
    transperitoneal approach, *94*
    open, 93
adrenal glands, 73–95
    adrenalectomy *see* adrenalectomy
adrenocortical carcinoma *see* adrenocortical carcinoma
adrenogenital syndromes, 76–7
    anatomy, 73–4
        blood supply, 73
        embryology, 74
        lymph drainage, 73
        microscopic, 74
        nerve supply, 73
    congenital adrenal hyperplasia *see* congenital adrenal hyperplasia (CAH)
    cortex
        adenoma, 88
        anatomy, 74
        embryology, 74
        physiology, 75–6, *76*
        zones, 74
    Cushing's syndrome *see* Cushing's syndrome
    incidentaloma, 90–2
    insufficiency *see* Addison's disease
    medulla
        anatomy, 74
        embryology, 74
        physiology, 74–5
    neuroblastoma, 90
    phaeochromocytoma *see* phaeochromocytoma
    physiology, 74–6
        adrenal cortex, 75–6
        adrenal medulla, 74–5
    primary aldosteronism *see* Conn's syndrome
    surgery *see* adrenalectomy; adrenal surgery
adrenal hyperplasia, familial ACTH-independent, 117
adrenaline production, 74
adrenal surgery
    outcome measures, 181
    standards, 181
adrenal vein, 73
adrenocortical carcinoma, 82–4
    diagnosis, 82–3

adrenocortical carcinoma (*Continued*)
  familial predisposition to, 116
  inherited susceptibility, 82
  prognosis, 83–4
  treatment, 83
adrenocortical disease, familial, 116–17
adrenocortical tumours, multiple endocrine
      neoplasia, 101
adrenocorticotropic hormone (ACTH), 75
  Addison's disease, 92
  carcinoid tumours, 148
  congenital adrenal hyperplasia, 76
  Cushing's syndrome *see* Cushing's syndrome
  ectopic secretion, 78
  Nelson's syndrome, 81
adrenocorticotropic hormone (ACTH)-oma, **122**, 139
adrenogenital syndromes, 76–7
AGES scoring system, thyroid cancer, 53
airway obstruction, thyroidectomy complications, 69
albumin, 40
aldosterone, 75
  Conn's syndrome *see* Conn's syndrome
  production, 74
  secretion, 89
aldosterone-secreting carcinoma, 88
aldosteronism, primary *see* Conn's syndrome
alpha-adrenergic blockers (alpha blockers),
      phaeochromocytoma, 86, 87
α-adrenergic receptors, 75
α-fetoprotein, rectal carcinoids, 171
α1α-hydroxylase, 15
alternative dispute resolution (ADR), 184
aluminium-binding agents, secondary
      hyperparathyroidism, 16
aluminium intoxication, 16
American Association of Endocrine Surgeons, 184
AMES scoring system, thyroid cancer, 53
amine precursor uptake and decarboxylation
      (APUD) cells, 121
aminoglutethimide, 81
ampulla of Vater, 155
anaemia, pernicious, 150
anaesthesia, phaeochromocytoma and, 88
anaplastic carcinoma
  parotid gland, 204
  thyroid gland, 57–8
androgens
  congenital adrenal hyperplasia, 76
  incidentaloma, 91
androstenedione, 76
angiography
  gastrinoma, 135
  midgut carcinoids, 160
  primary hyperparathyroidism, **9**, 12–13
  salivary glands, 194
  and venous sampling, **9**, 12–13
angiopathy, midgut carcinoids, 157
angiotensin-converting enzyme (ACE), 75, 89
angiotensin I, 75
angiotensin II, 75, 89
angiotensinogen, 89
antibiotics
  acute suppurative thyroiditis, 63
  bacterial parotitis, 196
  prophylactic, pituitary surgery, 81
antibodies, thyroid, 40, 63
anticholinergics, Frey's syndrome, 209
antithyroid drugs

hyperthyroidism, 60
  reaction to, 61
  see also specific drug
antrectomy, gastric carcinoids, 154
aorta, 73
aortic arches, 44
APC gene, 112
apologies, 183–4
appendectomy, 169
appendiceal carcinoids, 169, *169*
  incidence, 147
  occurrence, **148**
argyrophilia, 147
aromatase enzyme system, 76
arrhythmias
  carcinoid crisis, 167
  hypercalcaemia, 5
  phaeochromocytoma, 85
arteria lusoria, 44
arteriography
  calcium *see* calcium arteriography
  gastrinoma, **127**
  insulinoma, **127**, 128–9, *129*, 131
asthma, beta blockers, 61
atrophic gastritis, chronic *see* chronic atrophic
      gastritis (CAG)
atypical carcinoid syndrome, 152, 153
audit, risk management, 182
auriculotemporal nerve, 192
autoantibodies, thyroid-stimulating hormone (TSH)
      receptor (TRAbs), 40
autoimmune diseases
  malignant lymphoma, 58
  radiation exposure, 203
  salivary glands *see* Sjögren's syndrome
  thyroid gland *see* Hashimoto's thyroiditis
  thyroid peroxidase, 40
  ultrasonography, 194
autoimmune thyroiditis *see* Hashimoto's thyroiditis
autotransplantation, parathyroidectomy, 32–3, **33**
bacterial infections, salivary glands, 196
Bannayan-Riley-Ruvalcaba syndrome, 110–11
Bannayan-Zonana syndrome, 110–11
basal acid output (BAO), 132
battery, 182
Bayes' theorem, 108
Beckwith-Wiedemann syndrome, 82, 116
benign lymphoepithelial lesion, 197
Berry's ligament, 66, 67
beta-adrenergic blockers (beta blockers)
  hypertension, 86
  hyperthyroidism, 61
  phaeochromocytoma, 87
β-adrenergic receptors, 75
β-endorphins, 171
bicarbonate, 2
bilateral adrenal hyperplasia, 79, 89
bilateral neck exploration, primary
      hyperparathyroidism, 8
biochemical screening
  carcinoid syndrome, 159
  gastric carcinoids, 153
  multiple endocrine neoplasia type 1, **104**, 104–5
  multiple endocrine neoplasia type 2, 108–9
biopsy
  anaplastic thyroid carcinoma, 58
  gastric carcinoids, 153
  needle core *see* needle core biopsy

non-functional pancreatic endocrine tumours, 139
    Riedel's thyroiditis, 63
    salivary glands, 197
biotherapy, midgut carcinoids, 167–8
bisphosphonates, 6
    hypercalcaemia, 7
    neonatal severe hyperparathyroidism, 110
blood glucose, insulinomas, 124–6, *125*, **125**
Bolam test, 183, 186
bone(s)
    bones, stones and groans mnemonic, 3
    pain, secondary hyperparathyroidism, 16
    parathyroid hormone, 2
    resorption, parathyroid hormone, 15
botulinum toxin A, Frey's syndrome, 209
bowel contrast studies, 159
bradykinin, carcinoid syndrome, 158
brain metastases, 168
breast cancer, Cowden's syndrome, 110
breast disease, benign, Cowden's syndrome, 110
British Association of Endocrine and Thyroid Surgeons
    (BAETS), 178
bronchial carcinoid, 104
bronchoconstriction, carcinoid syndrome, 159
CA19–9, rectal carcinoids, 171
CA50, rectal carcinoids, 171
caecal carcinoids, 170
calcidiol (25-hydroxylated vitamin D$_{3}$), 15, 75
calcimimetics, secondary hyperparathyroidism, 16
calciphylaxis, secondary hyperparathyroidism, 16
calcitonin
    duodenal carcinoids, 156
    hypercalcaemia, 6, 7
    medullary thyroid carcinoma, 57
    multiple endocrine neoplasia type 2, 107
    parathyroid hormone antagonism, 2–3
    thyroid function investigation, 40
calcitonin gene-related peptide (CGRP), 56
calcitonin-secreting pancreatic endocrine tumour, **123**
calcitriol
    decreased synthesis, 15
    preoperative, 33
    secondary hyperparathyroidism, 15
calcium
    familial hypocalciuric hypercalcaemia, 109
    regulation, 2–3
    serum
      decrease in, 2
      elevated, 1, 4 (*see also* hyperparathyroidism)
      gastric carcinoids, 153
      ionised, 5
      screening, 3
    supplementation, secondary hyperparathyroidism, 16
calcium arteriography, insulinoma, 128–9, *129*,
    131, 139
calcium-channel blockers
    familial hyperaldosteronism, 117
    hypertension, 86
    hypoglycaemia management, 126
calcium:creatinine ratio, familial hypocalciuric
    hypercalcaemia, 109
calcium loading test, 5
calcium-sensing receptors (CSRs), 2
carbimazole
    goitre, 45, 62
    hyperthyroidism, 60
    in pregnancy, 61
carboxy-O-methyltransferase, 75

carcinoembryonic antigen (CEA)
    medullary thyroid carcinoma, 56, 57
    rectal carcinoids, 171
    thyroid function investigation, 40
carcinoid crisis, 167
carcinoid flush syndrome, 167
carcinoid polyps, 157
carcinoid syndrome
    atypical, 152, 153
    midgut carcinoids, 158–9, 161
carcinoid tumours
    classification, 147, **148**
    distribution by site, **148**
    gastrointestinal, 147–73
    octreotide, 126
    see also specific tumour
carcinoma
    acinic cell, 201, 203
    adenoid cystic, 201, 203–4
    adrenal, Cushing's syndrome, 78–9, *79*
    adrenocortical *see* adrenocortical carcinoma
    aldosterone-secreting, 88
    anaplastic *see* anaplastic carcinoma
    endocrine, 147, **148**
    follicular *see* follicular thyroid carcinoma
    medullary thyroid *see* medullary thyroid
      carcinoma (MTC)
    metastatic, of the thyroid, 58
    mucoepidermoid *see* mucoepidermoid carcinoma
    papillary *see* papillary thyroid carcinoma
    parathyroid *see* parathyroid carcinoma
    parotid gland undifferentiated, 204
    poorly differentiated neuroendocrine, 149, 152–3,
      154, 156
    primary hyperparathyroidism, 13, 14–15, *15*
    squamous cell *see* squamous cell carcinoma
carcinoma ex-pleomorphic adenoma, 204
cardiac arrhythmias *see* arrhythmias
cardiomyopathy, phaeochromocytoma surgery, 87
Carney-Stratakis syndrome, 115
Carney syndrome, 116–17
carotid body tumour, 114, 115
Casanova test, 34
catecholamines
    familial paraganglioma syndromes, 115
    neuroblastoma, 90
    phaeochromocytoma, 86, 87
    physiology, 74–5
    synthesis, 74–5
    von Hippel-Lindau syndrome, 113
cat-scratch fever, 196
causation, 187
cavernous lymphangioma, 204
C-cells, thyroid, 55–6
CD43, 201
cervical thymectomy, 102
cervicotomy, transverse, 31
chemoembolisation
    gastric carcinoids, 154
    midgut carcinoids liver metastases, 166
chemotherapy
    adenocarcinoids, 169
    anaplastic thyroid carcinoma, 58
    gastric carcinoids, 154
    gastrointestinal carcinoids, 148
    malignant pancreatic tumours, 141
    malignant thyroid lymphoma, 58
    medullary thyroid carcinoma, 57

chemotherapy (*Continued*)
midgut carcinoids, 167
neuroblastoma, 90
rectal carcinoids, 172
chest X-ray, Cushing's syndrome, 78
chief cells, 2, 14
children
Graves disease, 61
hypothyroidism, 63
neuroblastoma, 90
phaeochromocytoma in, 88
chloride:phosphate ratio, 4
choriomeningitis virus, 196
chromaffin cells, 74
chromaffin tissue, 84, *84*
chromogranin A
familial paraganglioma syndromes, 115
gastric carcinoids, 149, 153
midgut carcinoids, 159
non-functional pancreatic endocrine tumours, 138
chromogranin A staining
duodenal carcinoids, 156
gastrointestinal carcinoids, 148
midgut carcinoids, 160
poorly differentiated neuroendocrine carcinoma, 152
rectal carcinoids, 171
chronic atrophic gastritis (CAG)
gastric carcinoids, 149, **150**, 150–1, 153, 154
poorly differentiated neuroendocrine carcinoma, 152
cinacalcet, 16
classical carcinoids *see* midgut carcinoids
clinical governance, 177–82
agencies involved, 177–8
good practice definition, 179
key points, 177–9
risk management, 181–2
subspecialisation advantages, 179–81
colitis, colonic carcinoids, 170
colloid goitre, 44
colonic carcinoids, **148**, 170
colorectal adenocarcinoma, 159
communication issues, risk management, 182
complaints
handling, 183–4
local resolution of, 184
that turn into litigation, 184–5
computed tomography (CT) scan
adrenocortical carcinoma, 82
Conn's syndrome, 89
Cushing's syndrome, 78, 79–80, *79–80*, 81
dynamic, 160
fine-needle aspiration (FNA), 10
gastric carcinoids, 154
gastrinoma, **127**, 134–5, *135*, 138
incidentaloma, 91
insulinoma, 127, *127*, 128
malignant pancreatic tumours, 140, *141*
medullary thyroid carcinoma, 57, *57*
midgut carcinoids, 160
multiple endocrine neoplasia type 2, 107
neuroblastoma, 90
pancreatic tumours, 139
parotid gland, 193
parotid tumours, 205
phaeochromocytoma, 86
primary hyperparathyroidism, *9*, 10
rectal carcinoids, 171
retrosternal goitre, 49

single-photon emission, 12, *13*
thyroid gland, 42, *42*
von Hippel-Lindau syndrome, 113
conditional/contingency fees, 187–8
congenital adrenal hyperplasia (CAH), 76–7, *77*
characteristics, 76
management, 76–7
Conn's syndrome, 88–90, *89*
incidence, 89
vs. incidentaloma, 91
consent *see* informed consent
Convention on Human Rights: Biomedicine (1997), 183
cornstarch, hypoglycaemia management, 126
corticosterone, 75
corticotropin, 76
corticotropin-releasing hormone (CRH), 76
carcinoid tumours, 148
Cushing's syndrome, 81
cortisol, 75–6
Addison's disease, 92
Carney syndrome, 117
congenital adrenal hyperplasia, 76
Cushing's syndrome, 79
diurnal rhythm, 79
function, 74
twenty-four-hour urinary, 79
cortisone, carcinoid crisis, 167
Cowden's syndrome, 110–11
coxsackie viruses, 196
C-peptide, insulinoma, 125, **125**
cretinism, 63
Crohn's disease, colonic carcinoids, 170
cryopreservation, parathyroid tissue, 32, 33
Cushing's syndrome, 77–82
ACTH-dependent, 78, 80–1
ACTH-independent, 78–9, 79–80, *79–80*, 116
aetiology, 78–9
carcinoid tumours, 148, **148**
Carney syndrome, 116
diagnosis, 79
features, 77, 77–8, **78**, *78*
medullary thyroid carcinoma, 56
prevalence, 78
treatment, 81–2
vs. incidentaloma, 91
cutaneous flushing, carcinoid syndrome, 159
cyclic AMP (cAMP), parathyroid hormone, 2
cystadenomas, 203
cystic hygroma, 204
cytoreductive therapy, adenocarcinoids, 169
damage, 185, 187
DDX1, 90
dehydroepiandrosterone (DHEA), 74, 76
dehydroepiandrosterone sulphate(DHEA-S), 91
Department of Health, 177
depressor anguli oris paralysis, 210
de Quervain's thyroiditis, 62
desferrioxamine, secondary hyperparathyroidism, 16
dexamethasone
high-dose dexamethasone suppression test, 80–1
low-dose dexamethasone suppression test, 79, 117
dextrose, hypoglycaemia management, 126
dialysis
hypercalcaemia, 8
osteitis fibrosa cystica, 16
post-parathyroidectomy, 33
diarrhoea
carcinoid syndrome, 158–9

gastrinoma, 132
medullary thyroid carcinoma, 56
secretory, 158–9
diazoxide, hypoglycaemia management, 126
[111In]DTPA-octreotide, 168
dihydroxyphenylalanine (DOPA) receptors, 87
1,25-dihydroxyvitamin D, 2
diplopia, Graves' disease, 60
diuretics
calcium:creatinine ratio, 109
and hormonal assays, 89
hypercalcaemic crisis, 6
normocalcaemic hyperparathyroidism, 5
DMSA scanning, medullary thyroid carcinoma, 57
dopamine
neuroblastoma, 90
production, 74
double adenoma, 14, 14
doxazosin, phaeochromocytoma, 86
doxorubicin
anaplastic thyroid carcinoma, 58
medullary thyroid carcinoma, 57
dry mouth, 196
ductal adenoma of breast, 116
duodenal carcinoids, 155–6
gangliocytic paragangliomas, 155
gastrinomas, 155
neuroendocrine carcinomas, 156
occurrence, 148
pancreatic carcinoids, 156
somatostatin-rich carcinoids, 155
duodenal obstruction, midgut carcinoids, 157
duodenectomy, gastrinoma, 103, 136
duodenotomy
duodenal carcinoids, 155
gastric carcinoids, 154
gastrinoma, 136–7
duty of care, 185, 186
dynamic computed tomography (CT) scan, 160
dyshormonogenesis, 45
dysphagia, thyroid cancer, 52
ear lobe, hypoaesthesia of the, 209
echovirus, 196
ectopic parathyroid glands, 23, 23, 24
ectopic thyroid, 41, 41, 44
embolisation
hepatic artery see hepatic artery embolisation
liver, 166
embryology
adrenal glands, 74
parathyroid glands, 1–2
recurrent laryngeal nerve, 44
thyroid gland, 39
endocrine carcinoma
classification, 147, 148
see also carcinoid tumours; specific tumour
endoscopic parathyroidectomy, 27–9, 28, 29
conversion to conventional parathyroidectomy, 28
by lateral approach, 28, 28, 29
minimally invasive video-assisted (MIVAP), 28, 29
pure, 28
vs. conventional parathyroidectomy, 29
endoscopic transillumination, duodenal carcinoids, 155
endoscopic ultrasonography (EUS)
gastric carcinoids, 153, 154
gastrinoma, 127, 135
insulinoma, 127, 128
pancreatic neuroendocrine tumours, 114

primary hyperparathyroidism, 9, 10
rectal carcinoids, 170, 171
enterochromaffin (EC) cells
midgut carcinoids, 147, 156
rectal carcinoids, 171
enterochromaffin-like (ECL) cells
gastric carcinoids, 149
hyperplasia, 149, 151, 153
enterochromaffin-like (ECL) tumours, 101, 149–50
enteroglucagon, midgut carcinoids, 159
enteropancreatic islet tumours, 100–1, 102–3, 102–3
enucleation
gastrinoma, 137
insulinoma, 131
Warthin's tumour, 203
epidermal growth factor (EGF), thyroid cancer, 49
epinephrine see adrenaline
Epstein–Barr virus, 199
c-erbB2, 201
Escherichia coli, salivary glands, 196
etidronate, 6, 7
exocrine-endocrine carcinoma, 148, 148
exocytosis, 74
expert opinions, 187
external carotid artery, 192
external superior laryngeal nerve (ESLN), 65, 65, 68–9
extracorporeal shock-wave lithotripsy, sialolithiasis, 198
extragastrointestinal carcinoids occurrence, 148
extranodal marginal zone B-cell lymphoma
(EMZBCL), 204
extrathyroidal tumours, papillary carcinoma, 52
facial artery, 210
facial nerve
branches, 191
identification in parotidectomy, 206
injury after parotidectomy, 208
facial palsy, 193
faciohypoglossal transposition, 208
factitious hypoglycaemia, 124
familial ACTH-independent adrenal hyperplasia, 117
familial adenomatous polyposis (FAP), 112
familial adrenocortical disease, 116–17
familial endocrine disease, 99–117
see also specific disease/syndrome
familial glucocorticoid-suppressible hypoaldosteronism
syndrome, 88–9
familial hyperaldosteronism, 117
familial hypercalciuric hypercalcaemia (FHH), 30
familial hyperparathyroidism (FHP) syndromes,
25, 109–10
management, 110
presentation, 109–10
familial hyperparathyroidism-jaw tumour syndrome
(FHP-JT), 109, 110
familial hypocalciuric hypercalcaemia (FHH), 109
familial isolated hyperparathyroidism (FIHP), 109–10
familial non-medullary thyroid cancer syndromes,
110–12
familial non-MEN 2 phaeochromocytoma, 112,
112–16, 113
familial papillary thyroid cancer, 111
familial paraganglioma syndromes, 114–15
fatigue, primary hyperparathyroidism, 3
fibroblast growth factor (FGF), 49
fine-needle aspiration cytology (FNAC)
anaplastic thyroid carcinoma, 58
classification, 43
malignant thyroid lymphoma, 58

fine-needle aspiration cytology (FNAC) (*Continued*)
  medullary thyroid carcinoma, 56
  parotid tumours, 205
  salivary glands, 194–5, *195*
  submandibular gland tumours, 205
  thyroid cancer, 53
  thyroid gland, 42–3, **43**
  thyroid nodules, 46
fine-needle aspiration (FNA)
  computed tomography-guided, 10
  cytology *see* fine-needle aspiration cytology (FNAC)
  incidentaloma, 91
  preoperative localisation, 30
  ultrasound-guided, 10
fistulas
  salivary, 209
  thyroglossal, 43
fludrocortisone suppression test, 89
fluorodeoxyglucose (FDG) receptors, 87
flushing, cutaneous, 159
focal lymphocytic sialadenitis, 197
follicular thyroid carcinoma, *52*, 52–3
  clinical features, 53
  minimally invasive, 53
  pathology, 52–3
  treatment, 54–5
  widely invasive, 53
foregut carcinoids, 104
  classification, 147, **148**
  multiple endocrine neoplasia, 101
four-gland hyperplasia
  primary hyperparathyroidism, 8, 13, 14, *14*
  secondary hyperparathyroidism, 31, *31*
Frey's syndrome, 208–9
furosemide, 6
gallium nitrate, 6, **7**
gangliocytic paragangliomas, 155
gangrene, midgut carcinoids, 157
Gardner's syndrome, 112
gastrectomy, gastric carcinoids, 154
gastric acid
  gastric carcinoids, 153
  hypersecretion, 132, 133–4
gastric carcinoids, 149–54
  clinical evaluation, 153–4
    diagnosis, 153–4
    symptoms and patient history, 153
  histology, 149–50
  occurrence, **148**
  poorly differentiated neuroendocrine carcinomas, 152–3
  treatment, 154
  type 1: associated with chronic atrophic gastritis, **150**, 150–1, 154
  type 2: associated with ZES and MEN 1, **150**, 151, 154
  type 3: sporadic, **150**, 151–2, *152*, 154
gastric enterochromaffin-like (ECL) tumours, 101
gastrin
  gastric carcinoids, 149, 150, 153
  gastrinoma, 132
  multiple endocrine neoplasia, 105
  non-functional pancreatic endocrine tumours, 138
gastrinomas, 101, 102, 103, 132–8, 152
  diagnosis, 132–3, *133*
  duodenal, 136, *136*, 137
  duodenal carcinoids, 155
  features, **122**

gastric carcinoids, 149, **150**, 151
  incidence, 124
  localisation of, **127**
  malignant, 140
  management, 133–8
    medical control of gastric acid hypersecretion, 133–4
    multiple endocrine neoplasia type 1, 137–8
    preoperative tumour localisation, 134–5, *135*
    surgery for tumour eradication, 135–7, *136*
  occult, 139
  outcome, 138
  pancreatic, *136*, 137
  patient presentation, 132
gastrinoma triangle, 136
gastritis, chronic atrophic *see* chronic atrophic gastritis (CAG)
gastrointestinal bleeding, midgut carcinoids, 158
gastrointestinal carcinoids, 147–73
  see also specific tumour
gastrointestinal tract, calcium-sensing receptors, 2
general anaesthesia, thyroidectomy, 64
General Medical Council, 178
genetic counselling, 110
genetics
  familial paraganglioma syndromes, 114–15
  multiple endocrine neoplasia type 1, 99
  multiple endocrine neoplasia type 2, 105–6, *105–6*
  neurofibromatosis type 1, 116
  von Hippel-Lindau syndrome, 112–13, *113*
genetic testing/screening
  multiple endocrine neoplasia type 1, 101–2, 104
  multiple endocrine neoplasia type 2, 106, 108
  neonatal severe hyperparathyroidism, 110
  von Hippel-Lindau syndrome, 114
genitalia abnormalities, 76
glomus jugulare tumour, 114
glossopharyngeal nerve, 192
glucagon, rectal carcinoids, 171
glucagonoma, **122**, 139, *141*
glucocorticoids, 75–6, *76*
  congenital adrenal hyperplasia, 76
  Cushing's syndrome *see* Cushing's syndrome
  familial hyperaldosteronism, 117
  hypercalcaemia, 7, 8
  production, 74
  replacement therapy, 92
  see also specific glucocorticoid
glucose metabolism, glucocorticoids, 75
glycogen storage, 75
goblet-cell carcinoid, atypical, 169
goitre, 44–5
  classification, **44**
  colloid, 44
  diffuse toxic *see* Graves' disease
  environmental factors, 45
  multinodular, 47, *50, 52*, 59
  nodular, 45
  prevention and treatment, 45
  recurrent, thyroidectomy, 68
  retrosternal, 47–9, *51*
    thyroidectomy, 68
  simple, 44–5
  sporadic, 45
  toxic multinodular, 62
good practice, 179
G-protein receptor, 2
granulomatous diseases, salivary glands, 196–7
granulomatous thyroiditis, 62

Graves' disease
  children, 61
  neonatal hyperthyroidism, 62
  ophtalmopathy, 59–60
  ophthalmic, 62
  pregnancy, 61–2
  reaction to antithyroid drugs, 61
  recurrent, after surgery, 62
  subtotal thyroidectomy, 68
  thyroglobulin, 40
  thyroid peroxidase, 40
  thyroid-stimulating hormone receptor
      autoantibodies, 40
  toxic multinodular goitre, 62
  toxic solitary nodule, 62
  treatment, 60
GRFoma, **122**, 139
growth factors
  carcinoid syndrome, 158
  thyroid cancer, 49
growth hormone (GH), 153
growth hormone (GH)-secreting pituitary tumours,
      102, 104
growth hormone-releasing factor (GRF)-oma, **122**, 139
Gsα gene, 49
GTPase-activating protein (GAP), 116
guidelines, 178–9, 186
haemangiomas, parotid gland, 204
haematoma
  after parathyroidectomy, 26
  thyroidectomy complications, 69
haemodialysis
  hypercalcaemia, 8
  pruritus, 16
  secondary hyperparathyroidism, 16
  supernumerary parathyroid glands, 33–4
Haemophilus influenzae, 196
haemorrhage, thyroidectomy complications, 69
hamartomas, Cowden's syndrome, 110
Hashimoto's thyroiditis, 63
  malignant thyroid lymphoma, 58
  thyroglobulin, 40
  thyroid peroxidase, 40
Healthcare Commission, 177
heart valve fibrosis, carcinoid syndrome, 159
hemicolectomy, 170
hepatic artery embolisation
  gastric carcinoids, 154
  rectal carcinoids, 172
hereditary paragangliomatosis (HP), 114
herpesvirus, 196
high-dose dexamethasone suppression test
  Cushing's syndrome, 80–1
  overnight, 81
hindgut carcinoids, 147, **148**
Hirschsprung's disease, 105
histamine
  carcinoid syndrome, 152
  gastric carcinoids, 149, 152
H$_2$-receptor antagonists, 133–4, 167
histology, midgut carcinoids, 160
HIV (human immunodeficiency virus), parotitis, 196
HLA (human leucocyte antigen), 59
HMGA2, 201
hoarseness, 46, 49
Hodgkin's lymphoma, 204
homovanillic acid (HVA), 75, 90
House–Brackmann scale, 208

HRPT2, 109
human choriogonadotropin (hCG), 159
human immunodeficiency virus (HIV), parotitis, 196
human leucocyte antigen (HLA), 59
Hürthle cell lesions, 53, 55
hydrocortisone, 8
5-hydroxindoleacetic acid (5-HIAA)
  gastric carcinoids, 152
  midgut carcinoids, 159
21-hydroxylase, 76
25-hydroxylated vitamin D$_3$, 15
hydroxymethoxy mandelate (HMMA), 75
5-hydroxytryptophan (5-HTP), 152
25-hydroxyvitamin D, 2
hyperaldosteronism, familial, 117
hypercalcaemia
  aetiology, 5
  calls, 5
  differential diagnosis, 6
  hypercalcaemic crisis, 5–8
  lithium-induced, 34
  parathyroid carcinoma, 26
  post-parathyroidectomy, 110
  primary hyperparathyroidism manifestations, 3
  symptoms, 3, 5
  treatment, 5–8, **7**
hypercalcaemic crisis, 5–8
hypercalciuria
  idiopathic, 5
  normocalcaemic hyperparathyroidism, 5
  primary hyperparathyroidism, 4
hypergastrinaemia, 134
  gastrinoma, 132
  poorly differentiated neuroendocrine
      carcinoma, 152
hyperinsulinaemia, 121
hyperinsulinaemic hypoglycaemia, 121
hyperparathyroidism
  characteristics, 1
  familial *see* familial hyperparathyroidism (FHP)
      syndromes
  history, 1
  lithium-induced, 34
  prevalence, 1
  primary *see* primary hyperparathyroidism (PHP)
  secondary *see* secondary hyperparathyroidism (SHP)
  tertiary, 16, 34
hyperphosphataemia, 15
hyperplasia
  diffuse argyrophilic, of the non-antral
      mucosa, 150
  enterochromaffin-like (ECL) cells, 149, 151, 153
  four-gland, 8, 13, 14, *14*
  gastric carcinoids, 150, 151
  micronodular/adenomatoid, 150
  water-clear-cell, 24–5
hypertension
  neurofibromatosis type 1, 116
  phaeochromocytoma, 85, 86
hyperthyroidism, 58–62
  causes, 58–9
  clinical features, 59, 59–60
  follow-up, 62
  Graves' disease *see* Graves' disease
  investigation, 60, *60*
  medical treatment, 60–1
  neonatal, 62
  prevalence, 62

hyperthyroidism (*Continued*)
  recurrent, 62, 69
  special circumstances in Graves' disease, 61–2
  surgery, 61
hypoaesthesia of the ear lobe, 209
hypocalcaemia
  autotransplantation, 32
  post-parathyroidectomy, 26, 33
  secondary hypoparathyroidism, 15
hypoglossal nerve palsy, 210
hypoglycaemia
  factitious, 124
  hyperinsulinaemic, 121
  insulinomas, 124, 126
  medical management, 126
hypoparathyroidism
  parathyroid surgery risk, 25
  thyroidectomy complications, 69
hypophosphataemia, 4
hypothyroidism, 63–4
  causes, 64
  congenital, iodine deficiency, 44
  thyroidectomy complications, 69
hypoxia-inducible factor (HIF), 113
idiopathic hypercalciuria (IH), 5
imaging *see specific disease; specific technique*
immunoreactive insulin (IRI), **125**
incidentaloma, 90–2
Independent Complaints Advocacy Service, 184
inferior petrosal sinus catheterisation, Cushing's
  syndrome, 81
inferior phrenic arteries, 73
inferior thyroid artery
  embryology, 39
  parathyroidectomy, 21
inferior thyroid veins, 66
inferior vena cava
  adrenal glands, 73
  adrenocortical carcinoma, 82–3, *83*
influenza virus type A, 196
informed consent, 64, 182–3
insulin
  immunoreactive, **125**
  non-functional pancreatic endocrine tumours, 138
insulin-like growth factor I (IGF-I)
  gastric carcinoids, 153
  thyroid cancer, 49
insulinomas, 102, *102, 103*, 121–32
  diagnosis, 124–6
    nesidioblastosis, 126
    supervised standard fasting test, **123**, *123*, 124–6
  features, **122–3**
  incidence, 124
  localisation of, 126–9, **127**, *128, 129*
  malignant, 140
  management, 126–31
    laparoscopic surgery, 131
    medical management of hypoglycaemia, 126
    multiple endocrine neoplasia type 1, 131
    operative, 129–31
    preoperative tumour localisation, 126–9
  multiple endocrine neoplasia type 1, 124, 131
  occult, 139
  outcome, 131
  presentation, 121–4
  resection, 131
interferon α
  malignant pancreatic tumours, 141

midgut carcinoids, 167–8
rectal carcinoids, 172
International Cowden Syndrome Consortium, 110, 111
intestinal obstruction, midgut carcinoids, 158, 160
intraoperative ultrasonography (IOUS)
  gastrinoma, 136
  insulinoma, 129, 130
  occult pancreatic tumours, 139
intraperitoneal heated chemotherapy, 169
intrathyroidal tumours
  papillary carcinoma, 52
  parathyroid adenoma, 23
invasive fibrous thyroiditis, 63
iodine deficiency, simple goitre, 44
iodocholesterol scanning, Conn's syndrome, 89
ionised calcium, serum, 5
irradiation
  papillary thyroid carcinoma, 51
  primary hyperparathyroidism, 3
  salivary gland tumours, 199
  thyroid nodules, 45–6
  Warthin's tumour, 203
islet cell tumours
  incidence, 124
  metastases, 140
isotope scanning
  parathyroid glands, **9**, 11, *11*, 12, *12*
  phaeochromocytoma, 86, *86*
  thyroid function investigation, 40–1, *41*
  thyroid gland, 40–1, *41*
  thyroid nodules, 46–7
  von Hippel-Lindau syndrome, 113
isthmusectomy, thyroid cancer, 54
jejuno-ileal carcinoids *see* midgut carcinoids
JunD, 99
ketoconazole, Cushing's syndrome, 81
kidneys
  calcium-sensing receptors, 2
  see also entries beginning renal
Ki67 expression, rectal carcinoids, 171
Ki67 proliferation index, 147
  midgut carcinoids, 160
  salivary gland tumours, 201
Kocher manoeuvre
  gastrinoma, 136
  insulinoma, 130, *130*
L-amino acid decarboxylase, 152
lanreotide, 167
laparoscopic surgery
  adrenalectomy *see* adrenalectomy, laparoscopic
  adrenocortical carcinoma, 83
  insulinoma, 131
  phaeochromocytoma, 87–8
laparotomy
  midgut carcinoids, 160–1
  occult pancreatic tumours, 139
laryngeal nerve
  non-recurrent, 44, 66, 67
  palsy after parathyroidectomy, 26
  recurrent *see* recurrent laryngeal nerve (RLN)
legal aid, 185, 188
lesser petrosal nerve, 192
Lhermitte-Duclos disease (LDD), 110
Li-Fraumeni syndrome, 82, 116
lingual nerve, 209, 210
lingual thyroid, 43–4
lipomas
  multiple endocrine neoplasia, 101

parotid gland, 204
lithium-induced hyperparathyroidism, 34
litigation, 183
    see also medico-legal issues
liver
    embolisation, 166 (*see also* hepatic artery
        embolisation)
    lobectomy, midgut carcinoids metastases, 165
    metastases *see* liver metastases
    resection, midgut carcinoids metastases, 165
    transplantation, midgut carcinoids liver
        metastases, 167
    see also entries beginning hepatic
liver metastases
    duodenal carcinoids, 155
    gastric carcinoids, 152, 154
    gastrinoma, 134, 136
    malignant pancreatic tumours, 141
    midgut carcinoids, 158, 161, *161*, 164–7
        liver embolisation, 166
        liver transplantation, 167
        radiofrequency ablation, 165–6
        surgery, 165
    non-functional pancreatic endocrine tumours, 139
    rectal carcinoids, 171, 172
loop diuretics, 6, 7
low-dose dexamethasone suppression test
    Cushing's syndrome, 79
    familial hyperaldosteronism, 117
Lugol's iodide, thyroid crisis, 69
lung cancer, ectopic ACTH secretion, 78
lymphangioma, parotid gland, 204
lymphatic system, adrenal glands, 73
lymph node metastases
    duodenal carcinoids, 155
    gastric carcinoids, 151, 152, *152*, 154
    gastrinoma, 136, 137
    medullary thyroid carcinoma, 56
    midgut carcinoids, 157
    oesophageal carcinoids, 149
    rectal carcinoids, 171
lymph nodes
    parotid gland, 192
    parotid tumours, 205
    thyroid cancer, 52
    thyroidectomy, 54
lymphoepithelial lesion, benign, 197
lymphomas
    Hodgkin's, 204
    malignant, 58, *58*, 197
    MALT, 204–5
    non-Hodgkin's, 197, 204
    parotid gland, 204–5
    thyroid *see* thyroid lymphoma
MACIS scoring system, thyroid cancer, 53
magnesium
    familial hypocalciuric hypercalcaemia, 109
    hypertension, 86
magnetic resonance imaging (MRI)
    adrenocortical carcinoma, 82–3
    Conn's syndrome, 89
    Cushing's syndrome, 78, 80, *80*, 81
    gastrinoma, 134–5
    incidentaloma, 91
    insulinoma, 127, **127**, *128*
    malignant pancreatic tumours, 140
    medullary thyroid carcinoma, 57
    multiple endocrine neoplasia type 2, 107

neuroblastoma, 90
    parotid gland, 193–4, *194*
    parotid tumours, 205
    pleomorphic adenoma, 201
    primary hyperparathyroidism, **9**, 10–11
    retrosternal goitre, 49
    Sjögren's syndrome, 197
    submandibular gland tumours, 205
    thyroid gland, 42
    von Hippel-Lindau syndrome, 113, 114
magnetic resonance tomography (MRT)
    midgut carcinoids, 160
    rectal carcinoids, 171
malignant lymphoma, 58, *58*, 197
MALT lymphomas, 204–5
MAML2, 201
masseter muscle, 191
    hypertrophy, 193
Masson stain
    midgut carcinoids, 156
    rectal carcinoids, 171
MECT1, 201
median sternotomy at the same time as
    parathyroidectomy, 23–4
mediastinal adenoma, 23
mediation, 188
medical negligence *see* negligence
Medicine, Patients and the Law, 185
medico-legal issues, 182–8
    complaints
        handling, 183–4
        local resolution of, 184
        that turn into litigation, 184–5
    consent, 182–3
    damage, 187
    expert opinions, 187
    medical negligence, 185–7
    reforms, 187–8
medullary thyroid carcinoma (MTC), 55–7
    calcitonin, 40
    clinical features, 56
    diagnosis, 56–7
    familial, 105, 106
    follow-up, 57, *57*
    multiple endocrine neoplasia type 2, 105, 106, *107*,
        107–8
    pathology, 56, *56*
    prognosis, 57
    treatment, 57
membrane potentials, 5
MEN1 gene, 14, 151
    multiple endocrine neoplasia type 1, 99, 100, *100*
    screening, 104
MEN2 gene, 105–6, *105–6*
menin, 99–100
[131]Imetaiodobenzylguanidine (MIBG) scan
    familial paraganglioma syndromes, 115
    medullary thyroid carcinoma, 57
    neuroblastoma, 90
    phaeochromocytoma, 86, *86–7*
[131]Imetaiodobenzylguanidine (MIBG) therapy, 168
metanephrines
    familial paraganglioma syndromes, 115
    multiple endocrine neoplasia type 2, 108
    von Hippel-Lindau syndrome, 113, 114
metastases
    appendiceal carcinoids, 169
    brain, 168

metastases (*Continued*)
    gastric carcinoids, 151, 152
    gastrinoma, 101, 134, 136
    insulinoma, 129
    islet cell tumours, 140
    liver *see* liver metastases
    lymph node *see* lymph node metastases
    midgut carcinoids, *157*, 157–8, 158
    neuroblastoma, 90
    pancreatic tumours, 140
    parathyroid carcinoma, 26
    phaeochromocytoma, 88
    rectal carcinoids, 171, 172
    thyroid cancer, 52, 53
    thyroid carcinoma, 58
metastatic calcification, secondary
    hyperparathyroidism, 16
methimazole, hyperthyroidism, 60
methylmidazoleacetic acid (MelmAA), carcinoid
    syndrome, 152, 153
metyrapone, Cushing's syndrome, 81
MIBG scanning *see* [131]Imetaiodobenzylguanidine
    (MIBG) scan
micropapillary thyroid cancer, 51–2
middle thyroid vein, 39
midgut carcinoids, 156–68
    classification, 147, **148**
    clinical symptoms, 158–9
    diagnosis, 159–60
      biochemistry, 159
      histology, 160
      radiology, 159–60
    liver metastases, *164*, 164–7
      liver embolisation, 166
      liver transplantation, 167
      radiofrequency ablation, 165–6
      surgery, 165
    medical treatment, 167–8
    morphological features, 156–8, *157*, *158*
    prophylaxis against carcinoid crisis, 167
    radiotherapy, 168
    surgery, 160–4, *161–3*
    survival, 168
mineralocorticoid antagonists, 117
mineralocorticoids, 75
    congenital adrenal hyperplasia, 76
    production, 74
    replacement therapy, 92
    see also specific hormone
minimally invasive parathyroidectomy (MIP), 27–9
    broader context, 29
    contraindications, 27
    endoscopic *see* endoscopic parathyroidectomy
    open (OMIP), 27
    radioguided (MIRP), 27
    unilateral neck exploration, 27
mitotane
    adrenocortical carcinoma, 83
    Cushing's syndrome, 81
monoamine oxidase, 75
    carcinoid syndrome, 159
    midgut carcinoids, 158
MTCN oncogene, 90
MUC1, 201
MUC4, 201
mucoepidermoid carcinoma, 199, 201, 203
mucosa-associated lymphoid tissue (MALT) lymphomas,
    204–5

multidisciplinary team, 180
multiglandular disease, parathyroid glands
    minimally invasive parathyroidectomy, 27
    sporadic, *24*, 24–5
    see also four-gland hyperplasia
multinodular goitre, 47, *50*, *52*, 59
    toxic, 62
multiple endocrine neoplasia type 1 (MEN 1), 99–105
    adrenocortical carcinoma, 82
    clinical features, **100**
    diagnosis, 101–2
    duodenal carcinoids, 156
    familial hyperparathyroidism, 25
    functions of menin, 99–100
    gastric carcinoids, 149, **150**, 151, 154
    and gastrinoma, 137–8
    genetics, 99
    insulinoma, 124, 131
    management, 102–4
      enteropancreatic islet tumours, 102–3, *102–3*
      foregut carcinoids, 104
      pituitary tumours, 103–4
      primary hyperparathyroidism, 102
    presentation, 100–1
      adrenocortical tumours, 101
      cutaneous manifestations, 101
      enteropancreatic islet tumours, 100–1
      foregut carcinoids, 101
      pituitary tumours, 101
      primary hyperparathyroidism, 100
    prevalence, 99
    screening, **104**, 104–5
multiple endocrine neoplasia type 2A (MEN 2A), 105–9
    classification, 105
    familial hyperparathyroidism, 25
    genetics, *105*, 105–6, *106*
    management, *107*, 107–8
    medullary thyroid carcinoma, 56, *56*
    phaeochromocytoma, 85
    presentation, 106–7
    screening, 108–9
    tongue, 56
multiple endocrine neoplasia type 2B (MEN 2B), 105–9
    classification, 105
    genetics, *105*, 105–6, *106*
    management, *107*, 107–8
    phaeochromocytoma, 85
    presentation, 106–7
    screening, 108–9
mumps, 196
myxoedema, 63
myxomas, Carney syndrome, 116
NAG, 90
National Cancer Institute (NCI), 168
National Clinical Assessment Service (NCAS), 177–8
National Health Service Litigation Authority
    (NHSLA), 184
National Health Service (NHS), 177, 184
National Institute of Clinical Excellence (NICE), 177
N-cym, 90
neck exploration
    bilateral, 8
    unilateral, 27
necrolytic migratory erythema (NME), 139
needle core biopsy
    malignant thyroid lymphoma, 58
    midgut carcinoids, 160
    thyroid gland, 43

negligence, 183, 185–7
   breaching of duty of care, 185, 186–7
   damage, 185, 187
   duty of care, 185, 186
Nelson's syndrome, 81
neonatal hyperthyroidism, 62
neonatal hypothyroidism, 40
neonatal severe hyperparathyroidism (NSHP), 109
   genetic testing, 110
   management, 110
nephrolithiasis
   normocalcaemic primary hyperparathyroidism, 4
   primary hyperparathyroidism, 3
nesidioblastosis, 126
neuroblastoma, 90
neuroendocrine cells, 121
neuroendocrine tumours
   classification, 147, **148**
   poorly differentiated neuroendocrine carcinoma, 149,
      152–3, 154, 156
   see also carcinoid tumours; *specific tumour*
neurofibromatosis
   phaeochromocytoma, 86
   type 1 (NF1) *see* von Recklinghausen's disease
neurofibromin, 116
neuroglycopenia, 121, 125
neuroma, 209
neurone-specific enolase (NSE)
   carcinoid tumours, 148
   duodenal carcinoids, 156
   non-functional pancreatic endocrine tumours, 138
   rectal carcinoids, 171
neurotensin, 138
neurotensinoma, **123**, 139
NF1 gene, 116
NM23 protein, 201
nodular goitre, 45
non-Hodgkin's lymphoma, 197, 204
noradrenaline, 74
normetanephrines, 113, 114
normocalcaemic hyperparathyroidism, 4–5
no win, no fee, 187–8
occult pancreatic tumours, 139
OctreoScan
   gastric carcinoids, 154
   gastrinoma, **127**
   insulinoma, 127, **127**
   medullary thyroid carcinoma, 57
   midgut carcinoids, 160, 168
   rectal carcinoids, 171
octreotide
   carcinoid crisis, 167
   gastric carcinoids, 154
   hypoglycaemia management, 126
   malignant pancreatic tumours, 141
oesophageal carcinoids, **148**, 149
oesophagitis, 132
oestrogens, 76
omeprazole, gastrinoma, 133
oncocytes, 203
oncocytomas, 194, 203
oncogenes, thyroid cancer, 49
ophthalmopathy
   Graves' disease, 62
   hyperthyroidism, 59–60
organ of Zuckerkandl, 74
Orphan Annie cells, 52
orthopantogram, 109, 110

osseous lesions, secondary hyperparathyroidism, 16
osteitis fibrosa cystica, 16
osteoblasts, 2
osteoclasts, 2
osteomalacia, 15, 16
osteopenia, 3
osteoporosis, 3
oxyphil cells, 14
paclitaxel, rectal carcinoids, 172
pamidronate, 6, 7
pancreas
   surgery *see* pancreatectomy; pancreatic surgery
tumours *see* pancreatic tumours; *specific tumour*
pancreatectomy
   controversies, 178
   enteropancreatic islet tumours in MEN1, 103, *103*
   insulinoma, 129–31, 131
pancreatic carcinoids, **148**, 156
pancreatic islet-cell tumours, 113, 156
pancreatic neuroendocrine tumours, 114
pancreaticoduodenectomy *see* Whipple procedure
pancreatic polypeptide
   duodenal carcinoids, 156
   gangliocytic paragangliomas, 155
   midgut carcinoids, 159
   non-functional pancreatic endocrine tumours, 138
   rectal carcinoids, 171
pancreatic surgery
   controversies, 178
   outcome measures, 181
   standards, 181
pancreatic tumours, 121–41
   classification, 121
   functional, 121 *see also* (gastrinomas;
      insulinomas)
   malignant, 140–1
   non-functional, 121, 138–9
   occult, 139
   see also specific tumour
pancreatitis, 109
pantoprazole, gastrinoma, 134
papillary thyroid cancer (PTC), 111
papillary thyroid carcinoma, 51–2
   clinical presentation, 52
   extrathyroidal tumours, 52
   histology, 52
   intrathyroidal tumours, 52
   micropapillary cancer, 51–2
   pathology, 51–2
   treatment, 53, *54*
paragangliomas
   familial paraganglioma syndromes, 114–15
   gangliocytic, 155
parainfluenza viruses, 196
parathormatosis, 34
parathyroid adenoma, 8, 11, *11*, 12, *12*, 13–14
   double, 14, *14*
   intrathyroid parathyroid, 23
   localisation, 23
   mediastinal, 23
   recurrence, 30
   solitary, 24, *24*
   surgery, 31
parathyroid carcinoma, 13, 14–15, *15*
   failed parathyroid surgery, 30
   metastases, 26
   minimally invasive parathyroidectomy, 27
   recurrence, 26, 30

parathyroid carcinoma (*Continued*)
  surgery, 26
  survival, 26
parathyroid chief cells, 2
parathyroidectomy
  autotransplantation, 32
  conventional open
    associated with thyroid excisions, 26
    basic principles, 20–1
    continuation of exploration, *23*, 23–4
    evaluation of initial bilateral exploration, 22–3
    familial hyperparathyroidism, 25
    overall results, 26–7
    parathyroid carcinoma, 26
    search for inferior parathyroid, 22, *22*
    search for superior parathyroid, *21*, 21–2
    solitary parathyroid adenoma, 24, *24*
    sporadic multiglandular disease, *24*, 24–5
    vs. endoscopic parathyroidectomy, 29
  endoscopic *see* endoscopic parathyroidectomy
  familial hyperparathyroidism syndromes, 110
  gastrinoma, 137–8
  history, 1
  median sternotomy at the same time as, 23–4
  minimally invasive *see* minimally invasive
    parathyroidectomy (MIP)
  primary hyperparathyroidism, 20–32
  secondary hyperparathyroidism, 16, 32–4
  subtotal
    advantages and disadvantages, **33**
    PHP in MEN1, 102
    secondary hyperparathyroidism, 32–3, **33**
  with thyroidectomy, 26
  total
    advantages and disadvantages, **33**
    hyperparathyroidism in multiple endocrine
      neoplasia, 25
    PHP in MEN1, 102
    plus autotransplantation, 32–3, **33**
    secondary hyperparathyroidism, 32–3, **33**
parathyroid glands, 1–35
  adenoma *see* parathyroid adenoma
  anatomy, 1–2
  calcium regulation, 2–3
  carcinoma *see* parathyroid carcinoma
  ectopic, 23, *23*, **24**
  embryology, 1–2
  four-gland hyperplasia, 8, 13
  function, 2
  hyperparathyroidism *see* hyperparathyroidism
  hyperplasia, 8, 14, *14*
  inferior, 1, 2
    absent, 23
    ectopic, **24**
    localisation, 22, *22*
  location, 1–2
  multiglandular disease *see* multiglandular disease,
    parathyroid glands
  parathyroid hormone *see* parathyroid
    hormone (PTH)
  superior, 1, 2
    absent, 23
    ectopic, **24**
    localisation, *21*, 21–2
  supernumerary, 2, 33–4
  surgery *see* parathyroidectomy; parathyroid surgery
  in thyroidectomy, 66–7
  weight estimation, 10

parathyroid hormone (PTH)
  action, 2
  after parathyroidectomy, 26–7
  antagonism, 2–3
  bony resistance to, 15
  changes in set point, 15
  discovery, 1
  excessive *see* hyperparathyroidism
  hyperparathyroidism *see* hyperparathyroidism
  parathyroid carcinoma, 26
  production, 2
  regulation, 2–3
  serum
    elevated, 4 (*see also* hyperparathyroidism)
    gastric carcinoids, 153
  venous sampling, 12–13
parathyroid hormone (PTH)-like-oma, **123**, 139
parathyroid surgery, 20–35
  basic principles, 20–1
  controversies, 178
  hypoparathyroidism risk, 25
  in multiple endocrine neoplasia, 25
  outcome measures, 181
  primary hyperparathyroidism
    conventional open parathyroidectomy, 20–7
    minimally invasive parathyroidectomy, 27–9
    re-operation for persistent/recurrent, 29–32
  standards, 181
  see also parathyroidectomy
parotid duct stricture, 198
parotidectomy, 205–9
  extended, 207
  partial superficial, 207
  pleomorphic adenoma, 201–2
  postoperative complications, 208–9
  radical, 207–8
  retrograde, 207
  subtotal, 205
  superficial, 206
  total conservative, 205, 206–7
  Warthin's tumour, 203
parotid gland
  abscess, 196
  agenesis, 193
  anatomy, 191–2, *192*
  calculi *see* sialolithiasis
  cysts, 198
  developmental abnormalities, 192–3
  infection, 196
  investigation, 193–6
    clinical evaluation, 193
    fine-needle aspiration cytology, 194–5, *195*
    radiology, 193–4, *194*
    sialoendoscopy, 195–6
  lesions, 191, 193
  surgery *see* parotidectomy
  tumours *see* parotid tumours
parotid tumours
  benign epithelial, **199**, 201–3
    other, 203
    pleomorphic adenoma, 201–2, *202*
    Warthin's tumour, 202–3
  benign non-epithelial, 204
  malignant epithelial, **199**, 203–4
  management, 205–9
parotitis, 196
PegIntron, 168
Pendred's syndrome, 45

pentagastrin provocation test, 159
pentagastrin-resistant achlorhydria, 150
pentagastrin stimulation tests, 57
peptic ulcer disease, 132
peritoneal dialysis, 8
pernicious anaemia, 150
p53 gene
    poorly differentiated neuroendocrine carcinoma, 153
    salivary gland tumours, 201
    thyroid cancer, 49
PGP9.5, 148
phaeochromocytes, 74
phaeochromocytoma, *84*, 84–8, *85*
    adrenalectomy, 92
    clinical presentation, 85
    conditions associated with, 85–6
    diagnosis and preoperative management, *86*, 86–7
    familial non-MEN 2, **112**, 112–16, *113*
    malignant, 88
    medullary thyroid carcinoma, 56
    multiple endocrine neoplasia type 2, 105, 106, 108
    neurofibromatosis type 1, 115, 116
    in pregnancy and special circumstances, 88
    somatostatin-rich carcinoids, 155
    surgical removal, *87*, 87–8
    von Hippel-Lindau syndrome, 113
    vs. incidentaloma, 91
phenocopy, multiple endocrine neoplasia type 1, 100
phenoxybenzamine, phaeochromocytoma, 86
phenylethanolamine *N*-methyltransferase, 73, 74
phenytoin, hypoglycaemia management, 126
phosphate
    deprivation, 5
    hypercalcaemia, **7**, 8
    parathyroid hormone, 2
phosphate binders, secondary hyperparathyroidism, 16
phosphate-poor diets, secondary hyperparathyroidism, 16
pituitary gland
    adenoma, 78
    surgery, Cushing's syndrome, 81
    tumours *see* pituitary tumours
pituitary tumours
    growth hormone (GH)-secreting, 102
    multiple endocrine neoplasia, 101
    surgery, 103–4
PLAG1, 201
platelet-derived growth factor (PDGF), 158
pleomorphic adenoma, 201–2, *202*
plicamycin, **7**, 8
positron emission tomography (PET) scans
    midgut carcinoids, 160
    multiple endocrine neoplasia type 2, 107
    phaeochromocytoma, 87
    salivary glands, 194
    thyroid cancer, 55
    thyroid nodules, 47
post-irradiation sialadenitis, 198
postpartum thyroiditis, 40, 63
potassium iodide, 69
PPoma, **123**
PRAD1 oncogene, 14
prednisone, 8
pregnancy
    Graves disease, 61–2
    phaeochromocytoma in, 88
primary aldosteronism *see* Conn's syndrome
primary hyperparathyroidism (PHP), 3–15
    adenoma, 8

calcium-sensing receptors, 2
chloride:phosphate ratio, 4
clinical manifestations, 3
diagnosis, 3–4
elevated serum calcium, 4
elevated serum parathyroid hormone, 4
hypercalcaemic crisis, 5–8, *7*
hypercalciuria, 4
hypophosphataemia, 4
imaging and localisation, 8–13, **9**
    computed tomography, 10, *13*
    magnetic resonance imaging, 10–11
    parathyroid angiography, 12–13
    technetium–99m sestamibi scan, *11*, 11–12, *12*, *13*
    thallium–201-technetium–99m pertechnetate scan (Tl–^{99m}Tc scan), 11
    ultrasound, 10
    venous sampling for parathyroid hormone, 12–13
incidence, 3
irradiation, 3
multiple endocrine neoplasia, 25
    type 1, 100, 102
    type 2, 105, 106–7, 108
normocalcaemic, 4–5
operative strategy, 20–32 (*see also specific technique*)
pathology, 13–15
    adenoma, 14, *14*
    carcinoma, 14–15, *15*
    double adenoma, 14
    hyperplasia, 14, *14*
persistent/recurrent, re-operation, 29–32
    analysis of causes of failure, 29–30
    case history, 30, **30**
    confirmation of diagnosis, 30
    methods, *31*, 31–2
    preoperative localisation, 30
    results, 32
sporadic, 124
vitamin D deficiency, 3
primary pigmented nodular adrenal hyperplasia (PPNAD), 116
PRKAR1A gene, 116
proinsulin-like component (PLC), 125, **125**
prolactin, 103–4, 153
prolactinomas, 103–4
propranolol
    hyperthyroidism, 61
    thyroid crisis, 69
propylthiouracil
    hyperthyroidism, 60
    thyroid crisis, 69
prostaglandins, 158
protein metabolism, glucocorticoids, 75
protocol issues, risk management, 182
proton magnetic resonance spectroscopy (PMRS), 46
proton-pump inhibitors (PPIs), 102, 133–4
pruritus, secondary hyperparathyroidism, 16
psammoma bodies, 52, 155
psammomatous melanotic schwannoma, 116
PTEN gene, 111
PTH-like-oma, **123**, 139
pulmonary valve stenosis, carcinoid syndrome, 159
quick parathyroid hormone (QPTH) assay, 27, 31
radioactive iodine
    Graves' disease, 60
    hyperthyroidism, 60, 61
    post-thyroidectomy, 55

radiofrequency (RF) ablation
    gastric carcinoids, 154
    midgut carcinoids liver metastases, 165–6
radioimmunoassays
    thyroglobulin, 40
    thyroid hormones, 40
radioiodine uptake, thyroid gland, 41–2
radiological screening
    chest, 78
    Cushing's syndrome, 78
    multiple endocrine neoplasia, **104**, 104–5
radiotherapy
    anaplastic thyroid carcinoma, 58
    malignant thyroid lymphoma, 58
    medullary thyroid carcinoma, 57
    midgut carcinoids, 168
    multiple endocrine neoplasia type 2, 108
    post-parotidectomy, 205
    post-thyroidectomy, 55
    salivary gland tumours, 210
ranula, 198
Ras genes, 49
record-keeping, risk management, 182
rectal carcinoids, 170–2
    diagnosis and immunohistochemistry, 171–2
    occurrence, **148**
    outcome, 172
    presentation, *170*, 170–1
    recommendations, 172
    treatment, 172
recurrent laryngeal nerve (RLN)
    embryology, 44
    parathyroidectomy, 21, 25, 28, *28*
    sacrifice in thyroid cancer surgery, 54
    thyroid cancer, 52
    thyroidectomy, 65–6, *66*, 68
reflux oesophagitis, 133
renal arteries, 73
    stenosis, 116
renal failure
    secondary hyperparathyroidism, 15
    tertiary hyperparathyroidism, 16
renal transplant
    secondary hyperparathyroidism, 16
    tertiary hyperparathyroidism, 16
renal vein, 73
renin, 75, 89
respiratory function tests, retrosternal goitre, 49
RET gene, 40, 105–6, *105–6*
    multiple endocrine neoplasia type 2, 108
    papillary thyroid cancer, 111
    thyroid cancer, 49
retinoic acid, 55
retrosternal goitre, 47–9, *51*, 68
Riedel's thyroiditis, 63
risk management, 181–2
Royal Colleges, 178
Ruvalcaba-Mhyre-Smith syndrome, 110–11
saline, hypercalcaemia, 6, 7
salivary fistula, 209
salivary glands, 191–210
    anatomy, 191–2, *192*
    developmental abnormalities, 192–3
    granulomatous diseases, 196–7
    infections, 196–7
    investigation, 193–6
        clinical evaluation, 193
        fine-needle aspiration cytology, 194–5, *195*

        radiology, 193–4, *194*
        sialoendoscopy, 195–6
    obstructive disease, 197–8
    parotid *see* parotid gland
    Sjögren's syndrome, 197
    Stimulation, 197
    sublingual, 191, 192
    submandibular *see* submandibular gland
    surgery, 209–10
    tumours *see* salivary gland tumours
salivary gland tumours, 199–205
    aetiology, 199
    classification and staging, 199, **199–200**
    lymphomas, 204–5
    molecular biology, 201
    parotid neoplasms *see* parotid tumours
salmon calcitonin, 6, 7
sarcoidosis, 196–7
scintigraphy
    adrenocortical carcinoma, 83
    gastric carcinoids, 154
    pancreatic neuroendocrine tumours, 114
SDHA (succinate dehydrogenase complex
    subunit A), 114
SDHB *see* succinate dehydrogenase complex subunit B
    (SDHB)
SDHC (succinate dehydrogenase complex subunit C),
    114–15
SDHD *see* succinate dehydrogenase complex subunit D
    (SDHD)
secondary hyperparathyroidism (SHP), 15–16
    four-gland hyperplasia, 31, *31*
    operative strategy, 32–4
    pathogenesis, 15–16
    persistent/recurrent, 33–4
    presentation, 16
    recurrence, 33
    treatment, 16
    uraemia, 32–4
secretin stimulation test, 133
selective arterial secretin injection (SASI), 135
sentinel node assessment, thyroid cancer, 54
serotonin
    carcinoid syndrome, 158, 159
    duodenal carcinoids, 156
    gastric carcinoids, 152
    pancreatic carcinoids, 156
sestamibi scan *see* technetium–99m sestamibi scan
sex hormones, 75, 76
    production, 74
    see also specific hormone
short-bowel syndrome, 162
short Synacthen test, 92
sialadenitis
    focal lymphocytic, 197
    post-irradiation, 198
sialadenosis, 198
sialagogues, 197
sialectasis, 198
sialoendoscopy, 195–6
sialography
    magnetic resonance, 194
    parotid gland, 193
    sialolithiasis, 197
    Sjögren's syndrome, 197
sialolithiasis, 196, 197–8
simple goitre, 44–5
single nucleotide polymorphisms (SNPs), 106

single-photon emission computed tomography (SPECT), 12, *13*
Sistrunk procedure, 43
Sjögren's syndrome, 197
    bacterial infections, 196
    incidence, 197
    investigation, 193, 194
    primary, 197
    secondary, 197
skin flushing, 159
Smad3, 99
small intestinal carcinoids, **148**
smoking, Warthin's tumour, 203
sodium resorption, 75
solicitor's letter, litigation, 185
solitary parathyroid adenoma, 24, *24*
somatostatin
    gangliocytic paragangliomas, 155
    non-functional pancreatic endocrine tumours, 138
    rectal carcinoids, 171
somatostatin analogues
    midgut carcinoids, 167–8
    rectal carcinoids, 172
    VIPomas, 102
    see also specific somatostatin analogue
somatostatinoma, **122**, 139
somatostatin receptor scintigraphy (SRS)
    gastrinoma, 134–5, *135*, 138
    insulinoma, 127–8
    malignant pancreatic tumours, 140
    midgut carcinoids, 160
    non-functional pancreatic endocrine tumours, 139
somatostatin-rich carcinoids, 155
SPECT *see* single-photon emission computed tomography (SPECT)
splanchnic nerves, 73
splenectomy, insulinoma, 129–31
sporadic goitre, 45
squamous cell carcinoma
    parotid gland, 204
    thyroid, 58
staff issues, risk management, 182
Stafne cyst, 193
standard fasting test, 124–6, **125**, *125*
Staphylococcus aureus, 196
stenotomy, 198
Stensen's duct, 191
    obstruction, 193, 196
Streptococcus pneumoniae, 196
Streptococcus pyogenes, 196
Streptococcus viridans, 196
Sturge-Weber syndrome, 84
subacute thyroiditis, 62
subclavian arteries, 44
sublingual gland, 191, 192
submandibular gland, 191
    anatomy, 192
    calculi removal, 209, *209*
    excision, 209–10
    infection, 196
    radiotherapy, 210
    surgery, 209–10
    tumours, 205
subspecialisation, 179–81
substance P, 171
succinate dehydrogenase complex subunit A (SDHA), 114
succinate dehydrogenase complex subunit B (SDHB)

familial paraganglioma syndromes, 114–15
    phaeochromocytoma, 86
succinate dehydrogenase complex subunit C (SDHC), 114–15
succinate dehydrogenase complex subunit D (SDHD)
    familial paraganglioma syndromes, 114–15
    phaeochromocytoma, 86
sulphonylurea
    serum, insulinomas, 125
    urinary, insulinomas, 124
superficial temporal artery, 208
superior thyroid veins, 39
superior vena cava compression syndrome, 49, *51*
support services, risk management, 182
suppurative thyroiditis, acute, 63
Supreme Court Act (1981), 185
suramin, 83
surgeons
    clinical governance, 178
    guidelines, 179
    subspecialisation, 179–81
    training, 179
Synacthen test, 81, 92
synaptophysin immunostains
    duodenal carcinoids, 156
    gastrointestinal carcinoids, 148
    midgut carcinoids, 160
    poorly differentiated neuroendocrine carcinoma, 152–3
tachykinins, 158, 159
tachyphylaxis
    calcitonin, 6
    midgut carcinoids, 167
technetium–99m pertechnetate (^{99m}Tc) scan
    salivary glands, 194
    thallium–201-technetium–99m pertechnetate (Tl–^{99m}Tc) scan, 9, 11
    thyroid gland, 40–1, *41*
    thyroid nodules, 46–7
technetium–99m sestamibi scan
    dual-isotope subtraction scanning, 12, *12*
    primary hyperparathyroidism, 9, 11, *11*
    single-isotope dual-phase, 11, *11*
    single-photon emission computed tomography, 12, *13*
temporozygomatic branch of the facial nerve, 191
tertiary hyperparathyroidism, 16, 34
testosterone, 76, 91
thallium–201-technetium–99m pertechnetate (Tl–^{99m}Tc) scan, 9, 11
thiazide administration, urinary calcium excretion, 5
thionamides, 60
thymectomy, cervical, 102
thymus, embryology, 1
thyroglobulin, 40, 55
thyroglobulin autoantibodies (TgAbs), 55
thyroglossal cyst, 43
thyroglossal duct, 39
thyroglossal fistula, 43
thyroid antibodies, 40, 63
thyroid cancer, 49–62
    anaplastic carcinoma, 57–8
    familial non-medullary syndromes, 110–12
    familial papillary, 111
    follicular carcinoma, 52–3
    incidence, 49
    malignant lymphoma, 58

thyroid cancer (*Continued*)
  medullary carcinoma *see* medullary thyroid
    carcinoma (MTC)
  metastatic carcinoma, 58
  molecular biology, 49
  papillary carcinoma, 51–2
  risk of irradiation, 45–6
  scoring systems, 53
  squamous cell carcinoma, 58
  treatment of differentiated, 53–5
thyroid C cells, 55–6
thyroid crisis, 69
thyroid disease controversies, 178
thyroidectomy, 64–9
  bilateral subtotal
    hyperthyroidism, 61
    indications, **64**
  complications, 68–9
  guidelines, 179
  hyperthyroidism, 61
  multiple endocrine neoplasia type 2, *107*,
    107–8
  with parathyroidectomy, 26
  postoperative treatment, 55
  recurrent goitre, 68
  retrosternal goitre, 68
  subtotal, 68
  thyroid cancer, 53–5
  total, 68
    familial adenomatous polyposis, 112
    hyperthyroidism, 61
    indications, **64**
    medullary thyroid carcinoma, 57
    papillary thyroid cancer, 111
    thyroid cancer, 53
  unilateral total, 64–7
    general anaesthesia, 64
    incision, 64
    indications, **64**
    informed consent, 64
    patient position, 64
    procedure, 64–7, *65–7*
thyroid gland, 39–70
  anatomy, 39
  cancer *see* thyroid cancer
  cysts, 47
  developmental abnormalities, 43–4
    ectopic thyroid, 44
    lingual thyroid, 43–4
    non-recurrent laryngeal nerve, 44
    thyroglossal cyst, 43
    thyroglossal fistula, 43
  ectopic, 41, *41*
  embryology, 39
  function investigation, 39–43
    calcitonin, 40
    carcinoembryonic antigen, 40
    computed tomography, 42, *42*
    fine-needle aspiration cytology, 42–3, **43**
    magnetic resonance imaging, 42
    needle core biopsy, 43
    radioiodine uptake, 41–2
    thyroid antibodies, 40
    thyroid hormones and thyroid stimulating
      hormone, 39–40
    thyroid isotope scanning, 40–1, *41*
    ultrasonography, 42, *42*
  goitre *see* goitre

hormones *see* thyroid hormones; thyroxine (T_4);
  triiodothyronine (T_3)
hyperthyroidism *see* hyperthyroidism
hypothyroidism *see* hypothyroidism
inflammation *see* thyroiditis
lymphoma *see* thyroid lymphoma
nodules *see* thyroid nodules
surgery *see* thyroidectomy; thyroid surgery
thyroidectomy *see* thyroidectomy
thyroiditis *see* thyroiditis
thyroid hormones, 39–40
  metabolic effects, 40
  thyroid nodules, 47
  see also thyroxine (T_4); triiodothyronine (T_3)
thyroiditis, 62–3
  acute suppurative, 63
  autoimmune *see* Hashimoto's thyroiditis
  Hashimoto's *see* Hashimoto's thyroiditis
  postpartum, 40, 63
  Riedel's *see* Riedel's thyroiditis
  subacute, 62
thyroid lymphoma
  Hashimoto's thyroiditis, 63
  malignant, 58, *58*
thyroid microsomal antigen, 40
thyroid nodules, 45–7
  clinical assessment, 45–7
  environmental factors, 45
  examination, 46
  fine-needle aspiration cytology, 46
  history, 45–6
  isotope scanning, 41, *41*, 46
  occurrence, 45
  positron emission tomography scanning, 47
  risk factors, 45–6
  toxic solitary, 62
  treatment, 47, *48*, *49*
  ultrasonography, 46
thyroid peroxidase (TPO), 40
thyroid-stimulating antibodies (TsAbs), 59
thyroid-stimulating hormone (TSH)
  Graves' disease, 60
  hypothyroidism, 63
  simple goitre, 44
  stimulation, 44
  thyroid cancer, 49
  thyroid function investigation, 39–40
thyroid-stimulating hormone (TSH) receptor
  autoantibodies (TRAbs), 40
thyroid surgery
  guidelines, 179
  outcome measures, 180–1
  standards, 180
  see also thyroidectomy
thyrothymic ligaments, 22
thyrotoxicosis *see* hyperthyroidism
thyroxine-binding globulin (TBG), 40
thyroxine-binding prealbumin (TBPA), 40
thyroxine (T_4)
  Graves' disease, 60
  hypothyroidism, 63
  investigation of thyroid function, 39–40
  post-thyroidectomy, 55
  storage, 40
  thyroid nodules, 47
Tl–^{99m}Tc scan, 9, 11
tort civil law, 185

toxic multinodular goitre, 62
toxic solitary thyroid nodule, 62
toxoplasmosis, 196
TP53 gene, 116
tracheomalacia, 69
transforming growth factor β (TGF-β), 158
transrectal endosonography, rectal carcinoids,
    170, 171
tricuspid valve stenosis, 159
triiodothyronine (T₃)
  Graves' disease, 60
  hypothyroidism, 63
  investigation of thyroid function, 39–40
  storage, 40
Tru-cut biopsy, malignant parotid neoplasm, 205
tuberculosis, salivary gland, 196, 197
tuberosclerosis, 84
tumour suppressor genes, 49
tyrosine hydroxylase, 74
ultimobranchial bodies, 39
ultrasonography (US)
  Cowden's syndrome, 111
  endoscopic *see* endoscopic
    ultrasonography (EUS)
  familial adenomatous polyposis, 112
  fine-needle aspiration (FNA), 10
  intraoperative *see* intraoperative ultrasonography
    (IOUS)
  medullary thyroid carcinoma, 57
  midgut carcinoids, 160
  papillary thyroid cancer, 111
  parotid gland, 194
  pleomorphic adenoma, 201
  primary hyperparathyroidism, **9**, 10
  thyroid gland, 42, *42*
  thyroid nodules, 46
  Warthin's tumour, 203
undifferentiated carcinoma, parotid gland, 204
unilateral neck exploration, 27
uraemia, secondary hyperparathyroidism, 32–4
vanyllmandelic acid (VMA), 75, 90
vascular elastosis, 157
vascular endothelial growth factor (VEGF)
  salivary gland tumours, 201
  von Hippel-Lindau syndrome, 113
venogram, adrenocortical carcinoma, 82, *83*
venous sampling
  angiography and, **9**, 12–13
  Conn's syndrome, 89
  primary hyperparathyroidism, **9**, 12–13
vesicular monoamine transporter isoform 2
    (VMAT2), 149–50

VHL gene, 112–13, *113*, 114
VIPoma, 102, 139
  features, **122**
  malignant, 141
  octreotide, 126
viral infection, salivary glands, 196
virilisation, 76
vitamin B₁₂ malabsorption, 150
vitamin D, 2
  parathyroid glands, 2
  supplementation, secondary
    hyperparathyroidism, 16
vitamin D deficiency
  incidence, 3
  primary hyperparathyroidism, 3
vocal cord palsy, 49, 52
von Hippel-Lindau syndrome, 84
  age at presentation, **112**
  clinical characteristics, **112**
  diagnosis, 113–14
  frequency of expression, **112**
  genetics, 112–13, *113*
  pancreatic neuroendocrine tumours in, 114
  phaeochromocytoma, 86
  presentation, 113
  subtypes, 113
  surveillance and screening, 114
  treatment, 114
von Recklinghausen's disease, 84, *84*, 115–16
  gangliocytic paragangliomas, 155
  somatostatin-rich carcinoids, 155
Warthin's tumour, 199, 202–3
  incidence, 202
  investigation, 194
  presentation, 203
  surgery, 205
water-clear-cell hyperplasia, 24–5
Wharton's duct, 209, *209*
Whipple procedure
  duodenal carcinoids, 156
  enteropancreatic islet tumours, 103
  gastrinoma, 137
  insulinoma, 131
Woolf report, 188
wound complications, thyroidectomy, 69
woven bone, 16
xerostomia, 196
X-ray *see* radiological screening
Zollinger-Ellison syndrome *see* gastrinomas
zona fasciculata, 74, 75
zona glomerulosa, 74, 75
zona reticularis, 74, 75